Aloe Vera

Raymond

Health, wealth & happiness

– forever

Best wishes

Alasdair 24.1.05

ALOE VERA

Nature's Silent Healer

by

Alasdair Barcroft & Dr Audun Myskja

Foreword by Dr Tom Reynolds

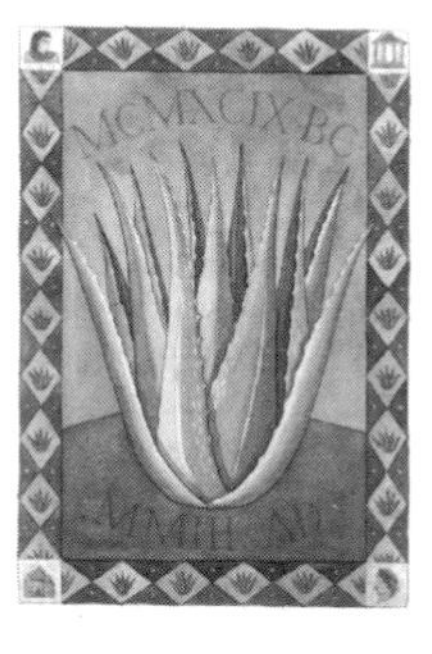

BAAM

First published in 2003 by BAAM
BAAM is the imprint of BAAM Publishing Ltd
42 Mexfield Rd
London
SW15 2RQ

Distributed by Gazelle Book Services Limited
Hightown, White Cross Mills, South Rd
Lancaster, England LA1 4XS

British Library Cataloguing in Publication Data
A catalogue record for this book is available from the British Library

ISBN 0-9545071-0-X

Typeset by Amolibros, Milverton, Somerset
This book production has been managed by Amolibros
Printed and bound by T J International Ltd, Padstow, Cornwall, UK

Quotations

Four vegetables are indispensable for the well being of man:
Wheat, the grape, the olive and aloe.
The first nourishes him, the second raises his spirit,
The third brings him harmony, and the fourth cures him.

Christopher Columbus (1451–1506)

You ask me what were the secret forces which sustained me during my long fasts. Well, it was my unshakeable faith in God, my simple and frugal lifestyle and the Aloe whose benefits I discovered upon my arrival in South Africa at the end of the nineteenth century.

Mahatma Gandhi (1869–1948)

During the twenty years that I have been treating my patients with Aloe, I have found that there are many diseases described by the doctors of antiquity which disappear rapidly when I administer Aloe in the form of granules or powder. Therefore, the good results which I have always obtained allow me to quote the adage of Roger Bacon:

'Do you wish to live as long as Noah? Then take some pills of Aloah!'

Francois Vincent Raspail (1794–1878)

O love what hours were thine and mine,
in lands of palm and southern pine,
in lands of palm, of orange blossom,
of olive, aloe and maize and wine.

Tennyson, 'The Daisy'

The doctor of the future will give no medicine but will interest his patients in the care of the human frame, in diet and in the cause and prevention of disease.

Thomas Edison (1847–1931)

All that mankind needs for good health and healing is provided in nature…the challenge to science is to find it.

Paracelsus, the father of pharmacology

Those who do not find a little time every day for good health, must sacrifice a lot of time one day for illness.

Father Sebastian Kneipp

It is my firmly held belief that with an adequate intake of micro-nutrients – essential substances we need to nourish us – most chronic diseases would not exist. Good nutritional therapy is the medicine of the future. We have already waited too long for it.

Dr Carl Pfeiffer

Let food be your medicine and medicine your food.

Hippocrates (5 BC)

Nature is doing her best each moment to make us well. She exists for no other end. Do not resist. With the least inclination to be well, we should not be sick.

Henry David Thoreau

Dedication

THIS BOOK, my third, is dedicated to the memory of my father, Drew Barcroft, who during his lifetime touched the lives of countless millions of people around the world.

When my dad died suddenly and very unexpectedly not long after I had started my second book project, I simply could not focus on completing what I had started several months before his death. However, now that I am able to reflect on his life and what he achieved and I am able to consider the countless number of people all over the world who benefited from his work, he continues to inspire me. My first thank you is to him, his memory, his humility and his fighting spirit, his values and ethics and his enthusiasm, all of which have proved to be such an inspiration to my family and me since his death.

Few people can look back at their lives and genuinely say, 'I made a difference.' He really did.

We all, both family and friends, miss you, your love, your support, your common sense, your wisdom, your integrity, your guidance and your friendship. Your spirit is always with us.

> You will live beyond the stars,
> You will live in the land of the moons,
> Happiness and friendship will always be yours,
> And the love and laughter of those you left behind,
> Will always rise to you.
>
> *Old Aboriginal prayer*

Disclaimer

ALL PERSISTENT symptoms, of whatever nature, may have underlying causes that may need, and should not be treated without, professional elucidation and evaluation. It is therefore essential that, if you intend to use this book for self-help, only to do so in conjunction with duly prescribed conventional or other therapy. In any event, read the advice carefully and pay particular attention to the advice and warnings.

The publisher makes no representation, express or implied, with regard to the accuracy of the information contained in this book, and legal responsibility cannot be accepted by the author or the publisher for any errors or omissions that may be made or for any loss, damage, injury or problems suffered or in any way arising from the use of aloe vera.

Acknowledgements

I SHOULD like to thank everyone who has contributed to making this book possible.

Firstly to Audun Myskja for agreeing to co-author this book with me, and I look forward to working with him in many different countries as we test the resolve of our translators.

Dr Tom Reynolds, of the Jodrell Laboratory, Royal Botanical Gardens, Kew, for his kind comments on my first book, for the interesting paper on aloe vera he sent me subsequently and for kindly agreeing to provide the foreword.

Rex Maughan, who through his vision, commitment and persistence has established and cemented aloe vera's reputation as a globally available health, nutrition, beauty and skin-care product.

Dustin Greene for his hard work and 'stickability' in helping to pioneer the development of the UK and European markets for aloe vera.

Gene Hale of the International Aloe Science Council (IASC) for his support and his ongoing work and commitment to establishing worldwide benchmarks for quality, purity, efficacy and professional standards in the aloe vera industry worldwide.

Hazel Courteney, for writing those articles in her pioneering health column – 'What's the Alternative' – in both the *Daily Mail* and *The Sunday Times*, and for placing aloe vera firmly on the map through her now legendary article in the *Daily Mail* on 14th February 1995. We all owe her a great debt of gratitude.

Dr Gregg Henderson, chiropractic physician, for his contribution to this book and my previous one and his inspirational and instructive talks and audio- and videotape presentations, and for his initiatives in using aloe vera in his practice.

Susanne and Neil for their unflagging support and critical input at the most challenging times, and for their friendship and belief over the years.

Sandy, Reidun and Audun for their friendship and support over the years.

Deborah for her 'quiet inspiration' and friendship and Richard for his 'larger than life' inspiration.

David Urch for his commitment to helping me with my book, providing some great pictures, and for writing what is now undoubtedly the definitive book on aloe vera and animal care in veterinary practice, available anywhere in the world. A big thank you for being a great pioneer in the veterinary world.

Babbi Wallenberg for her leadership, courage, indomitable spirit, selfless example and support – we all miss you.

Sunil, Brenda, Jennifer, Bronte, Carrie and Michael, Diane, Sarah and the many other people who have made important contributions to this book.

Dr Peter Atherton for his ongoing commitment to making a positive impact on his ex-colleagues in allopathic medicine

Patrick Holford, founder of the Institute for Optimum Nutrition (ION) and prolific author, speaker and broadcaster on diet, health matters and nutritional issues. I would also like to recognise his contribution to this book and his commitment to optimum nutrition.

My mother, Daphne, for being so supportive at a time of great personal tragedy and sadness for herself and also for the guidance, support and love she has given me over the years.

Finally, my biggest thank you is to my fantastic and continually supportive and loving wife, Mary, especially for her support in the dark days after my dad's death. She's always there like a lighthouse in a storm, a shining beacon, guiding, encouraging and showing the best way forward. She's an irrepressible and irreplaceable little Leo!

I also thank her for her lightning speed on the keyboard – with the keyboard itself struggling to keep pace with her 'flying fingers' at times!!

My three incredible kids, Angus, Hamish (my IT consultant par excellence!) and Helena, also deserve special mention for putting up with all the trials and tribulations and the occasional bouts of short temper (as I missed yet another deadline!) during the time I have been working on this book. They are a source of great love, joy, pride and affection to both of us. Their academic and sporting achievements are a continual inspiration to us. They are just great to be with.

Alasdair Barcroft

Acknowledgements for Colour Plates

Colour Plates, Nos 1-4, reproduced with the kind permission of Forever Living Products.

Colour Plates, Nos 5-8, reproduced with the kind permission of Bronte, Carrie and Michael Holmes.

Colour Plates, Nos 9-14, reproduced with the kind permission of Ruth Dwornik.

Colour Plates, Nos 15-16, reproduced with the kind permission of Dr Mike Wyndham.

Colour Plates, Nos 17-20, reproduced with the kind permission of Philippa Jackson-Cox.

Colour Plates, Nos 21-24, reproduced with the kind permission of Kate Fields.

Contents

List of Colour Illustrations

Meadow – Sarcoid

17: Shows Sarcoid growing between forelegs, prior to application of aloe vera.
18: Shows Sarcoid – during application of aloe vera.
19: Shows Sarcoid prior to falling off – tissue healing underneath.
20 & 20a: Meadow – totally healed.

Sevenge – leg injury

21: Protruding wound with proud flesh– one month after accident.
22: Two weeks later – wound healing and all proud flesh has gone.
23: Four weeks later – wound area has decreased by fifty per cent.
24: Sevenge – totally recovered.

Foreword by Dr Tom Reynolds

Former director of the Jodrell Laboratory, Kew Gardens

TOM REYNOLDS BSC, MSc, DIC, ARCS is a graduate of Imperial College, London where he trained in research under Professor H K Porter. He has been active in plant biochemistry at the Royal Botanic Gardens, Kew since 1966 and at present occupies the position of Senior Research Fellow in the Jodrell Laboratory at Kew. Dr Reynolds has also edited another book on 'aloes' in the series Medicinal and Aromatic Plants-Industrial Profiles *due to be published in 2003.*

"Of making many books on aloes there is no end" (Ecclesiastes **12**, 12 with addition). This is not surprising because the genus *Aloe* presents so many different areas of interest from the academic to the purely decorative. Aloes are a large genus of about 400 species, confined to sub-Saharan Africa and parts of Arabia, together with a few neighbouring islands, although a few species have been carried in cultivation for decorative or medicinal purposes around the world from the West Indies to China and Japan.

Their curative powers are legendary and multitudinous, many it is true being unsubstantiated folk remedies but it would be surprising if there were not a lot of true efficacy among the many cures claimed. Two parts of the aloe plant have been used. When a leaf is cut a yellow-brown exudate appears dripping from the outer tissues, which eventually solidifies to a gum. This is the traditional bitter aloes with a powerful purgative activity, little used nowadays because of its tendency to produce griping. The inner part of the leaf contains colourless tissues containing a gelatinous material, abundant in some species, notably *Aloe vera,* and referred to as the gel. This has numerous curative properties especially for inflammatory disorders, typically those of the skin but perhaps potentially much more wide-ranging.

Aloes as a group are the subject of fascinating scientific study and are also of immense attraction to the non-scientific public, especially in warmer countries. The leaf exudate, bitter in some but not all species, has proved to be chemically very interesting and over the 400 species, around at least 80 chemical compounds, many new to science have been recognized recently, although many of them have as yet been determined. Their biological activity also remains largely unexplored, so some may prove to have novel medicinal uses. The part the chemicals play in the life of the plant remains unknown. The chemistry and biology of the inner gel is another story. As a show plant aloes are unrivalled. Many streets and public buildings in frost-free parts of the world are adorned with aloes while flowering *Aloe ferox* is a symbol of South Africa. Collectors are so avid for some of the rarer species that strict conservation measures have had to be imposed. The general public can always enjoy the plants' beauty in their own gardens using nursery-grown stock

This book contains a very wide-ranging description of all those things about aloes which you don't find in the more erudite textbooks and yet are so vital for a proper appreciation of these fascinating plants. A glance at the contents list leaves one wondering if there will ever be any more information and anecdotes for people to write about.

A mighty tome on aloe science is about to be published and the present book will complement it nicely. The author has delved far and wide seeking all the things you really want to know about aloes. So this beautiful and worthy plant will become well known and not just a subject for puns in cosmetic supermarkets.

Tom Reynolds
Jodrell Laboratory
Royal Botanic Gardens, Kew.

Introduction

It started with my chronic sinus infection – Alasdair Barcroft

MY 'LOVE affair' with aloe vera began in earnest in the 1990s. It was actually in 1994 and I had been suffering from a chronic sinus infection for over three years – I had picked up a 'bug' while on holiday in the Middle East. Despite taking numerous medications (antibiotics and nasal sprays) and frequent and ongoing treatment, including two painful operations, more than three years later I still had the sinus infection.

Someone I knew (Susanne), who had been a corporate lawyer in the City, came to see my wife Mary and me to talk to us about this 'amazing plant' called aloe vera. I said that I had used aloe vera for years topically in suncreams and shampoos, etc. but was not aware of its medicinal properties and benefits when taken internally. I decided to try the products (after three years of suffering, I was prepared to try anything!), so I used an aloe vera nasal spray, drank the aloe vera gel drink (and also took another of the products she showed us – bee propolis – a natural antibiotic from the beehive). Within less than four months, the sinus infection had disappeared and I was a totally changed person. Although sinus problems aren't exactly life-threatening, they can be extremely debilitating and can cause severe disruption to one's work and personal life.

It was then that I realised the enormous potential that such quality products offered in terms of healing benefits for a whole range of disorders and ailments. I decided to spend some time trying other products and researching the properties and benefits of aloe vera when taken internally. With a background in press, public relations and marketing communications, I felt that such 'ground-breaking' information should be shared with the media and health journalists in particular, and that's how I got to know Hazel Courteney. I had contacted many newspapers and Hazel was one of the first people to reply. She told me she was familiar with aloe vera as an effective treatment for sunburn – she had used it frequently while living in the Caribbean – but she did not know about its benefits when taken internally.

In mid-1994, through her 'What's the Alternative' column in the *Daily Mail*, Hazel ran the first of several articles on aloe vera drinking juice and its benefits for ulcerative colitis and other ailments. Subsequent articles she wrote also included irritable bowel syndrome (IBS), eczema, ulcerative colitis, animal care and so on and also mentioned topical uses of aloe vera. We continued to liaise and discussed the opportunity to do a feature-length article on aloe vera in the *Daily Mail* and, in late 1994, just before she went on holiday to the Caribbean, I sent her a copy of a book called *Aloe Vera – The Natural Healer*. This book had been written by someone that I knew called Paul Hornsey-Pennell. On her return, Hazel and I spoke several times. She said she had found the book very informative and she also asked me for the names of any doctors I knew who might be prepared to talk about aloe vera as her editor now wanted her to write a feature-length article on aloe vera.

One name I gave Hazel was that of Dr Peter Atherton, who is now the medical advisor to the largest aloe vera company in the UK and is himself an author of another book on aloe vera, called *The Essential Aloe Vera*. The subsequent article that Hazel wrote in the 'Good Health' section of the *Daily Mail* – 'The cactus drink that may help cure millions' – was a watershed in the aloe vera industry in the UK. Suddenly millions of people became aware of the benefits of drinking aloe vera. The rest is history and the UK aloe vera industry is now worth tens of millions of pounds every year.

In 1999, I received a phone call from a Dr Audun Myskja and his wife Reidun who had read my first book on aloe vera and had seen my website. He had apparently used a particular aloe vera herbal spray on a sports injury and had himself experienced highly significant benefits in relation to healing and the speed of healing. We had several phone conversations and I agreed to fly to Norway to discuss how we could work together. I flew to Oslo, met them and spent time with them and we have all worked closely together ever since. Several years later, and now with two books about aloe vera between us, this new book is driven by our joint desire to provide people all over the world with the most definitive book on aloe vera ever written. We hope that our readers are able to determine very quickly that aloe vera is truly one of 'nature's miracle healers' and that whether they use aloe vera orally as a drink or topically on their skin it can have significant benefits in terms of accelerated healing and improved general health and well-being.

Over the last six years, I have become increasingly convinced that the future of maintaining good health and well-being is about creating the optimum health environment within our own bodies. Creating the optimum environment in terms of nutrition is about increasing our intake of 'positively beneficial' substances that help us boost our health and eliminate altogether the substances that don't!

Unfortunately today, modern medicine is more concerned with the 'quick fix' and treating the symptoms rather than the causes. Many drug treatments may be effective – albeit in the short-term – but they do little or nothing to address the causes of disease. With diet-linked diseases accounting for as much as seventy per cent of cancers and other serious diseases, one of the major factors that drugs can do nothing for is the 'poor nutritionional levels' that many people exist on in relation to what they eat and drink. Today, all of us consume thousands of toxins, such as fertilisers, pesticides, herbicides, food additives, oxidants, drugs and many, many other noxious substances through the food we eat, the water we drink and the air that we breathe. We are, knowingly and unknowingly, producing a chemical cocktail in our bodies that is wreaking havoc with our health and well-being. To survive and maintain good health in the twenty-first century, we must all be more pro-active with regard to nutrition and we must increase our intake of bio-available adaptogens and anti-oxidants – vitamins, minerals, amino-acids, essential fatty acids and other 'health-giving' and 'free radical scavenging' substances.

Aloe vera is not only a powerful adaptogen, it also enhances the bio-availability of essential nutritional and health-giving substances like vitamin C and vitamin E ('Effect of aloe vera preparations on the human bio-availability of vitamins C and E', Joe A Vinson, Hassan Al Kharrat and Lori Andreoli, Department of Chemistry, University of Scranton, PA, USA, 2002).

Having been involved in the aloe vera business for nearly a decade and having both experienced and witnessed the healing and health-giving benefits of this remarkable plant, I am still amazed when I consider its complexities and its 200-plus constituents and the synergistic actions they have. Aloe vera contains many powerful nutrients and has many proven benefits. It improves collagen repair in the skin, helping to heal burns and other skin damage, prevents wrinkles and helps to regenerate new tissue. Aloe vera also contains biologically active compounds called anthraquinones, which have antiseptic, anti-fungal, anti-viral and anti-bacterial properties. Aloe vera can also stimulate the healing of wounds and help prevent conditions like sepsis. It is also a powerful detoxifier and has anti-oxidant and immune-boosting properties and improves digestion. Drinking a high-quality aloe vera gel/juice every day is now widely accepted as having powerful benefits as a healing and health tonic for the body and the nervous system. Aloe vera also has 'soapy substances' (saponins) that help cleanse wounds of debris and kill microbes and 'woody substances' (lignins) that help soften tough skin and provide aloe vera with its renowned penetrative properties, allowing the healing agents to penetrate deep into the tissue.

Exactly why everyone who is interested in health should use aloe vera as an integral part of their ongoing health regime is the subject of this book. It explores the history, the science and the evidence that enhances the credibility of this remarkable plant and puts aloe vera firmly on the map as an important and integral part of everyone's mission to attain optimum health. Enjoy the journey. It is a story that has its roots in ancient times, it is a story of legends over the millennia, from ancient myth to the modern day, it is a miracle medicine that has fascinated me for many years.

I wish you all hours of happy and informative reading and the best of health.

Alasdair Barcroft

Dr Audun Myskja

Why would a doctor raised in the land of the midnight sun write a book about a semi-tropical plant? The road to this project has indeed been long and winding. In the early seventies I started my therapeutic career with an interest in Norwegian medicinal herbs and traditional forms of healing. To my surprise I found that I was linking into a strong therapeutic tradition in rural Norway. My roots lie in a craggy coastal landscape where doctors were few and far between. Traditional healers and 'herb women' were the main therapists and they often used a combination of a laying-on of hands and local herbs, where plant combinations had been used since ancient times. My father had frequent throat infections as a child and there was never any question of seeing a doctor. The chosen treatments were poultices for topical problems, and herbs like sage and thyme were frequently used both topically and internally. The old Norwegian herbal remedies I found were a fascinating source of knowledge about a rapidly vanishing tradition.

The depression in the 1930s and wartime in the 1940s in Norway led to a scarcity of food and the revival of old traditions, extending even into using bark as an ingredient in bread and nettle soup and these as a staple of daily food during the summer.

The development of modern antibiotics and new effective drugs from World War II onwards made the old herbs seem old-fashioned, even redundant. An old doctor I knew referred to the fifties as the 'golden age' of modern medicine. Although most contemporary doctors would disagree with him, he stated that modern medicine seemed to have all the answers to the problems of illness and disease, given more time for research. This was the age of innocence. We didn't know about antibiotic-resistant bacteria, nor did we even consider that many of the new 'wonder' drugs could have serious or even fatal side effects. During this period, much of the traditional knowledge of healing plants was lost. People were saying, why use sage and thyme for a sore throat when penicillin could fix it quicker and easier? The 'green wave' of the seventies in Norway created a renewed interest in natural forms of healing and a revival in the knowledge and benefits of herbs and edible plants.

The public were increasingly concerned about the often serious side effects of the effective synthetic drugs. An old Indian saying became popular in herbal circles I frequented around this period: 'When you isolate separate ingredients from a plant, you keep the knowledge, but throw out the wisdom.' To a certain extent this saying expresses a slight dilemma for modern drug treatment. Single ingredients can have a powerful effect, like the substance taxol from the bark of a tree, that in its natural state has only weak pharmacological effects in the body. In concentrated form, taxol is one of our most powerful chemotherapeutic drugs, used in the treatment of many forms of cancer. I saw enough of acute hospital medicine and chronic illness to know that, when serious disease strikes, there is no question that modern drugs are an essential part of such treatment. Many of the patients I saw in the acute ward at the hospital with heart failure could be helped by digitalis, a drug substance isolated from the plant foxglove (Latin name *Digitalis purpurea*). Giving the same patients a herb tea extract from foxgloves would not have had a powerful enough effect on their heart muscle to make any difference. Natural forms of healing can seldom replace modern medical treatment in such instances.

But as they say, 'an ounce of prevention is worth a ton of cure,' and I felt that a diet based on vegetables, supplemented by healing plants and herbs could be important ingredients in a more holistic approach to preventative medicine and of individualised programmes to restore well-being. When I started gathering herbs and medicinal plants in the early seventies, many of the old sources of knowledge I had in my Norwegian tradition were lost. I had to seek foreign sources, like the old *Culpepers Herbal* from Elizabethan times, one of the most fascinating documents in the history of herbal medicine. I sought exact knowledge in the almost pedantic descriptions found in books from the Deutsche Naturheilkunde, carried by a centuries-old *gesundheit* tradition. At the same time I enjoyed the sheer sensuality of Messeguè's more poetic French herbals. I was pleasantly surprised to discover that both Messeguè's recipes and the old healing herbs described by the venerated Culpeper worked on my modern-day

Norwegian patients. My practice as a herbalist was steadily growing, but to my dismay I found that the same patients had problems using my carefully gathered and dried herbal mixtures – it was often time-consuming, complicated and messy.

Norway was a moderately poor country that struck it rich when oil was discovered in the mid-1970s. This new-found wealth led to people demanding all the trappings of a modern society and the lifestyle that went with it. Out with the old and in with the new! Most people had more money in their pockets but less time on their hands. My time-consuming herbal powders in canvas bags had to give way to pills and other medications bought from the modern health food stores and pharmacies. I never got the same results from the modern tablets, sold over the counter in health food shops, as from my own herbal mixtures. No small surprise, in the light of all the time, effort and tender loving care I had put into my carefully prepared dried herbal mixtures. Natural remedies were now presented and taken in much the same way as prescription pills and I presumed that the separate ingredients found in the herbal combinations had too weak an effect in themselves, compared to modern synthetic drugs. There was little research on the effects of herbs to be found in the late seventies and early eighties and I became slightly disillusioned by the claims of medical healings reported in weekly magazines. In the magazine stories, a great number of patients, many of whom had been suffering from serious conditions, were apparently 'healed' by herbs. However, I could not find any evidence to support these claims in my practice or from other people I spoke with.

During the eighties and early nineties many patients sought my help in a different way. They did not come to me in order to obtain natural medicines or herbs but for advice on the proper use of the bagfuls of natural remedies they had bought, often not knowing or remembering why they had bought them or how they were meant to work. I was finding it increasingly hard to help my patients as much as I wanted through the use of supplements and plant remedies, so instead I concentrated on working in regular medicine as a hospital doctor. I also specialised in medical music therapy, voice-work and therapeutic touch as a concept of self-healing for the patient, and I continued to work with Bach flower remedies, which I had used since the mid-seventies. Although they seemed to work mainly on the emotional and mental areas, they could also sometimes have an effect on bodily health and physical ailments.

It is often hard to leave your first love completely. I kept investigating herbs with healing potential, like ginger and garlic. I had only a cursory interest in aloe vera, until someone gave me an aloe vera plant in 1988. A visitor to our house had a severe burn and I'd heard about the use of aloe vera on burn injuries.

I applied the inner gel from one leaf of the plant and let our friend continue to apply the gel thereafter. I had often worked with burns patients in acute surgery wards and knew the normal span for the healing of such injuries. I was amazed to see that her hands were completely healed within two days and there was no trace of the severe burn damage. Over the years, I had often seen the beneficial effects of using plant remedies on various ailments, but these effects were general and often long-term. They were more of 'an increased well-being' over a span of months than concrete effects on physical symptoms. In contrast I found, to my surprise, that aloe vera's effect on burns was:

- fast acting
- tangible – with a visible effect within a few hours
- working relatively consistently from one person to the next, when I tried it on several other similar cases

Since aloe vera seemed to have a general effect on skin repair, I tried it on different skin ailments. But I was confused by the great number of preparations and companies and had difficulties finding which preparations were most effective. At one point, I bought a large batch of aloe juice from a company on the Canary Islands to use on my patients, only to find that the whole batch was 'rotten' and had to be discarded when it arrived.

As with so many people, it was a personal experience in the late nineties that was the turning point for me regarding aloe vera and its healing potential. I had played soccer on an asphalt surface and had been tackled hard and suffered a severe knee injury. I had severe pain and was not able to walk or move the joint. I had had a similar injury some years earlier and prepared myself for three weeks of painful and protracted recovery. A friend offered me an aloe vera herbal spray that he often used on injuries – with good results. The spray consisted of aloe vera as the main ingredient, supplemented by other herbs with skin-penetrating and anti-inflammatory properties. When I first used the spray – and it was only after a couple of applications – I was surprised to feel the pain subsiding almost immediately. After further use of the spray the pain had disappeared entirely. The next morning I saw that the deep wounds in the knee area were also visibly reduced. With renewed enthusiasm I applied the spray several times during the day and could almost 'watch' the tissue healing. Within two days I was able to walk normally and, within only a week, there was no trace of the injury. After this episode I started to look more deeply into the research literature concerning aloe vera. To my surprise I found that it must be one of the most thoroughly investigated medicinal plants in modern research, with the possible exception of garlic, another traditional plant that has made a significant impact in health and medical use in the last few years. Not all of the research on aloe vera is recent and neither is all of it of the highest quality, but nevertheless it is there and there also seems to be thousands of years of anecdotal evidence. When I review the case histories and testimonials I receive every month from people using aloe vera, there is no doubt in my mind that we have to take the healing capacities of this plant very seriously.

The use of aloe vera has been growing steadily over the last three decades, while many other natural remedies have had their 'day in the limelight' and then faded.[1]

About that time I also contacted Alasdair Barcroft who ran an organisation called the Aloe Vera Centre in London and had already written a book on aloe vera called *Aloe Vera – Nature's Legendary Healer.* We met soon after in Oslo and we have now been working together for several years. This book is something of a culmination of our wish to pool our resources and share our passion for this plant with all of our readers – wherever they live and whatever language they speak.

This ancient plant with seemingly legendary powers has a deserved reputation as a natural healer and is making a spectacular comeback in modern society. This book aims to tell you why.

Dr Audun Myskja

The day that really launched aloe vera in the UK – 14th February 1995

On 14th February 1995, the feature article, 'The cactus drink that may help cure millions' by Hazel Courteney, appeared in the 'Good Health' section of the *Daily Mail.* The article focused on the benefits of taking aloe vera juice for IBS and led to a massive increase in both awareness and demand for aloe vera products in the UK. That article really did more than anything else before had ever done to put aloe vera (as a drinking juice) and its benefits on the map in the UK. It also helped create what has now become a multi-million-pound industry, with tens of thousands of people deriving benefits, on a daily basis, from drinking aloe vera juice and using topical aloe vera products. It is pleasing to know that we were instrumental in bringing about that article and that it has had such a massive impact in the UK. People are now beginning to realise that aloe vera *really* can make a positive impact to their overall health and well-being.

It is hard to believe that it is now nearly twenty years since I first witnessed the incredible healing properties of aloe vera, when, like Hazel Courteney, my younger sister was badly burnt while sunbathing on holiday in the Caribbean. My elder brother and a friend of his immediately treated her with the raw gel from a fresh aloe plant when they saw what had happened. My sister, who had been in considerable pain, said that the relief was almost instantaneous when the raw gel was rubbed on. She felt that the healing properties were 'miraculous' because there was little blistering, the pain subsided and the redness disappeared. Within only a few days she had totally recovered. This was one of those many lifetime incidents one simply files away in the memory and does not think much of, though, as a family, we had travelled extensively and lived in the Far East and Africa for many years and had been regular users of products containing aloe vera.

In the years since being involved in the aloe vera business and establishing the Aloe Vera Centre, a retail mail order and advice centre based in London (see Appendix 1.1), we have seen and heard of thousands of people benefiting from taking products made from this amazing plant. Sometimes I have to pinch myself at what has happened in such a short space of time. I am still continually amazed at the impact this plant has had and continues to have on so many people's (and indeed animals') daily lives and how their overall health, general well-being and quality of life has improved as a direct result of taking aloe vera, either internally, topically or both.

The medical fraternity is still sceptical – but changing!

Although many doctors (including the ones referred to and featured in this book) are themselves now witnessing the benefits of herbal plants like aloe vera, I also know how sceptical many of the so-called conventional medical fraternity have been and indeed still are whenever they have heard of or have been exposed to anything like aloe vera. I have had doctors – people I know personally – laugh when I tell them about aloe vera and what it has done for people. Reactions such as these are, I believe, either due to ignorance or fear or a combination of the two! This is especially the case with plants like aloe vera that often seem to have almost 'panacea-like' or sometimes almost 'inexplicable' healing properties and benefits, or that the plants or plant extracts or products have not been clinically trialled in the UK.

However, it's a fact that you and I will use complementary therapies and natural remedies. Not least because we have become more aware that conventional medicine (which includes the use of pharmaceutical drugs) does not and will never hold all the answers to ill health and doctors like anyone else can also be fallible. Very often such natural remedies, which sometimes have thousands of years of healing history behind them, may not have gone through 'official' clinical trials, but that does not mean to say they do not have a part to play in maintaining good health and improving overall well-being. Many drugs that have gone through these 'official' trials have had to be withdrawn at a later date because of the damaging or toxic side effects they have had. It is important to note that the vast majority of the world's population still, to this day, relies on natural remedies and herbal medicines for the treatment of illnesses and diseases. To my knowledge there is no documentary evidence anywhere that would suggest that taking aloe vera might be harmful in any way to humans or animals, provided the product is of the highest quality and is used correctly.

In writing this book, I had the same difficulties as before in choosing the case histories (see Chapter 5). This is because there are so many examples of people whose conditions and lives have changed and improved significantly as a result of taking aloe vera, either orally or topically or both. One should always remember that whatever aloe vera's remarkable healing history – it dates back over 4,000 years – it cannot and should never be regarded as some magical panacea for all ills. Aloe vera products should never be promoted or sold as a 'cure' and should be used as an integral part of a healthy lifestyle regime.

Aloe vera gel is a natural herbal plant extract with proven healing properties and benefits.

The properties of 'fresh' aloe vera

When the gel is used fresh from the leaf or when it is properly stabilised and processed to retain the essential 'freshness and efficacy' of the raw gel, it has

- potent healing
- immune boosting
- anti-viral, anti-bacterial, anti-fungal
- anti-inflammatory
- nutritional, general health-giving and rejuvenating properties

for a wide range of ailments and disorders in both humans and animals alike.

Although common folklore would have us believe that aloe vera has 'magical' healing properties, it should never be regarded as a cure-all. It does however seem to have significant and highly positive benefits when taken internally (as a drink), topically on the skin or both simultaneously on a wide range of seemingly unconnected ailments and disorders. These range from skin conditions such as acne, athlete's foot, cold sores, eczema, dermatitis and psoriasis to arthritis (both rheumatoid and osteoarthritis), asthma, candida, colitis, conjunctivitis, Crohn's disease, diabetes, diverticulitis, hiatus hernia, IBS, lupus, chronic fatigue syndrome (ME), ulcerative colitis, ulcers, and many, many more, and that's just the human story. It is no less impressive to see the incredible range of disorders affecting animals that aloe vera can help with, from the smallest domestic pets to the largest commercial animals. For animals the list of ailments and benefits seems as endless as it is for humans! For a fuller explanation of how aloe vera can also be used extensively on animals too, see Chapter 7.

Aloe vera – used for centuries

It's amazing to think that aloe vera was used for many centuries by different civilisations to treat a wide range of both internal and external ailments, long before the advent of the more modern medical practices and the development of the pharmaceutical based treatments now practised throughout the world. In the eighteenth and nineteenth centuries, aloe vera was widely used in countries like England and France by both doctors and vets. Despite this, its seemingly 'magical' properties have increasingly been dismissed as folklore and myth by the vast majority of the conventional medical fraternity.

This (in my view) rather misguided assessment, on the grounds that there is no significant clinical evidence to support the hundreds or even thousands of years of documented use and the growing wealth of existing and new anecdotal evidence, should be reconsidered given the now growing evidence of the benefits being derived by users of high quality aloe vera products, and the fact that there is well documented evidence going back to the 1930s relating to aloe vera's healing properties.

Despite this 'resistance' to old established, natural healing plants (much of which is no doubt encouraged by pharmaceutical manufacturers), there has been a move, since the 1980s (by both the medical profession and the general public) towards a more natural, open and holistic approach to general health, well-being and healing.

There is now a groundswell of support for the use of natural products and herbal remedies, in parallel with a greater acceptance of the need for and the role of alternative or complementary therapies. Nowadays it is becoming increasingly common to find complementary therapists working alongside conventional doctors in medical centres and surgeries in the UK and many other so-called developed countries. Also many doctors are now training to become homeopaths and other types of complementary practitioners – something that was almost unheard of twenty years ago.

The market for complementary therapies and the use of nutritional supplements, herbal remedies and natural products has exploded in recent years, as the general public becomes more concerned about the long-term side effects of some 'over-prescribed' medications and realises the role and significance of improved nutrition. More and more people are now beginning to take more control of their own health and realise that 'prevention is better than cure' in terms of developing and maintaining a healthier lifestyle. There is no doubt that over the last thirty years that what started as a rather fringe interest in the USA has become a worldwide trend for improved health and nutrition. There is also no question that aloe vera products, provided they are of the highest quality, can play a significant and highly beneficial role in the development and maintenance of improved health and general well-being for millions of people around the world.

I have written this book to provide an updated, accessible, highly readable and factual introduction to aloe vera, its properties, features, benefits and uses. For those who are interested in more detailed research, there are scores of references at the back of this book in Appendices 2 and 3.

My objective is to make more people aware of the 'miracle' of aloe vera and to provide the general public, both lay-people and health professionals throughout the world, with a book that is both interesting and informative and easy to read. I intend this book to be both factual and educational. I hope it provides you with sufficient information about aloe vera and its properties and benefits to give you the opportunity to make an objective judgement about aloe vera's potential uses and benefits. I'd like to think that armed with this book, you'll feel confident in taking or using aloe vera products internally or topically, whether from a nutritional/health point of view, cosmetically or both.

What Aloe Vera – Nature's Silent Healer *is about*

The aim of this book is to explain in layperson's terms:

- what aloe vera is
- aloe vera's history
- what aloe vera contains
- aloe vera's properties and benefits
- the importance of quality assurance and control in the growing, harvesting, processing and manufacturing of aloe vera products
- case histories of aloe vera users

- comments by doctors, vets, therapists, nutritionists and other health/complementary practitioners
- why aloe vera has an important role in diet and nutrition today
- references to research papers and studies
- objective advice on what you should know before purchasing aloe vera products
- the type of aloe vera products now available worldwide
- what aloe vera can be used for
- how to use aloe vera products and some handy hints and tips

While it is not my intention to promote a particular brand of aloe vera and no branded products are mentioned by name, it has become increasingly obvious in the last few years that the growing awareness and subsequent increase in demand for aloe vera products has led to a rash of poorer quality products being introduced that have little or no therapeutic benefits. These products, which contain much less aloe vera (as a percentage by volume), are being marketed on the back of the extensive and positive publicity that has often not only been initiated by the companies with much higher quality products but also feature case histories using those same higher quality products.

Unfortunately, it is not always obvious from these press articles that there is a huge disparity in quality, potency, purity and efficacy between the different brands of aloe vera currently being sold throughout the UK, Europe, the USA, the Far East, Australasia and other parts of the world. Hence my desire to educate people about what to look for before making the decision to purchase aloe vera products. We have tried to ensure that no specific brand names appear in this book. Any references to aloe vera products are generic and are generally confined to those chapters describing doctors', therapists' or individuals' own experiences with a particular product and its benefits. Many of them have tried different brands of aloe vera and have found them to be ineffective or less effective than the products they have used and may have referred to in this book.

Discern the quality aloe product from the inferior product

I would hope that by reading this book you will be able to discern more easily the difference between the quality of aloe vera products on offer. Say, for example, you read an article in the media, which referred to a case study using aloe vera (or any other such natural remedy), I would maintain that the only way the reader can ensure the maximum chance of gaining similar benefits is to obtain the same brand of aloe vera that was featured. We would suggest referring to the article, telephone number, etc., as given, or writing away for the information to the address listed. Having said that, the reader can still do independent research and can always ensure that what is bought is the best available. This is an important and highly significant point when you consider that the largest producer of aloe vera in the world and the company whose products are most often featured in the media sells its products only direct to the end user. In other words, they are not available through shops. They are available only through appointed distributors. This is also increasingly the case as more and more people purchase nutritional supplements, natural products and herbal remedies on a direct sales basis from manufacturers/suppliers or through the internet.

Consumers everywhere are becoming more discerning about quality and are much more brand conscious than ever before. However there is still a long way to go before all the poorer quality products are forced out of the marketplace through consumer pressure and lack of demand. Bear in mind the old saying, 'you pays your money and you takes your choice.' The use of the words 'aloe vera' could simply mean there is a small percentage by volume in that particular product. It is certainly not an indicator of purity, potency, quality or efficacy, nor does it offer the potential buyer any guide to the amount of aloe vera contained in the product. Very often there is simply not enough aloe vera content to be of any real therapeutic benefit but the very presence of the two magic words – 'aloe vera' – on the label is often enough to sell the product. I will refer to a comment that I made in my first book. It is clearly still relevant five years later. Potential buyers should take heed of the words of a well known US grower of aloe vera who, when asked to comment on the huge proliferation of aloe vera drinks on the market (and this is now very evident in the UK and many other countries in Europe), said,

> If it looks like water, smells like water and tastes like water, then it probably is mostly water.

Please note, there is a difference between water and the naturally occurring liquid in aloe vera's inner gel. Having tried well over fifty different aloe vera drinks in the UK, the USA and Europe myself, I know there is a huge disparity in the stabilised aloe vera gel content, the polysaccharide content and the purity, quality and strength of the products currently being sold (both drinks and topical products). Nowadays, many of the best brands of aloe vera and other nutritional supplements and herbal remedies are sold direct (and not necessarily through shops) and I would suggest that anyone wanting to try aloe vera does a little research before buying a product. I feel that it is important for you as a potential consumer of aloe vera to receive good, objective and ongoing advice about the aloe vera you are buying, whether it's a drink or a topical product.

Additional criteria to consider are the IASC seal of approval (see Chapter 3) and other guarantees. For example, the sixty-day, unconditional money-back guarantee offered to its customers by the world's largest aloe vera grower, manufacturer and distributor, gives those customers total confidence in the quality, efficacy and purity of that company's products. If other manufacturers are serious about their commitment to quality and quality assurance, they should also offer their customers this level of 'security'.

I hope that you find this book informative and educational. I also hope that it provides you with a unique insight into this incredible plant – one of nature's true miracle healers – and the role it can play in helping both you and me to attain better health, immunity and improved overall well-being.

Aloe vera is really only now coming of age

The reason for this is undoubtedly that the words 'aloe vera' are now so much in the public consciousness. The general public and more and more doctors, vets, therapists and other health professionals all over the world are realising that aloe vera can make a significant and powerful contribution to the improved health and general well-being of millions of people. Multinational corporations are now adding to the aloe vera momentum. Many are now including aloe vera in such products as baby wipes, washing powders and washing-up liquids, tissues, safety razors and even toilet paper! Why? Because they too understand the 'marketing power' of including aloe vera in their products, all of which are heavily advertised on TV and in the national press and consumer media. This is just adding to the public awareness of aloe vera, though it is debatable whether the quantity of aloe vera used in such products has any therapeutic value.

There is absolutely no doubt that using aloe vera internally and externally can improve your general health, well-being and skin. Unfortunately, there are still many people, including some complementary and alternative practitioners (plus the allopathic doctors, dentists and vets) who seem to be 'locked in the Dark Ages' when they talk negatively about the safety of drinking or using aloe vera. It is a shame that these negative practitioners don't seem to have kept pace with the developments in the aloe vera industry. Or that they simply give no consideration or credibility to Ayurvedic medicine, Chinese herbal medicine or British herbal medicine, where the references to the uses of aloe vera, both orally and topically are plentiful.

Their opinions and observations are based more on ignorance, possible prejudice or vested interest, rather than any factual information. There is no question that, provided you always use a high quality product, it is not only perfectly safe but it is positively health enhancing. We are only now really beginning to understand the true potential of aloe vera as we rediscover the potent health-giving properties of one of 'nature's true legendary healers'.

1

Aloe vera – ancient myth or modern day miracle?

THROUGHOUT THE ages, copious volumes have been written about aloe vera and its healing properties, uses and benefits. Its reputation as a natural healer has led to it being given a host of names all associated with its beneficial properties. Aloe vera is sometimes known as the 'medicine plant', the 'burn plant', the 'first-aid plant', the 'miracle plant', the 'wand of heaven' and many other equally apt descriptions. In Spanish it's known as 'sa'vila', in Sanskrit it's 'gbrita-kumari', in Malay it's 'jadam', in Chinese it's 'lu-hui' and in Portuguese 'erva-babosa'. These different names, from all parts of the globe, show how great an impact this plant has had over the centuries as more and more civilisations and cultures discovered its wide-ranging healing benefits.

For centuries, aloe vera has been used extensively by many cultures because of its apparently magical properties and effectiveness in treating burns, healing wounds and relieving aches and pains and a whole range of internal and external disorders. Historical documentation from the Egyptians, Romans, Greeks, Algerians, Moroccans, Tunisians, Arabians, Indians and Chinese reported its use for both medicinal and cosmetic applications.

Earliest record of aloe vera – circa 2100 BC

No one can really say for certain when aloe vera's healing powers were first discovered or for how long it has been used in this context. However one of the earliest recorded medicinal uses of it can be found on an ancient Sumerian clay tablet dating back to 2100 BC, and there are even reports (unproven) of drawings of the plant on the walls of temples in ancient Egypt which date back even further, to 4000 BC. Because of its potent properties, aloe vera's prowess as a healer has been the stuff of legend. Through the ages, it was revered by many civilisations and cultures, so much so that it acquired almost divine status.

Whatever the reality about its first recorded use, there is absolutely no doubt – it is too well chronicled – that aloe vera played a significant role in the pharmacopoeia of many early civilisations, both BC and AD. There is well documented and irrefutable evidence of its use as a broad-spectrum healing agent in areas of the world as far apart as southern Europe, Asia, North Africa, the Americas and the Far East.

Egyptian use of aloe vera

One of the earliest and most detailed accounts of aloe vera's use appears in the Egyptian *Papyrus Ebers*, which dates back to 1550 BC. This ancient document (the originals of which are located in Leipzig University in Germany) stated that aloe vera had many medicinal values and that they were widely acclaimed and had been for many centuries before.

The plant of immortality

The ancient Egyptians revered aloe vera and called it the 'plant of immortality'. Part of the myth and legend that surrounds aloe vera are the claims (highly disputed!) that the two famous Egyptian queens, Nefertiti and Cleopatra, used extracts of the plant in their beauty regimes. Whether or not either of these two queens was beautiful is open to question but such stories added to aloe vera's status.

Mesopotamian use of aloe vera

The ancient peoples of Mesopotamia were said to have used the plant to ward off evil spirits from their homes (maybe the spirits didn't like the taste!!).

Arabs name aloe vera the 'desert lily'

Aloe vera had apparently reached Persia and India by 600 BC – it was probably introduced there by Arab traders. The Arabs, who called the plant the 'desert lily', had been using it for a range of both internal and external disorders, and had developed a process to separate the inner gel and sap from the outer leaf or rind. This involved using their bare feet (similar to the old way of crushing grapes) to crush the leaves before placing the resulting pulp into goatskin bags. These were then set out in the sun until completely dried and the contents ground to a powder.

You will doubtless all be relieved to know that today's leading manufacturers of aloe vera products now use much more sophisticated extraction and stabilisation techniques (as I mentioned in my first book)!! To this day, the Bedouin tribes and Tuareg warriors of the Sahara know the plant as the 'desert lily', though with the increasing urbanisation of so many of these cultures and their ways of life, people soon forget the importance of natural 'plant medicine'.

Aloe vera and Alexander the Great

From around 500 BC onwards, the island of Socotra, which lies off the Horn of Africa, developed a reputation as a centre of aloe vera cultivation. Another of the aloe vera legends was that Alexander the Great was persuaded to conquer Socotra in order to gain control of the aloe vera plantations, thus ensuring a continuous supply of plants for his wounded soldiers during his extensive military campaigns. This legend is again highly disputed by historians because there is apparently no record of Alexander ever having ventured that far south during his military campaigns, though it does sound a plausible if rather romantic story!

There are reputed to have been at least five aloe vera plantations on Socotra and these were probably the source of the reported aloe trade with countries as far away as Tibet, India and China. It is even feasible that Alexander the Great (if indeed he did use aloe vera) obtained supplies from this same Socotran source but not in the manner as described above.

Hindus and Chinese use of aloe vera

The Hindus believed that aloe vera grew in the Garden of Eden and called it the 'silent healer'. Ancient Chinese doctors and physicians considered it to be one of the plants that had major therapeutic properties and called it the 'harmonic remedy'.

Dioscorides – the first written account

Much of this may be part of the 'legend' of aloe vera, and it is to a famous Greek physician of the first century AD that we must turn for the first real benchmark in our present day understanding of the general use of aloe vera medicinally. Dioscorides in his *De Materia Medica* (AD 41–68) writes that the aloe vera plant,

> Has a leaf like squill, thick, fat, somewhat broad in its compass, broken or bowbacked behind and both sides of the leaf are prickly, appearing thin and short. All of it has a strong scent and is very bitter to the taste. It has the power of binding, of inducing sleep, of drying, of thickening of the body, it loosens the belly and the cleansing of the stomach by drinking two spoonfuls with cold water or warm milk.

Dioscorides developed both his skills as a physician and his knowledge of aloe vera's remarkable healing properties while accompanying the conquering Roman armies of the time. His writings included a commentary on the use of aloe vera for a broad range of applications. These included the treatment for boils and haemorrhoids, for healing the foreskin, to help soothe dry and itchy skin, for ulcerated genitals, for irritations to the tonsils, gums and throat, to help heal bruising and to stop the bleeding in wounds.

Pliny the Elder, AD 23–79

Another famous physician of that era, Pliny the Elder (AD 23–79), confirmed in his *Natural History* the findings of Dioscorides. However, he went a stage further by establishing that aloe vera could also help with numerous other ailments, including leprous sores. He also stated that aloe vera could also reduce perspiration (could aloe vera have been the world's first anti-perspirant or deodorant?). Apparently honey and rose oil were often mixed with aloe vera to counteract the bitterness. At that time people probably did not understand how to remove the major part of the bitter sap content and quite possibly because no one, even then, believed that the plant, on its own, could be such a powerful and effective healer!

The quality issue in the first century

Interestingly even in those days (first century AD), both Dioscorides and Pliny warned of the difference between high quality aloe vera and some of the other lesser quality products that were available. The subject of quality is nothing new! The huge disparity in the quality, efficacy, purity and potency of aloe vera and aloe vera products has been a major concern and a talking point for those using aloe vera for nearly 2,000 years!

The Roman physicians

By the end of the second century AD, it seems that aloe vera had become an important part of the developing pharmacopoeia of the age and was used by physicians such as Antyllus, Aretacus and Galen (AD 131–201) – the latter of whom was the physician to the Roman emperor, Marcus Aurelius. Galen's formidable reputation developed not only from his prodigious work as an author (he is said to have written hundreds of books and his influence on both herbal and conventional medicine over the ages was considerable) but also from his important role as the physician to Rome's gladiators.

He is reputed to have drawn many of his ideas from the works of both Hippocrates (BC 460–377) and Aristotle (BC 384–322), who themselves had been influenced by the writings of both Egyptian and Indian 'medical writers'. Galen's works soon became the benchmark for medical practice and the treatment of illnesses and his influence also spread to the Arab world. Even as late as the sixteenth and seventeenth centuries, his writings were still being quoted by medical practitioners in Europe and the Middle East.

Chinese use of aloe vera in the seventh century

Aloe vera was used extensively throughout the Arab world to treat a variety of internal and external disorders and was also an important trade commodity. In the seventh century, the Chinese *Materia Medicas* made particular mention of aloe vera's healing powers for conditions like sinusitis (I will definitely attest to that) and numerous skin and internal disorders, including worm fever and convulsions in children.

Elixir of Jerusalem

Many years later, the Knights Templar were said to have developed a brew or concoction of palm wine, aloe vera pulp and hemp – an elixir that they called the 'elixir of Jerusalem' and to which they attributed their health, strength and longevity.

This elixir may have similar healing and health-giving properties to the drink mentioned by Michael Peuser in his book, *Aloe – Empress of the Healing Plants*, referred to in Chapter 4 of this book.

Middle Ages and the Renaissance

During the Middle Ages and the Renaissance, the medicinal use of aloe vera spread across the world and northwards into the colder parts of Europe. Because the plant was a native of hotter climates, it was not fully understood by the northern Europeans, though it grew widely in Spain, Portugal and Italy where it was held in high regard as a healer. More of the 'legends' of aloe vera surround the stories that the famous explorers Marco Polo and Christopher Columbus both wrote concerning its healing properties. They were reputed to have used it on their respective voyages and explorations to China and the West Indies (as they are now known).

Knowledge of the 'miracle plant' was passed down through the generations by word of mouth (folklore), and where it grew indigenously it was revered for its potent medicinal properties and its seemingly 'magical' powers of healing. Ancient priests used it in many religious rites, and royal physicians wrote of its properties and wide-ranging uses and benefits in their medical records. To local, indigenous peoples, aloe vera was a traditional remedy for numerous ailments either used raw from the leaf itself or processed in some way by boiling or drying.

The use of aloe vera in the fifteenth century

In the fifteenth century, a time that heralded a massive explosion in exploration by the then leading maritime powers, namely Spain, Portugal, Holland, France and Britain, it was the Jesuit priests of Spain who were instrumental in bringing aloe vera to the New World, as they called it. As highly educated physicians and scholars, they were familiar with the famous Greek and Roman medical texts and the writings of such people as Dioscorides and Pliny the Elder. They understood aloe vera's healing properties and powers and began to use it extensively when they accompanied explorers to new countries. The Spanish are credited with introducing aloe vera not only to their New World possessions but also for its spread through what is now known as Central America, the West Indies, California, Florida, Texas and so on.

Aloe vera spreads through the Caribbean and the Americas

Aloe vera spread rapidly throughout Central and South America and the Caribbean and became an important source of local, 'indigenous' healing in the Caribbean, in both the French- and English-speaking areas. It is a plant that has developed a formidable reputation as a potent healer and general tonic, and in Jamaica it's known as 'Sinckle Bible'. Most people in the Caribbean are familiar with aloe vera's legendary healing powers and it is something that is used on a daily basis by locals for general health and well-being.

People use aloe vera for their skin and for numerous topical ailments, as a health tonic and even as a shampoo. It is also sold in a fresh form (as fresh whole leaves – the same as my sister was given) or a bottled form to European, American and other tourists as a potent healer for sunburn!

Why aloe vera fell from grace

Strangely there seem to be few mentions of aloe vera for the next two centuries, except for medical references to 'bitter aloes', and in the northern European countries where it was generally used as a powerful and highly effective purgative remedy. This must have been where the sap was used in its entirety or the whole leaf was used with the sap content intact. It was really its fearsome reputation as a purgative, rather than its potent healing properties and use as a rejuvenating tonic, that stuck for so many years and still, to this day, clouds the opinions of the less enlightened and less well informed observers! Over the last three decades, the aloe vera industry has moved on in leaps and bounds. The inner-gel-based, high quality, pure, potent and efficacious aloe vera products that have gained so much in reputation and popularity in recent decades are totally different from the 'bitter aloe' products that were often referred to as purgatives.

Ironically, it may have been its deserved reputation as a healing plant that was ultimately its undoing and contributed to its failure to perform in the more temperate climates. In colder climates, where aloe vera was imported, it never demonstrated the same degree of healing that was apparent in the countries where it grew naturally and was available as a completely fresh plant. The main reason was the availability of fresh aloe vera leaves. As aloe vera's reputation as a healer spread throughout different regions of the world (including those where it did not grow naturally), so the demand for the leaves increased. However, there was little or no understanding of the necessity to use fresh leaves in the balms and other medications and healing products of the time, in order to ensure their purity, efficacy, potency and indeed safety. It was therefore impossible to reproduce, to anything like the same degree, the seemingly 'magical' healing properties of aloe vera when fresh leaves were unavailable. As a result, and perhaps rather unfairly it would seem, aloe vera's reputation faltered.

Over the years more and more people became convinced that the amazing healing powers of which they had heard so much were rooted more in myth and folklore than in fact and reality. So, although in the hotter parts of the world, where aloe vera grew in abundance, the plant continued to be used as widely as ever for wounds and a host of other internal and external disorders, in Europe and North America it was discarded by the medical profession. This move gathered pace after World War II with the rapid advancement and availability of pharmaceutical drugs. The once mighty aloe vera was superseded by the rapid advances in so-called modern medicine and the introduction of synthetic drugs and soon lost its reputation as a natural healer.

Aloe vera fights back in the 1950s

However, soon after, in the 1950s, there was a growing realisation among the scientific community that more work had to be done to understand the impact of oxidation and how detrimental it was to the quality and effectiveness of the inner leaf gel extract.

Scientists at last discovered how the oxidation process vastly reduced the medicinal properties and overall healing benefits of fresh aloe vera. For aloe vera to stand any chance of making a comeback in the face of the monopoly and stranglehold that conventional medicine and synthetic drugs had on medical practice and the health industry in the post-World War II era, a method had to be found to ensure that the efficacy and integrity of the plant's healing properties were totally maintained, post-harvest. This would require the development of a process to both stabilise and preserve the inner gel and thus ensure it could be utilised in a pure form by people throughout the world and not just by those who were fortunate enough to have sufficient mature plants in their immediate neighbourhood.

Over the years, many different processing techniques and stabilisation methods were tried but were found to be ineffective. The reasons for continued failure were mainly the result of the use of excessive heat that effectively destroyed many of the active ingredients and nutrients and so unwittingly compromised the plant's unique healing properties. The other main reason was that some techniques used the whole leaf, which at the time resulted in contamination of the inner gel extract. Whichever technique was used, there remained a higher than acceptable percentage of the bitter substance called aloin – apparently discovered in 1851 by a Scotsman in Edinburgh called Smith (another first for Scotland!). Aloin is the bitter purgative agent found just below the hard green rind. Although most people now accept that its presence in very small amounts (measured in ppm or parts per million) is actually beneficial, in those days there was little knowledge of either its benefits or, indeed, of ways of ensuring that extraction techniques ensured only the minimum amount remained.

'Silent healer' and other common names for aloe vera

Nowadays, it is also known as the 'silent healer' in the USA, and the Russians, echoing the ancient Egyptians, call aloe vera the 'elixir of longevity'. In the Americas, the plant was used by native Indians, including the Mayans (Yucatan, Mexico) and the Seminoles (Florida) for its moisturising, healing and rejuvenating powers. The Mayan women are reputed to have used the bitter tasting sap to help wean their babies off the breast.

Aloe vera in the USA

The history of this remarkable plant can be traced back to the 1820s when a number of aloe vera preparations were listed in the US pharmacopoeia. Like so many references of the time, most potential uses were related to the laxative 'benefits' of aloe. By the 1920s, there were over twenty-five different 'popular preparations' and the commercial cultivation of the plant had started. It wasn't until the ground-breaking work of Collins and Collins in 1935 that the healing powers of fresh aloe vera were established in the modern era. Since then, the USA has been at the forefront of both research into the benefits of aloe vera and its wide ranging healing properties and its development as a commercial crop to supply the burgeoning international demand for products made from this remarkable plant. Worldwide the aloe vera industry (this includes all finished products containing aloe vera) is now estimated to be worth in excess of US$42 billion.

'Fresh' aloe vera in a bottle – 1970s to 1990s

The breakthrough for 'fresh aloe vera available to anyone, anywhere' came in the 1970s when scientists in the USA found an effective way of separating the aloin and the rind and then stabilising the inner leaf gel (using natural ingredients and cold processing techniques). This technique at last provided consumers around the world with a product that was 'essentially identical' to the inner gel from a fresh leaf even when consumed or used several years later. The technique was patented and paved the way for a new and exciting chapter in the 'legend of aloe vera' story and one that has resulted in the aloe vera industry developing into a multi-billion dollar global business over the last twenty years.

Aloe vera products, and especially those that are 'essentially' the same as fresh aloe vera, are now making an even greater impact on overall health and general well-being. This is because more and more health professionals realise the true value of this remarkable plant and the significant contribution it can make to complement the role of allopathic medicine. As we move further into the new millennium, myth and folklore have now been replaced by the growing realisation that plants like aloe vera (and other natural products) can play an integral part in prevention as well as improved health and nutrition. High quality aloe vera products now have a very real and important role to play in the ongoing development and management of good health and in combating numerous internal and external disorders and diseases.

Aloe vera in the new millennium

We are witnessing a dramatic change in the health of many young people in the developed and more affluent parts of the world. Young people are now overfed, undernourished and lead more sedentary indoor lives than ever before – bombarded by advertising for sugary/salty snacks, processed/fast food and computer games. Diet plays a major factor in this frightening new scenario. Fatty, processed foods, with high salt, sugar and other 'unhealthy' substance contents are beginning to take their toll on young people. More and more health professionals, including doctors, medical specialists, nutritionists and dieticians are realising that more and more young people are beginning to suffer from obesity, heart disease, diabetes and numerous digestive disorders – illnesses and ailments normally associated with older people. Young people also take much less exercise than they did in previous generations.

The warning signs are there and unless we all take more responsibility for our own health and that of our children, we will become part of that ticking time bomb, if not directly then indirectly through higher taxes to pay for a huge increase in the healthcare costs of more chronically ill young people. Some health professionals talk about the potential for these types of diseases in almost 'epidemic' scale proportions. No one is suggesting that taking aloe vera can address the causes of such problems. I would suggest that by educating more people about health and diet – a fairly simple and straightforward task – we can promote the role of natural health drinks such as aloe vera and their potential role as an integral part of an improved health regime and a better lifestyle.

We have started this new millennium with potentially one of the most exciting trials that has ever been undertaken involving aloe vera drinking juice. In 2001, the world's first ever randomised, placebo-controlled, double-blind, crossover clinical trial, using an aloe vera gel drinking juice in the treatment of IBS, was launched at the Morriston Hospital/University of Wales, Swansea. The trial, under the supervision of Professor Baxter (the professor of surgery) and his team (including Professor Williams), will involve over 200 patients – all of whom have not responded to conventional treatments – and it is expected to last about three years. IBS is a common and debilitating problem and a great deal is known about the disease but effective treatment has remained elusive. Although there has been considerable anecdotal evidence that drinking aloe vera juice can help manage IBS, this is the first time that a rigorous scientific trial has been undertaken anywhere in the world. In the UK alone, IBS is the most common disorder seen by gastroenterologists and is estimated to affect around twenty per cent of the people in the developed world at some time during their lives.

In 2002, research funded by the IASC and undertaken at the University of Scranton in the USA (see Chapter 8) has found that the bio-availability of essential vitamins, such as vitamins C and E, can be enhanced by as much as 350 per cent when taken with aloe vera juice compared to water. Other trials using aloe vera for arthritis, burns and many other ailments, diseases and problems are expected to be undertaken in the near future. The legend lives on.

2

Aloe vera – the true aloe

Botany and anatomy

ALOE VERA (L) Burm f (the same as Aloe Barbadensis Miller), is just one of a large genus, of over 400 species, of succulent plants originally from Africa and Arabia. They were once classified in the liliaceae but now have their own family, the aloaceae. Aloe grows typically in semi-arid regions but a few have been found in true desert, some in wetter regions and even one species adjacent to a waterfall.

The gel of several species, including aloe vera and aloe arborescens, have been found to have significant healing and therapeutic properties. Of these, aloe vera has been more widely used, probably because the gel is more abundant, being easier both to grow and to extract commercially. Aloe vera is also known as Aloe Barbadensis Miller, though apparently the first name is acknowledged to have priority by about ten days (Newton, 1979). However, the commonly accepted name now seems to be Aloe Barbadensis Miller and that is the description that you will find in most media articles about aloe vera and on the labelling of most aloe vera products.

Aloe vera – the 'true aloe'

It is now irrefutable that the most potent of all the aloe species, rich in minerals, vitamins, amino acids, enzymes, mono- and polysaccharides and many other constituents, is Aloe Barbadensis Miller, commonly known as aloe vera or 'true aloe'. Aloe vera is now grown commercially in many parts of the world, including the Americas, the Caribbean, Asia, southern Europe, Africa and Australasia. Aloe vera is also the species with which this book is concerned and any reference to aloe means aloe vera, unless otherwise specified. While the writer accepts that other species of aloe may have healing properties it is not the intention of this book to discuss or describe these. Some confusion exists, but it is thought that the word 'aloe' is derived from an old Arabic word 'alloeh', meaning 'shining, bitter substance', while 'vera' is the Latin word for true, because in ancient times this particular species was regarded as the most effective for general therapeutic and medical use.

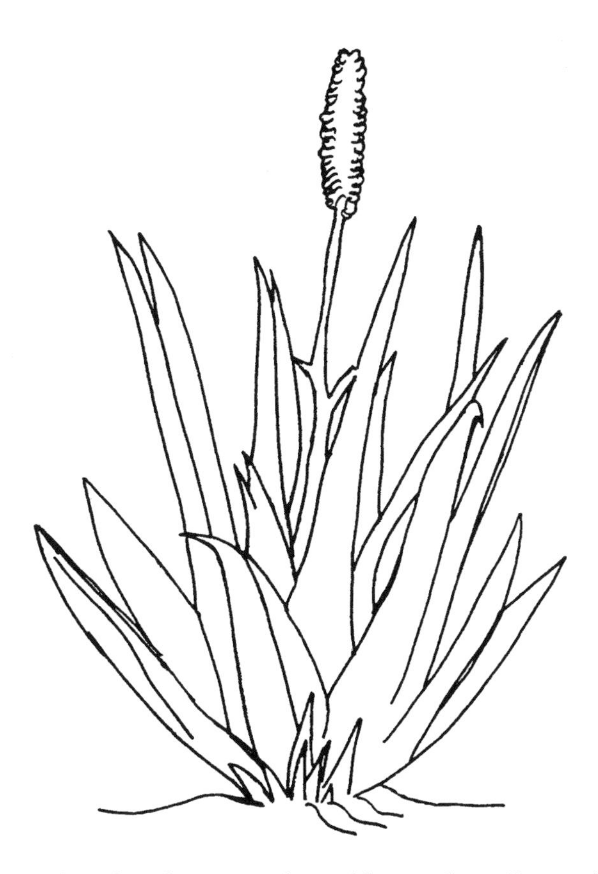

Diagram 1 – the aloe vera plant (drawn by a Barcroft child!).

Not a cactus but a perennial succulent

Although some people consider that aloe vera resembles a cactus, it is in fact a perennial succulent. It is a member of the aloaceae and is related to the liliacea family, which includes the onion and garlic (both of which have well documented and potent healing and health-giving properties), the asparagus, the lily and the tulip. The aloe vera plant is characterised by long, hard, sword-shaped, fleshy, green leaves, with sharp points and an array of barbed spikes on each leaf edge. Each plant can have between twenty and thirty leaves and these leaves grow in a rosette pattern straight out of the ground. When the plant blooms, its bright yellow flowers appear on a central leafless stem high above the gel-bearing leaves (see Colour Plate 1).

The genus 'aloe' belongs to a larger class of plants known as 'xeroids', so called because of their ability to open and close their stomata (minute openings in the epidermis of the leaf) to ensure that water is retained when necessary within the plant. This ability to conserve precious water allows members of the xeroid group to survive long periods of dry weather and even drought conditions when other plants would undoubtedly wither and die.

Aloe vera also has the apparently 'miraculous' ability (due to its special chemical and physical make-up) to close up any wound or damage to its outer skin almost instantly, thus preventing the loss of precious water and nutrients from the plant. It is this incredible power to heal itself that may have given ancient civilisations the clue to the potential healing and curative powers of this remarkable plant. You should try and see for yourself how quickly such activity takes place. If you have an aloe vera plant, try cutting off the tip or even slicing into one of the larger, more mature leaves and then observe how quickly the plant's in-built response and healing mechanisms take to seal over the freshly cut leaf. The healing action is both fast and highly effective – providing a totally airtight seal.

When cultivated for commercial use, the plant takes three to four years to mature (this is a vital factor and one that is described in detail in Chapter 3). At this stage, the gel contained within the tough green outer leaf is at its optimum potency in terms of nutritional content and potential therapeutic value.

The dimensions of a mature plant

When fully grown the outer leaves can reach a height of around sixty to ninety centimetres (two to three feet or more), are generally about seven and a half to ten centimetres (three to four inches) in width at their widest point, and weigh approximately one and a half to two kilograms (three to four pounds) each. The rosette-like growing pattern means that the larger, thicker, harder and more mature outer leaves protect the newer growth and the younger leaves, growing from the centre of the plant. The plants also produce tiny replicas of themselves (similar to the common household plant known as the 'spider plant'), called pups, which are carefully removed to avoid damaging the leaf or root and then planted out in special nursery areas or beds. Every step of the cultivation and harvesting process (including the removal and replanting of pups) is carried out by hand to avoid damaging the leaves. If the leaves are damaged during the harvesting or collection processes and the gel is exposed to the elements, it will start to oxidise and thus begin to lose its unique nutritional and therapeutic properties.

Leaf structure

The aloe vera leaf is made up of four layers,

- the rind – the tough outer protective layer
- the sap – the bitter layer may be a natural chemical protection from animals
- the mucilage
- the gel or parenchyma layer (this is the material that is filleted out for inner gel-based products)

The structure of the aloe vera leaf (as seen in Diagram 2) shows the hard green outer rind (around fifteen cells thick), which is important because of its

Diagram 2 – leaf structure

Four key layers in the leaf structure.

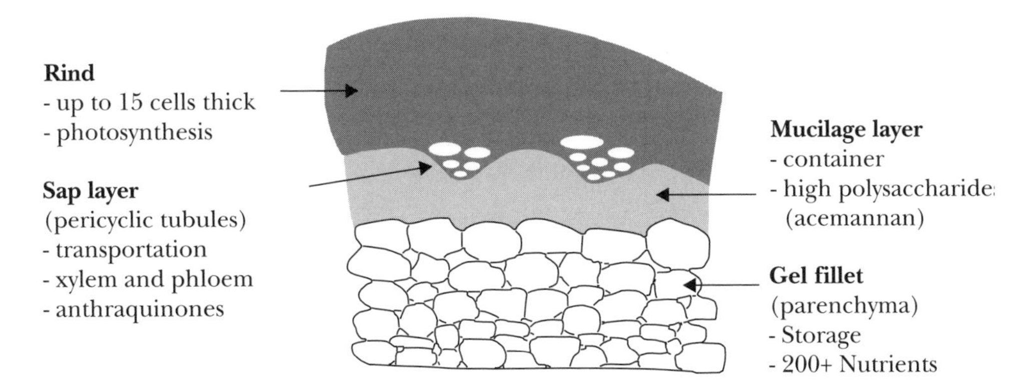

physical protective properties. Additionally, it is this layer that contains all the photosynthetic materials and where the synthesis of all the naturally occurring nutrients (currently over 200 have been identified) found in aloe vera, takes place. This layer contains vascular bundles running the length of the leaf, and closely associated with these bundles are elongated cells known as 'aloin' cells, in which phenolic substances are either synthesised or stored or both. Below the rind layer is the sap, which has a yellowish colour and a very bitter taste (this is the layer in which the anthraquinones are found – the importance of these are discussed later in this chapter).

When an aloe vera leaf is cut, an exudate arises from this area and tends to drip out when the leaf is held up. This substance was probably the origin of 'bitter aloes', well known in many pharmacopoeiae for their purgative properties. Below the sap is the mucilage layer (this is the layer rich in the long-chain sugars, known as polysaccharides, including acemannan – the important role of acemannan is discussed in detail later in this chapter), which effectively holds in the next layer, the parenchyma or gel. The parenchyma or gel layer, in the middle, is the largest section of the leaf and is full of a gelatinous gel. When exposed, this layer resembles a 'raw fish fillet' – it has a structure and is transparent. The inner gel is both sterile (hence it can be used immediately, safely and effectively as a freshly cut leaf on wounds, burns, etc.) and where most of the nutrients are stored.

KEY TIP

The most effective manufacturing and extraction techniques, as pioneered and used by the world's largest aloe vera grower and processor, ensure that the gel is filleted to retain the mucilage layer (with the polysaccharides), the sterile gel or parenchyma layer (with all the nutrients) and only small traces of anthraquinones from the sap layer.

KEY TIP

The Food and Drug Administration (FDA) in the USA is reported to have classified aloe vera juice, with or without the sap, as a vegetable juice, provided that the juice does not contain more than fifty ppm of aloin (more details about stabilisation and processing in Chapter 3).

Nature's treasure chest

Aloe vera is a veritable treasure chest of nutritional ingredients. Since Smith and Stenhaus (in 1851) showed that aloin was the principal ingredient responsible for aloe's laxative effects, an ever increasing number of biologically active compounds have been identified. To date, more than 200 have been identified by scientists, though this number is likely to rise as more and more research is carried out to try and unlock the plant's many secrets.

The list of amino-acids, enzymes, minerals, polysaccharides, vitamins and other key categories of naturally occurring ingredients reads like a *What's What* of nutrition. Aloe vera undoubtedly contains a unique spectrum of 'micronutrients' and research continues apace to discover what it is that makes aloe vera work and thus determine what the ingredient is that gives this plant such 'magical' healing properties.

> KEY TIP
> The opinion of the many 'aloe gurus' who have painstakingly investigated aloe vera over the years seems to conclude that there is no one single, so-called 'magic bullet' or 'ingredient'. Rather, it is the synergistic way in which all of the nutritional components work that gives aloe vera its incredible healing and nutritional properties and health-giving benefits.

The natural chemical constituents of aloe vera can be categorised in the following main areas:

- Amino acids
- Anthraquinones
- Enzymes
- Lignin
- Minerals
- Mono- and polysaccharides
- Salicylic acid
- Saponins
- Sterols
- Vitamins

All these are described in more detail below:

The 'what's what' in aloe vera

Amino acids

Amino acids are the building blocks of protein and affect brain function, including emotions. Twenty amino acids are considered necessary for good health (in human beings) and the body is able to 'manufacture' only twelve, all except the eight 'essential' (essential because the body does not manufacture them itself) amino acids, which we have to introduce through our food and drink intake. All of the eight essential amino acids can be found in aloe vera and they are:

- Isoleucine
- Leucine
- Lysine
- Methionine
- Phenylalanine
- Threonine
- Valine
- Tryptophan

The non-essential amino acids are:

- Alanine
- Arginine
- Asparagine
- Cysteine
- Glutamic acid
- Glycine
- Histidine
- Proline
- Serine
- Tyrosine
- Glutamine
- Aspartic acid

Isoleucine

Research would suggest that an isoleucine supplement may help with symptoms of ME because it reduces levels of tryptophan (a precursor to sleep) in the brain. Isoleucine is found in such foods as cheese, oats, gelatine and sunflower seeds.

Leucine

Again this helps to inhibit the level of tryptophan in the brain and when taken in combination with isoleucine it can reduce chronic fatigue. It is found in the same food sources as isoleucine.

Lysine

In studies it has been shown to help with the symptoms of the herpes virus. In trials, people taking a lysine supplement have seen a reduction in the frequency of outbreaks of cold sores and genital herpes. It is found in such foods as tofu, beans, lentils, broccoli and potatoes.

Methionine

In studies this has been found to help combat allergies, such as hay fever, as it reduces histamines. In order for it to be metabolised effectively, it should be taken in conjunction with B vitamins (i.e. B12 and folic acid). It is found in such foods as Brazil nuts, sesame seeds and oats.

Phenylalanine

It is used in the production of adrenal and thyroid hormones. Through its production of natural painkillers – known as endorphins – it has been found to help reduce persistent pains caused by backache and arthritis. It also seems to act as a natural anti-depressant. It is found in such foods as gelatine, cheese, peanuts, almonds and oats.

Threonine

A study found that low levels of threonine were found in patients with clinical depression, and of those supplemented with it the majority had reduced symptoms. It is found in such foods as peanuts, almonds, gelatine, cheese and fish.

Valine

This has been shown to help reduce the symptoms of ME by inhibiting the levels of trypotophan in the brain. It is recommended to be taken in conjunction with isoleucine and leucine. It is found in such foods as gelatine, cheese, peanuts, oats, fish and sunflower seeds.

Tryptophan

This produces serotonin in the brain and is used in common with anti-depressants. Low levels of serotonin can cause insomnia, depression, food cravings and attention deficit disorder. A double-blind study on a group of twenty obese patients using 900 milligrams per day of tryptophan resulted in significant weight loss in all patients and a dramatic reduction in food cravings, especially for carbohydrates, over a twelve-week period. It is found in such foods as sunflower seeds, cheese, oats and Brazil nuts.

The non-essential amino acids are:

Alanine

People on low-fat or high-protein diets or who do a lot of exercise need more alanine, as do diabetics, who need higher amounts in order to produce enough glucose. Alanine is found in such foods as gelatine, red meat, fish, sunflower seeds, almonds, peanuts and oats. There are no alanine food supplements.

Arginine

This is used mainly to make muscle tissues and sperm as well as relaxing blood vessels. Recent research has found that L-arginine helps in reducing angina, high blood pressure and glaucoma. Supplementation has also been found to help increase muscle mass for weight trainers. Arginine is found in such foods as gelatine, peanuts, almonds, Brazil nuts, red meat, fish, oats and grains.

Asparagine

Closely related to aspartic acid, asparagine is required by the nervous system to maintain equilibrium. It is also required for amino acid transformation from one form to the other, which is achieved in the liver. Asparagine is found in such foods as dairy and beef products and poultry and eggs.

Cysteine

Research has shown that cysteine can be used when an overdose of paracetamol has been taken, because it helps to break down toxins in the liver. It is also helpful for cancer patients undergoing chemotherapy, as well as helping to remove excess heavy metals from the body. It is found in such foods as sunflower seeds, oats, eggs, wheat flour and Brazil nuts.

Glutamic acid

Its main use is in the production of folic acid, which is necessary in healthy people, especially women. However, too much glutamic acid in the body can sometimes promote epilepsy and seizures. People need to make sure that they keep their vitamin B6 levels high in order to combat the high levels of glutamic acid, which is broken down by an enzyme supported by vitamin B6. Glutamic acid is found in such foods as cheese, sunflower seeds, almonds and wheat flour. There is no need for supplements because we get plenty from food, and levels may even need to be reduced if you are susceptible to epilepsy.

Glycine

People suffering from gout may be helped by glycine supplements because it helps to break down uric acid in the kidneys. Several scientific studies have found that supplementation can also reduce the symptoms of schizophrenia. Glycine is found in such foods as gelatine, buckwheat flour, walnuts, almonds and sunflower seeds.

Histadine

Its main function is for making histamines that cause allergies and hay fever, so sufferers should make sure their intake is not too high. Research has shown that people with rheumatoid arthritis have very low levels of histadine and that supplementation reduces joint inflammation. Taken alongside standard anti-inflammatory painkillers, it also helps to reduce the main side effect of the painkillers, which is gastric inflammation. Histadine is found in such foods as gelatine, dairy products, peanuts and sunflower seeds.

Proline

This has been shown to slow down the progression of a condition called gyrate atrophy or lesions of the eye. It needs to be taken with vitamins B3 and C. It is also believed to speed up wound-healing. Proline is found in such foods as gelatine, cheese, wheat, oats and sunflower seeds.

Serine

Research has found that supplementation with serine can improve memory function with regard to numbers, names and lists in the over-sixties by as much as twelve years, because it helps to release two crucial memory neuro-transmitters, acetylcholine and dopamine. It is found in such foods as eggs, walnuts, gelatine and almonds.

TYROSINE

This makes the neuro-transmitter dopamine, which is low in people with Parkinson's disease. Used alongside conventional treatments, there have been better results than with drugs alone. It can also help to reduce stress levels because it increases the production of the hormone noradrenaline, which is depleted by stress. It is found in such foods as peanuts, cheese, almonds, sunflower seeds and eggs.

GLUTAMINE

Studies have shown that supplementation with L-glutamine can hasten the repair of stomach linings damaged by excessive alcohol consumption, as well as slowing down the body's cravings for alcohol. L-glutamine is found in such foods as potatoes, barley and cabbage.

ASPARTIC ACID

Research has shown that aspartic acid is beneficial for cancer patients who have undergone radiotherapy because it helps red-blood-cell-producing organs to regenerate after radiation exposure. It can be found in such foods as walnuts, gelatine, almonds, sunflower seeds, meat and fish.

Much of the information in this section on amino acids has been sourced from the excellent book by Linda Lazarides called *The Amino Acid Report.*

Anthraquinones

There are twelve anthraquinones found in the sap layer of aloe vera, which are:

- Aloetic acid (antibiotic)
- Aloe emodin (bactericidal)
- Aloin (analgesic, anti-bacterial, anti-viral)
- Anthracene (antibiotic, anti-inflammatory)
- Anthranol (antibiotic)
- Barbaloin (analgesic, antibiotic)
- Chrysophanoic acid (fungicidal for the skin)
- Emodin (bactericidal and skin problems)
- Ester of cinnamic acid (analgesic, anaesthetic)
- Ethereal oil (analgesic)
- Isobarbaloin (analgesic, antibiotic)
- Resistanol (bactericidal)

Anthraquinones have traditionally been regarded as powerful laxatives and researchers have found that when used in relatively high concentrations on their own these substances can be toxic to cells. However when present in the gel and in low concentrations of less than the widely accepted level of fifty ppm, the anthraquinone fraction can demonstrate highly beneficial and potent properties, which include: acting as a tonic for the digestive system by strengthening the digestive muscle; being effective natural analgesics (painkillers) and having powerful virucidal, anti-bacterial and anti-fungal properties. When the anthraquinones are present in properly stabilised, pure aloe vera drinks, these beneficial properties are demonstrably evident without the other less desirable side effects such as the laxative/purgative effect.

Enzymes – the keys to life

Enzymes are critical to both human and animal life and their function is quite simply to break down the proteins in the food we eat into amino acids. These are then absorbed by the body and converted back by the enzymes into body protein. Essentially, enzymes turn the food we eat into fuel for every cell in our body, so enabling those cells to function and our body to operate efficiently. However what is it that fuels the enzymes and allows this ongoing and complex chemical process to continue? The answer is vitamins and minerals, without which the whole process would come to a grinding halt. For example, the body cannot break down or utilise protein without zinc and vitamin B6, and vitamins B1, B2, B3 (niacin) are essential for the production of energy.

Just as aloe vera's powerful healing properties seem to be attributable to the highly complex and synergistic action of all of its nutritional components, so the body is a complex mix of ongoing and continual chemical processes and nutrient interactions. A good example of this is in the movement of muscles. In order for this to take place effectively the body needs fuel – oxygen and carbohydrate – plus an array of minerals and vitamins, including calcium, magnesium, phosphorous and iron, and vitamins B1, B2, B3 and B5. The vitamins A, C and E (the so-called ACE or anti-oxidant vitamins), plus the minerals zinc and selenium, are potent antioxidant nutrients. Vitamins B3, B5 (pantothenic acid), B6 and B12, in combination with choline, calcium, magnesium, zinc, manganese, chromium, selenium and the vitamins A, C and E, have a positive effect on brain function.

The main enzymes found in aloe vera are:

- Amylase (one of the two main digestive enzymes, with protease, breaks down sugars and starches)
- Bradykinase (stimulates immune system, analgesic, anti-inflammatory)
- Catalase (prevents accumulation of water in the body)
- Cellulase (aids digestion – cellulose)
- Lipase (aids digestion – fats)
- Oxidase
- Alkaline phosphatase
- Proteolytiase (hydrolyses proteins into their constituent elements)
- Creatine phosphokinase (aids metabolism)
- Carboxypeptidase

Lignin

This is a cellulose substance that seems to give aloe vera its powerful penetrative properties and, so far, no other particular properties or benefits have been established.

Minerals

To date, many different minerals have been found in aloe vera, the most important being the following:

Calcium	essential for the healthy formation of teeth and bones and in muscle contractions and heart function
Chromium	helps to balance blood sugar through GTF – glucose tolerance factor – and helps in protein metabolism
Copper	essential component of red blood cells, pigmentation of skin and hair
Iron	essential component of haemoglobin in red blood cells, involved in the transportation of oxygen
Magnesium	helps strengthen teeth and bones, helps maintain healthy muscles and nervous system, helps to activate enzymes
Manganese	helps activate enzymes, helps form healthy bones, nerves and other tissues
Potassium	helps regulate and maintain fluid balance in the body

Phosphorous	helps form and maintain bones and teeth, aids metabolism, helps maintain body pH
Sodium	helps regulate body fluids, aids nerve and muscle function, aids in the transport of nutrients into body cells
Zinc	present in most tissue and scores of enzymes, essential for good health, accelerates healing of wounds, essential for growth, mental alertness, aids healthy teeth and bone growth, is essential in the normal functioning of the skin, immune, digestive and reproductive systems

Mono- and polysaccharides

Aloe vera contains simple sugars that include glucose, fructose and mannose and are known as monosaccharides and more complex, long-chain sugars, known as polysaccharides. The monosaccharides are simple structures that are readily broken down by enzyme action and then absorbed by the body.

The more complex, long-chain sugars, where glucose and mannose are linked, are known as polysaccharides or gluco-mannans. It is these unique long-chain sugars that researchers such as Dr Ivan Danhof in the USA (see references to him later in this chapter) and medical practitioners, such as Dr Gregg Henderson (he has been using aloe vera for over twenty years), Dr Peter Atherton, a UK doctor, and David Urch, a UK veterinarian (the latter two have both been using aloe vera for over seven years) and many others in the USA, the UK, Europe and other parts of the world, believe are the key to aloe vera's unique healing and immuno-stimulating properties.

KEY TIP

These complex structures (i.e. polysaccharides) have the ability to retain their structure and are thus not broken down but absorbed whole by cells in different parts of the body, e.g. in the digestive tract. This process is known as pinocytosis and means that the polysaccharides, with all their healing and immuno-stimulating properties and actions enter the blood stream intact.

One polysaccharide in particular – acemannan – has now been shown to have significant health-giving properties. It:

- restores and boosts the immune system
- is anti-viral
- stimulates the production of macrophages (large white blood cells)
- increases the capacity of T-lymphocytes by up to fifty per cent

The ongoing confusion that seems to exist about polysaccharides and the so-called and often quoted term – 'mucopolysaccharides' – needs to be addressed. It is important to note that aloe vera does *not* contain mucopolysaccharides. The situation may have arisen through confusion between the terms mucinous polysaccharides (which are characteristic of aloe vera) and mucopolysaccharides (nitrogen containing polysaccharides found in animals and bacteria), which has been misused in the promotion of some aloe vera products. All scientists working with aloe vera would agree that plants do not contain mucopolysaccharides.

Given the scientific agreement that aloe vera does not contain mucopolysaccharides and the fact that the methanol precipitable solids (MPS) test does not measure polysaccharides, it would be prudent to look very carefully at those products that are promoted using the respective 'mucopolysaccharide' content, especially based on the MPS test.

See the paper by Ronald P Pelley, PhD, MD, Department of Pharmacology and Toxicology, the University of Texas Medical Branch, entitled 'The story of aloe polysaccharides', produced by the IASC.

Salicylic acid

Aloe vera also contains salicylic acid. This substance is similar in its properties to aspirin in that it helps to reduce fever and inflammation by lowering the body's temperature. This is what helps give aloe vera its anti-pyretic properties.

It is thought that thousands of years ago the Greek physician Hippocrates discovered that a concoction using the bark and leaves of the willow could help relieve the aches and pains of childbirth and lower fevers. What he didn't know was that this potion contained salicin, part of the salicylate family of drugs that includes the common aspirin – acetylsalicylic acid. Modern researchers believe that because of its anti-inflammatory and anti-clotting properties, aspirin may help with a broad range of medical problems including:

- fever and pain
- heart attacks
- stroke
- cancer
- pre-eclampsia in high-risk women
- dementia
- Alzheimer's
- diabetes (those diabetics with cardiac or vascular complications)

Saponins

These are natural soapy substances that have both cleansing and antiseptic properties.

Sterols

These are naturally occurring plant steroids with analgesic, anti-inflammatory and antiseptic properties. The main sterols in aloe vera are:

- beta sitosterol
- lupeol
- campesterol

Vitamins

Aloe vera contains many vitamins and the main ones are:

Vitamin A	beta carotene and retinol	essential for healthy skin and tissue, bones, sight, anti-oxidant, boosts immune system, one of the so-called ACE or anti-oxidant vitamins that helps combat free radicals.
Vitamin B1	thiamine	essential for tissue growth, energy, brain function.
Vitamin B2	riboflavin	essential for energy production, healthy skin and tissue.
Vitamin B3	niacin	essential for energy production, brain function, helps regulate the metabolism.

Vitamin B6	pyridoxine	essential for brain function, hormone balance (PMS, menopause), metabolism.
Vitamin B12	cyanocobalamin	essential in the utilisation of proteins, energy production. B12 is mainly found in meat and dairy products and rarely in plants (vegans/vegetarians please note). Lack of B12 can lead to anaemia.
Vitamin C	ascorbic acid	essential to the immune system, helps in the production of collagen, helps to maintain healthy skin, joints, tissue and bones, helps fight infections, cancer and heart disease, one of the so-called ACE or anti-oxidant vitamins, essential to combat free radical damage. Vitamin C is the most important of the immune boosting nutrients and helps in the production of T-cells that in turn help destroy cancer cells.
Vitamin E	tocopherol	essential for healthy skin and tissue, aids fertility, promotes tissue healing, one of the three so-called ACE or anti-oxidant vitamins, essential to combat free radical damage.
Folic acid		essential for healthy nerve and brain function and in the production of red blood cells, critical in pregnancy to reduce the risk of birth defects such as hare lip and spina bifida.

Anti-oxidants and free radicals

The subject of anti-oxidants and their vital role in combating oxidants or free radicals will be covered in more detail in Chapter 6.

Healing properties

When one first hears, reads or is told about the almost 'miraculous' and diverse properties of aloe vera, it seems almost unbelievable. In the past aloe vera (or parts of it) have been used as a laxative and now people take it because of its wide ranging benefits, including immune boosting, anti-microbial and wound-healing properties. These very diverse 'benefits' also help to explain its wide range of both general and clinical applications. Initially, it is easy to be highly sceptical and disbelieving simply because it is hard to accept that aloe vera can be so beneficial. Unless you have used aloe vera, it is difficult to understand how one plant can have so many healing properties and benefits. Generally, in the past, your doctor's response to aloe vera may have tended to verge on the scathing and dismissive. It is only once you try aloe vera for yourself (either internally or topically) that you can really begin to experience the real potency and power of this plant – which is truly one of nature's many gifts.

> KEY TIP
> Most of the doctors and practitioners who now write about and promote the healing benefits of aloe vera came to know about this amazing plant through personal first-hand experience.

Many people, including most doctors, vets and dentists, often ask how can a single plant have such a wide range of benefits. How can aloe vera be:

- one of the most efficient detoxifying agents
- a powerful immune system stimulant
- a strong anti-inflammatory agent
- an analgesic
- a stimulator of cell growth
- an aid to the acceleration of tissue healing
- an antiseptic
- a rich source of nutrients
- a powerful aid to the digestive system
- and be adaptogenic?

How can aloe vera be all of these things simultaneously and without any toxic side effects?

Properties of aloe vera

Through the ages aloe vera has been used for many different purposes – both internal and external. In many parts of Europe and the USA in the nineteenth century, one of the most popular uses of aloe vera (with the aloin fraction included) was as a laxative and purgative. Modern day processing methods have tended to focus on extracting this fraction so that only a minute percentage remains. The two most important of these anthraquinones, namely emodin and aloin, do have anti-microbial, anti-viral, anti-bacterial and painkilling properties. Since the 1930s, when modern day research began to unlock some of the secrets of aloe vera and its healing properties, a wide spectrum of therapeutic benefits have been identified. These include the following benefits-actions that have all been testified to and witnessed by medical practitioners, veterinarians, dentists, complementary therapists, nutritionists and laypeople throughout the world.

The key to aloe vera's extraordinary properties and powers is, according to Dr Bruce Hedendal of the Hedendal Chiropractic and Nutrition Center, in the USA the fact that the plant is a rich source of the long-chain sugars known as polysaccharides. In his opinion these polysaccharides are as vital to the body as bricks are to a house. So what do these polysaccharides do? What functions do they perform in the body? Most agree that these polysaccharides must act synergistically with all the other nutritional constituents found in aloe vera in order to make such a positive health impact.

KEY TIP

Some of the latest thinking is that this essential component (i.e. the polysaccharides) of aloe vera may work by lubricating our joints and lining the colon, thus preventing the re-entry of toxic waste and providing a natural barrier against microbial invasion of the body's cells.

Acemannan and the anti-viral effect

Aloe vera is especially rich in one such polysaccharide, known as acemannan. This polysaccharide works, it is believed, by interacting with the immune system, boosting it rather than overriding it. It is a potent stimulator of macrophages (white blood cells that destroy bacteria, tumour cells, viruses and so on) to produce immune agents such as interferon and interleukin.

In 1990, at the Third International Conference on Antiviral Research in Brussels, it was reported that acemannan had been found to inhibit the growth of implanted sarcoma in mice. Also, when tested (i.e. injected acemannan) on cats suffering from feline leukaemia, over seventy per cent of the animals recovered – a complete reversal of the prevailing statistics for this disease. Feline leukaemia, like AIDS, is caused by a retro-virus and previously, seventy per cent of cats would normally die within six to eight weeks of being diagnosed. As a result of this research, in 1991, the US Department of Agriculture (USDA) approved the use of acemannan in the treatment of fibrosarcoma in dogs and cats. Previously there had been no effective treatment for this cancer, but when exposed to acemannan the cancerous tissue is encapsulated and the tumour killed off, thus facilitating surgical removal.

KEY TIP

The unique mechanism of this key active ingredient (i.e. polysaccharides), coupled with its direct anti-viral activity, may explain why aloe vera shows such exciting potential in treating a wide range of both human and animal diseases and ailments.

Acemannan has been isolated and extracted from aloe vera by a company in the USA – Carrington Laboratories. The product, called Carrisyn™ is licensed for the treatment of feline leukaemia and has apparently also been used in tests and trials in the treatment of HIV/AIDS in humans. Acemannan has also been shown to demonstrate 'significant antiviral activity against other viruses including the influenza virus and measles virus'. (Source: *Pharmacology of Natural Medicines*, Michael T Murray, ND, Joseph E Pizzorno Jr, ND.)

Aloe vera, as we have said before, seems to have wide ranging healing and therapeutic properties and benefits, much of which it is believed is due to the synergistic way in which all its 200-plus identified nutritional constituents work together.

Adaptogen

Aloe vera is widely accepted as having adaptogenic properties and this is one of its most extraordinary qualities. Aloe vera seems to have the ability to act appropriately on the specific problem or problems of the individual using it, and this is one reason why people respond to it in so many different ways. You might, for instance, discover that while taking aloe vera (as a drink) for your arthritis, asthma or IBS, that your skin has improved or your gums have stopped bleeding or that you have more energy. Effectively this means that, for example, if someone was drinking aloe vera, the body would be able to benefit whether the person was suffering from one or more of the following conditions, e.g. IBS, arthritis, asthma and so on.

This means that aloe vera can help with many different problems at the same time and that the body seems to be able to take from aloe vera what it needs, when it needs it and where it needs it!

This 'holistic healing and therapeutic effect' seems to bemuse many conventional medical practitioners, whether doctors, dentists or vets. These are just some of the truly amazing properties of this apparently miraculous plant. One could also add that it helps maintain liver and kidney function and can even help correct hepatic dysfunction. It can also have a beneficial effect on people with diabetes, working to reduce blood sugar levels and to restore the natural release mechanism. I have also heard of people suffering from thyroid problems – both under-active and overactive – who say that their condition seems to be more stable than previously.

I am very pleased that since I started writing on aloe vera (1996–97) several highly positive and illuminating research studies or projects have been undertaken in the UK and the USA. I am confident that as the realisation of the significance of aloe vera's wide ranging healing properties grows, coupled with the fact that there are no serious side effects, more research will be undertaken. I am greatly encouraged when I hear of more people benefiting from using aloe vera, but the real test will come when the results of the research projects, currently taking place, are published. Day by day, more and more evidence appears about the benefits of aloe vera. It cannot be long now before the mainstream medical profession and everyone else will see the true scale of the potential of natural products like aloe vera in fighting disease, boosting the immune system and promoting and maintaining a greater sense of overall well-being.

You don't have to be ill to take aloe vera

Aloe vera can be taken orally simply as a health tonic or used topically on the skin to moisturise and condition the skin. It is not something that one uses only when one is unwell.

KEY TIP
Aloe vera can also contribute to an improvement in overall general health, as well as acting to help both prevent and manage many ailments, disorders and diseases.

The studies, which focused on the use and benefits of aloe vera for both animals (see Chapter 7) and humans (see Chapter 5), are documented later in this book.

Anti-ageing

Dr Ivan Danhof is one of the world's leading authorities on aloe vera, its properties, uses and benefits. He is a former professor of physiology at the University of Texas and is president of North Texas Research Laboratories. Dr Danhof has conducted many studies to discover the secret of aloe vera's rejuvenating ability.

KEY TIP
He believes that one of the main reasons lies in the plant's unique ability to increase production of human fibroblast cells between six and eight times faster than normal cell production.

Fibroblast cells are found in the dermis of the skin and are responsible for the fabrication of collagen, the skin's support protein that keeps skin firm, supple and 'youthful' looking. During exposure to the sun and through the normal ageing process (and exposure to free radical damage), fibroblasts slow their collagen production and, as we grow older, the quality of collagen is reduced and the wrinkling in the skin becomes deeper as the skin loses its suppleness and flexibility.

Dr Danhof found that aloe vera not only improved fibroblast cell structure but also accelerated the collagen production process. He also believes the clue to aloe vera's 'unique' anti-ageing properties may lie, once again, with the 'magic' polysaccharides and their moisture-binding properties.

KEY TIP
Don't forget that many skin products that promise anti-ageing benefits do little more than temporarily rehydrate the skin. They do not have any positive effect on the stimulation of the production of natural collagen and any existing facial and other lines tend to remain as before.

Collagen production is not aloe vera's only contribution to the body's anti-ageing battle. As people grow older, most tend to develop ageing spots on their hands, due to a complicated chemical process in the body, as well as to external factors like sunlight.

> KEY TIP
> Aloe vera however contains a potent blocker that can actually help reverse the ageing process by providing the skin with the necessary components to rejuvenate itself at cellular level. This can lead to softer, more pliable and younger looking skin.

Dr Danhof himself tested the effects on his own hands by daily applications of aloe vera to one hand, leaving the other hand untreated. The difference was remarkable: the untreated hand had numerous ageing spots, while the treated hand had no blemishes whatsoever and resembled the hand of a much younger person!

Anti-inflammatory

Aloe vera acts as a powerful anti-inflammatory because of the presence of the naturally occurring plant sterols, anthraquinones and other naturally occurring substances, and the synergistic way in which all the constituents, including the polysaccharides, act together.

Aloe vera has been shown, in a number of studies (see references at the end of this chapter: 2, 4, 5, 14, 28–31), to exhibit a number of anti-inflammatory properties through its ability to 'block the generation of inflammatory mediators such as bradykinin and thromboxanes' (source: *Pharmacology of Natural Medicines*). It is thought that it is a combination of glycoproteins, some anthraquinones and salicylates that both inhibit and break down the bradykinin, which is one of the 'major mediators' of pain and inflammation. Aloe vera is widely used by people in the treatment and management of inflammatory conditions such as arthritis (both osteo- and rheumatoid) where it has a steroid-like action, without the side effects. It can also reduce the redness, pain and swelling associated with such conditions as muscular pain, sprains, strains, bruising and tendonitis.

As I mentioned in the introduction, I have both seen and experienced aloe vera's effectiveness with sunburn and many writers report its wide ranging uses and benefits. In her book, *Herbal Medicine: The Natural Way to Get Well and Stay Well*, Dian Dincin Buchman advocates using aloe vera on burns, stings, insect bites, poison ivy blisters, acne and so on.

> KEY TIP
> In fact rashes of all kinds will generally be soothed by an application of aloe vera gelly to the inflamed area.

Anti-microbial (anti-fungal and anti-bacterial)

Aloe vera has been shown to demonstrate significant activity against many common bacteria and fungi. As far back as 1949 (RY Gottschall), the anti-microbial properties of aloe vera were recognised. Gottschall found aloe vera to have anti-bacterial activity against mycobacterium tuberculosis. In a subsequent paper by Gottschall ('Antibacterial substances in seed plants active against tubercule bacilli', published in the *American Review of Tuberculosis*), he confirmed his original findings about aloe vera's properties.

In 1964, in the *Journal of Pharmaceutical Sciences*, Lorenzetti, Salisbury, Beal and Baldwin, in their paper 'Bacteriostatic property of aloe vera' agreed with Gottschall's findings and further concluded that aloe vera was a broad spectrum germ controlling agent and was also effective against e-coli, salmonella and streptoccus.

In 1982, Robson et al (source: Robson, MC, Heggers, JP, Hagstron, WJ, 'Myth, magic witchcraft, or fact? Aloe vera revisited', *Journal of Burns Rehabilitation*, 1982; 3: 157–62) demonstrated the anti-microbial properties of an aloe vera extract with silver sulfadiazine (a powerful antiseptic used in the treatment of extensive burns). The anti-microbial effects of aloe vera compared favourably with the conventional treatment. The anti-microbial activity of the aloe vera extract in a cream base performed better than silver sulfadiazine in agar well diffusion studies.

In numerous studies, the following percentage content of aloe vera extracts were found to be bactericidal against common bacteria.

A sixty per cent aloe vera extract was bactericidal against Pseudomonas aeruginosa, Klebsiella pneumoniae, Serratia marcescens, Enterobacter cloacae, Streptococcus pyogenes and Streptococcus agalactiae. A seventy per cent aloe vera extract was bactericidal against Staphylococcus aureus, while an eighty per cent extract was bactericidal against Escherichia coli (E coli) and a ninety per cent extract was bactericidal against Streptococcus faecalis and Candida albicans. These anti-microbial properties have been further endorsed by Dr Gregg Henderson, a chiropractic physician who is director of the Fallbrook Chiropractic Center in California and has been using aloe vera as an integral part of his treatment programmes for over twenty years (see Chapter 4).

Table: Anti-microbial effects of aloe vera extract in cream base compared with silver sulfadiazine in agar well (6mm) diffusion (Index 14)

Organism	*Aloe vera*	*AgSD*
Gram-negative		
E coli	16	12
Enterobacter cloacae	14	12
K pneumoniae	14	6
P aeruginosa	17	12
Gram-positive		
S aureus	18	12
S pyogenes	16	12
S agalactiae	16	12
S faecalis	6	11
B subtilis	19	14

Inhibition zones measured in mm

Anti-oxidant

Aloe vera is a potent anti-oxidant, helping the body scavenge dangerous free radicals (cancer forming agents) through the actions of its anti-oxidant constituents, including the so-called ACE vitamins, i.e. vitamins A, C and E and other naturally occurring nutrients. Free radicals are toxic and potentially carcinogenic compounds that are absorbed by all of us on a daily basis through pollution and the food we eat, and are also created by our natural body processes. It is vital that we ingest sufficient amounts of anti-oxidants in our diets to counteract such damaging substances.

KEY TIP

We can absorb anti-oxidants through our skin as well as through our stomachs. So using aloe vera, both topically and internally can help in this process.

Cancer and the immune system

Dr Danhof reports that aloe vera causes the release of tumour necrosis factor alpha, which blocks the blood supply to cancerous growths.

In Japan, at the University of Okinawa's department of epidemiology, it was reported in a study that daily doses of aloe vera could help prevent the onset of lung cancer in smokers. As mentioned earlier, encouraging results have been obtained when treating cancer in animals with aloe vera and it has been widely reported that some cancer patients have experienced benefits from drinking aloe vera gel (a potent, proprietary, unflavoured drinking juice). It is important to note however that aloe vera should never be 'promoted' or 'marketed' as a cure for cancer, whatever the level of anecdotal evidence available.

In general, aloe vera seems to have a remarkable and sometimes almost unbelievable effect on the immune system: stimulating, supporting and modulating. More specifically, it has proved highly beneficial to AIDS sufferers, helping to restore the T and B lymphocyte balance. It is also known to protect the immune function of the skin against ultraviolet radiation. A study at the MD Anderson Clinic at the Medical Center in Houston, Texas, considered the effects of damaging ultra-violet exposure on the skin and it was found that when an aloe vera gelly (topical gel) was applied to the skin before testing, the immune cells were fully protected.

Detoxifying agent

When taken internally as a drink, high quality aloe vera juice or drinking gel acts as a gentle cleanser and detoxifier. It does not – contrary to what one often reads in the columns of some newspapers – act as a purgative (providing the aloin concentration or parts per million of aloin is within the accepted levels, i.e. a maximum of fifty ppm).

In Japan, for example, which is one of the largest markets for aloe vera products in the world, including aloe vera drinks, there is a reported fifty ppm limit or standard. At the time of writing this book, I am not aware of any such standard in the UK, Europe or the USA. However, we are aware that the company that dominates global sales of aloe vera is also the largest supplier of aloe vera products to the Japanese market and as such conforms to Japanese standards.

Aloe vera works right through the digestive system and carries its healing properties throughout the epithelial tissue of the body. It has the ability to flush out dead skin cells and it helps to generate new cell growth and promotes healthier tissue, thus accelerating the healing of wounds, lesions and ulcers. It will also have this effect when applied externally to cut, burnt (including the damage caused by radiotherapy) or otherwise damaged skin tissue.

Digestive function

One of the curses of the modern so-called developed world is that in many of these highly industrialised countries we have totally forgotten the basic need to eat good, natural and nutritious food. The vast majority of people in such countries eat food with a high degree of processing, containing many chemicals and few bio-available nutrients (and with the additional concerns of genetically modified foodstuffs) and the worst offenders, in terms of food types, tend to be packeted, heavily processed, convenience foods.

Is it really any wonder that so many people in these 'developed' countries suffer from digestive conditions such as IBS and other ailments and diseases that can be linked to immune deficiency problems, stress and diet? In the UK alone, it is estimated that one in five people (around 12,000,000 people), suffer from IBS (statistics show that more than two thirds of all IBS sufferers are women) or some digestive tract problem like ulcers, colitis, ulcerative colitis, diverticulitis, Crohn's disease and so on during their lives. You will undoubtedly know someone with one of these problems.

> KEY POINT
> Apparently in the UK, IBS is one of the most common reasons for patients being referred to gastroenterologists by their GPs.

What is even more concerning is that, according to Dr Peter Atherton (he was a GP for over twenty years) in his book *The Essential Aloe Vera*,

> conventional treatment is not very effective and depends on dietary change, usually with an increase in fibre, anti-diarrhoea or bulking agents, anti-spasmodic drugs, anti-depressants and psycho/hypnotherapy, etc.

According to Dr Mark Hamilton (as reported in *Good Housekeeping*, February 2003 (UK version)), medical adviser to the Digestive Disorders Foundation and a consultant gastroenterologist at London's Royal Free Hospital, IBS is a positive diagnosis and not just a convenient get-out when doctors don't know what's wrong. He says,

> We use clear, internationally agreed criteria to diagnose IBS. It's a combination of abdominal pain, variations in bowel habit, bloating and distension, in the absence of anything else going on…IBS isn't curable, so treatment focuses on relieving your particular symptoms…some people develop IBS after an infection such as salmonella and research shows that these people have abnormalities in the chemical transmitters in the gut. Something seems to have been altered by the infection.

KEY POINT
Dr Ivan Danhof, who has acted as a consultant to many of the world's leading pharmaceutical research institutes and has advised organisations such as the US FDA, believes that aloe vera is beneficial to the whole gastro-intestinal system.

He maintains that due to its magnesium lactate content, aloe vera is able to lower activity in the stomach and is effective in reversing both occasional and chronic symptoms in the upper gastro-intestinal tract.

In their book, *Pharmacology of Natural Medicines*, Michael T Murray, ND, and Joseph E Pizzorno Jr, ND refer to the study by Dr Jeffrey Bland and relate the effect of aloe vera juice on the inhibition of gastric acid secretion. Apparently using Heidelberg gastric analysis, the aloe vera juice was shown to increase gastric pH by an average of 1.88 units. This would support the findings of other researchers that aloe vera gel, when taken orally as a drinking juice, can inhibit the secretion of hydrochloric acid. The test also suggested that the consumption of aloe vera juice could slow down gastric emptying with the possible benefit of improved digestion.

In his paper, 'Effect of orally consumed aloe vera juice on gastro-intestinal function in normal human beings', published in the US magazine *Prevention* in 1985, Dr Jeffrey Bland, of the Linus Pauling Institute of Science and Medicine in California, concluded from the results of a clinical trial that aloe vera helps in the following ways:

- it improves the digestion without causing diarrhoea
- it acts as a buffering agent to normalise the pH (rather like an alkalising agent)
- it reduces yeast content and promotes a more favourable balance of gastro-intestinal symbiotic bacteria

- it can help specifically with disorders such as indigestion, IBS, colitis and stomach acidity

KEY POINT
Dr Bland also found that aloe vera could improve bowel regularity and participants in the trial reported both an increase in energy levels and an overall sense of improved well-being (these are commonly reported benefits of people drinking high quality aloe vera gel or juice).

KEY POINT
Other research would indicate that aloe vera penetrates the wall of the digestive system, flushing out harmful bacteria and helping to repopulate the system with beneficial flora.

KEY POINT
Aloe vera also helps reduce inflammation, promotes healing and enhances the uptake of nutrients.

Healing agent

As far back as 1934–35, the first accepted medical study on the healing properties of aloe vera was conducted in the USA by C E Collins and his son. Collins and Collins wrote of the use of aloe vera to treat fifty patients suffering from radiation injuries. One particular patient who had developed severe Roentgen dermatitis as a result of having had a depilatory x-ray treatment (in 1932) was told she would have to have a skin graft because of the condition she had developed and the resultant damage. Yet within five months of being given regular topical applications of fresh aloe vera, the area was completely healed (further details of this and many other examples of research and trials are outlined in Chapter 8).

KEY TIP
We have already discussed aloe vera's ability to promote tissue regeneration. This property makes it a powerful healing agent for all types of wounds, both internal and external.

Dr Danhof notes that it can also accelerate the healing of broken or fractured bones by stimulating the uptake of both calcium and phosphorous – two minerals which are essential for healthy bone growth. Aloe vera is also known to help regenerate healthy skin tissue much more quickly than is the norm. Dr Danhof also found that under laboratory conditions, the presence of aloe vera could effect up to an eight-fold increase in the replication of human fibroblast cells – the cells that are closely linked with the production of new collagen in the body.

As a natural antiseptic, antibiotic and bactericide, aloe vera can also help clear up a wide range of infections, including those of a fungal nature. Professor Patrick Pietroni in his *The Family Guide to Alternative Care* advocates its use for such conditions as athlete's foot, thrush and vulvitis.

Ross Trattler, author of *Better Health Through Natural Healing*, recommends the use of aloe vera to help treat haemorrhoids, warts and verrucae. Dian Buchman has also found that by applying aloe vera regularly to patches of hard skin on the elbows, hands and feet, the tissue softens and any cracked skin is healed.

Dr Peter Atherton's paper, 'Aloe vera: magic or medicine', which appeared in the July 1998 issue of the *Nursing Standard*, describes in detail the clinical trial he undertook to examine the benefits of how topically and orally administered aloe vera in patients with chronic venous leg ulcers may aid healing. This paper is covered in more detail in Chapter 8.

Heart conditions

Heart disease is reputed to be the number one killer of both men and women in the UK (it may have a similar significance in the USA and many other developed countries). This one disease costs the UK and other countries billions of pounds every year in terms of medical treatment and the loss of highly trained and skilled people.

It is a disease that could be materially improved with fundamental changes to methods of prevention, which include diet or nutrition and exercise. Obviously many people may be predisposed, genetically, to heart disease but much more could be done to help reduce the incidence of this 'killer'.

KEY TIP

Again, Dr Danhof has found that calcium isocitrate salts in aloe vera can help people with heart problems or with a history of heart disease in the family. He suggests a daily intake of high quality aloe vera drinking juices for those most at risk.

This finding has apparently been endorsed by other researchers. In 1985, at the annual meeting of the American College of Angiology, a paper presented by Dr OP Agarwal summarised the results of a five-year study of 5,000 people diagnosed as having angina pectoris. After aloe vera and the husk of 'isabgol' were added to their diets, they showed a marked reduction in serum cholesterol and the frequency of angina attacks was also noticeably reduced. Five years later, all the patients were still alive and no adverse side effects had been reported. Interestingly, fifty per cent of those involved in the study also had diabetes and the results demonstrated that aloe vera could also help in the control of blood sugar levels in diabetics. Other studies have shown that daily doses of aloe vera can help lower blood cholesterol significantly and that blood pressure can also be lowered within weeks. What it is that causes this effect has not yet been identified, though some believe that it could be related to some ingredient in aloe vera that helps emulsify cholesterol, thus enabling the body to eliminate it. Further research would have to be conducted to determine the extent to which aloe vera could be used universally to achieve such results.

Moisturiser and cohesive agent

Anyone who uses aloe vera on their skin (and by that I mean a high quality topical preparation where aloe vera and not water is the main ingredient) on a regular basis will see a gradual improvement in condition, quality and consistency.

> KEY TIP
> If aloe vera is used regularly, the skin will look better, feel better and will offer improved protection against damage caused by harmful rays.

Aloe vera is a uniquely effective moisturiser and healing agent for the skin (both human and animal!!). It works in three main ways. The first, through its ability to carry nutrients and moisture through the layers of the skin, thus facilitating penetration and absorption. Secondly, through its polysaccharides, by creating a barrier that helps prevent moisture loss from the skin. Because of this and the fact that it also contains an anti-histamine and has antibiotic properties, it is beneficial for people with dry, sensitive and damaged skin. Thirdly, it enhances the production of fibroblasts that are involved in the natural collagen generation process (as detailed earlier in this chapter) and also helps protect the skin from damaging rays.

> KEY POINT
> All these properties contribute to its increasingly formidable reputation as a potent healing, moisturising, protective and cohesive agent.

Bio-availability

In a recent randomised, double-blind crossover trial, supported and funded by the IASC and run by the department of chemistry at the University of Scranton, PA, USA, and approved by its Institutional Review Board in accordance with the Declaration of Helsinki ('Effect of aloe vera preparations on the human bio-availability of vitamins C and E', Joe A Vinson, Hassan Al Kharrat and Lori Andreolli, department of chemistry, University of Scranton, PA, USA, 2002), tests were conducted to determine the effect of two samples of commercially available aloe vera drinks (selected and certified by the IASC) on the bio-availability of vitamin C (500 milligram tablets) and vitamin E (420 milligram capsules). Previously there have been no literature references describing the effect of the consumption of aloe vera liquid preparations (one based on the inner leaf gel product, 'AVG', and one on the whole leaf product, 'AVL') on the absorption of water or fat-soluble vitamins.

The number of people taking vitamin supplements is increasing due to a greater awareness of the benefits. In the USA alone, it is currently estimated that between fifty-one and sixty-one per cent of the population consumed supplements (refs 1, 2 – see below). The elderly population is greatly increasing as a percentage of the overall population in developed countries and this age group is especially vulnerable to vitamin deficiency due to age-related decreases in absorption, reduced food intake and increased drug use (ref 3 – see below). Vitamin C (ascorbic acid) is a water soluble vitamin essential to good health and to prevent scurvy. It is one of the most common supplements because there is epidemiological evidence that vitamin C reduces the risk of cancer, diabetes, cataracts and Alzheimer's disease. Vitamin C has also been proven to greatly enhance the absorption of iron and improve poor iron status (ref 4 – see below).

A recent report showed that helicobacter pylori infection significantly impairs the bio-availability of vitamin C (ref 5 – see below) and this bacterium infects half of the world's population (ref 6 – see below) and is especially common in peptic ulcer patients (refs 7, 8 – see below). Individuals with kidney problems are deficient in vitamin C and hemodialysis further decreases ascorbate levels (ref 9 – see below). The US government has recently increased its guidelines for the consumption of vitamin C to seventy-five milligrams and ninety milligrams per day for women and men respectively, with a warning that smokers need to add an additional thirty-five milligrams per day because their metabolic turnover of vitamin C is more rapid as is their rate of oxidative stress (ref 10 – see below). In a comprehensive study of its pharmokinetics in humans, it was suggested that the amount be increased to 200 milligrams per day, a figure that represents the maximum bio-availability (ref 11 – see below). This amount can be obtained by eating a minimum of five servings of fresh fruit and vegetables per day. Since the majority of pëople in the USA and other developed nations do not consume five servings (ref 12 – see below), then it is recommended that either a supplement of vitamin C or ingestion of an agent that can increase absorption of vitamin C may be needed.

Vitamin E, a lipid soluble vitamin, is needed in much smaller amounts than vitamin C. It is mainly found in oils that are often avoided by those with weight problems or those trying to diet. Vitamin E can reduce cognitive decline (ref 13 – see below) and improve the immune system (ref 14 – see below) in elderly people. Higher intakes of vitamin E were recently shown to be associated with a lower risk of Alzheimer's disease (ref 15 – see below) and prostate cancer (ref 16 – see below). Age-related cataract and age-related macular degeneration are delayed by consumption of antioxidant nutrients such as vitamins C and E (ref 17 – see below).

Epidemiological studies indicate that vitamin E may also reduce the risk of cardiovascular disease, though results from supplementation studies are mixed (ref 18 – see below). Dietary fibre (ref 19 – see below) and low fat meals (ref 20 – see below) reduce the bio-availability of E as do the long-term consumption of orlistat (a fat absorption inhibitor used for weight loss) and olestra, a fat substitute (refs 21, 22 – see below).

The study was designed as a randomised, double-blind crossover trial and on study days, at least one week apart, each volunteer, after an overnight fast, had a baseline blood sample taken. They then consumed in a random fashion 500 milligrams of vitamin C tablet or 420 milligrams of vitamin E capsule with either 60 millilitres (2 ounces) of either water (control) or one of the two aloe vera preparations (inner leaf gel or whole leaf), which was slowly sipped over five minutes. Further blood sampling was after one, two, four, six, eight and twenty-four hours (fasting) post-dosing. Subjects were allowed to eat their normal lunch and evening meals. One week and two weeks later, the other liquid was consumed with vitamin C or vitamin E and the sampling repeated. Blood was converted to plasma, mixed with metaphosphoric acid preservative only for vitamin C and stored at minus eighty degrees centigrade.

The results were significant and indicated that the aloe vera preparations improve the absorption of both vitamin C and vitamin E by up to 369 per cent. The absorption is slower and the vitamins last longer in the plasma with the aloe vera preparations. Aloe vera is the only supplement known to increase the absorption of both of these essential vitamins and should be considered as a complement to their use.

Eight subjects consumed 500 milligrams of ascorbic acid alone (control) or with 60 millilitres of aloe vera juice (AVG, gel; or AVL, whole leaf extract). (Data are mean standard error of the mean.)

Figure 1

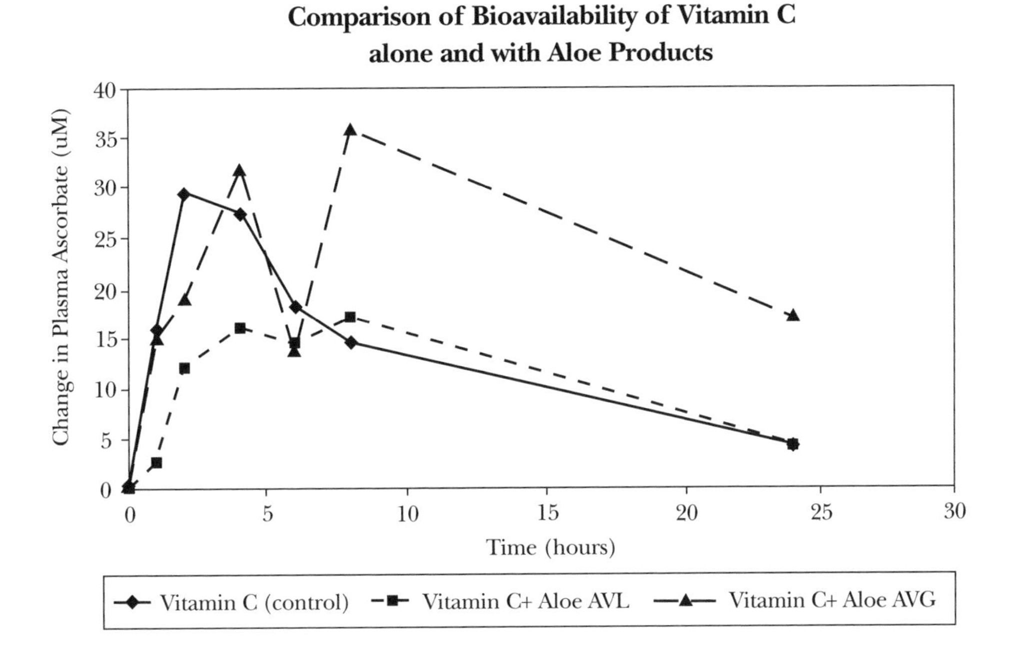

Ten subjects consumed 400 milligrams of tocopherol acetate alone (control) or with 60 millilitres of aloe vera (AVG, gel; or AVL, whole leaf extract). (Data are mean standard error of mean.)

Figure 2

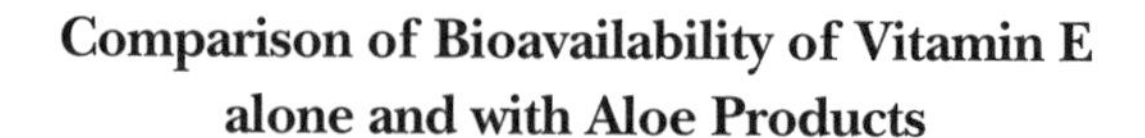

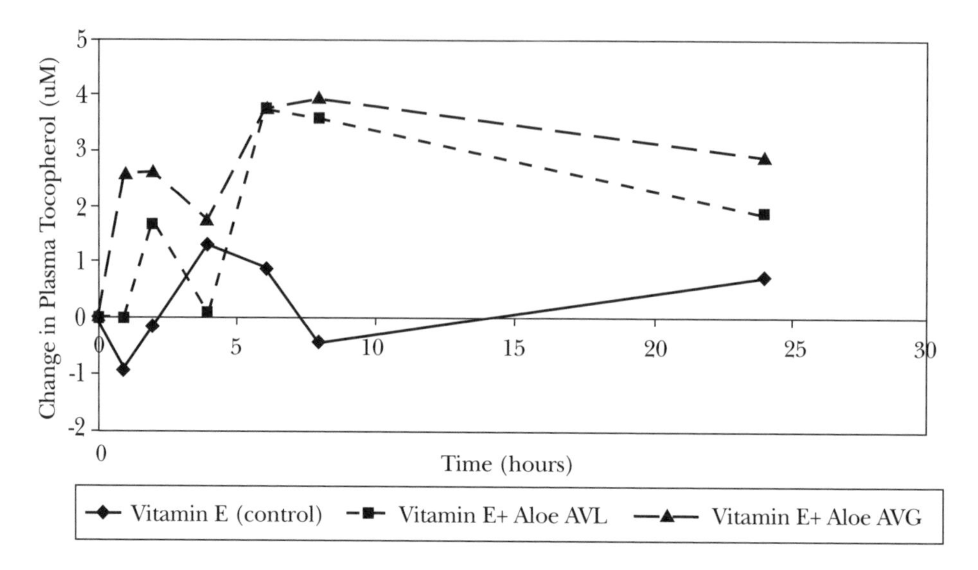

This section on bio-availability was extracted from the paper 'Effect of aloe vera preparations on the human bio-availability of vitamins C and E', Joe A Vinson, Hassan Al Kharrat and Lori Andreoli, department of chemistry, University of Scranton, PA, USA, 2002. The work was supported and funded by the IASC.

References, anti-inflammatory

1 Klein, A D, Penney, N S, 'Aloe vera', *Journal of the American Academy of Dermatology*, 1988, 18: 714–19.
2 Grindlay, D, Reynolds, T, 'The Aloe vera leaf phenomena: a review of the properties and modern use of the leaf parenchyma gel, *Journal of Ethnopharmacy*, 1986, 16: 117–51.
3 Shelton, R W, 'Aloe vera, its chemical and therapeutic properties', *International Journal of Dermatology*, 1991, 30: 679–83.
4 Robson, M C, Heggers, J P, Hagstron, W J, 'Myth, magic, witchcraft or fact? Aloe vera revisited', *Journal of Burn Care Rehabilitation*, 1982, 3: 157–62.
5 Davis, R H, Shapiro, E, Agnew, P S, 'Topical effect of aloe with ribonucleic acid and vitamin C on adjuvant arthritis', *Journal of American Podiatrists' Medical Association*, 1985, 75: 229–37.

6 Davis, R H, Parker, W L, Samson, R T, Murdoch, D P, 'Isolation of a stimulatory system in an aloe extract', *Journal of American Podiatrists' Medical Association*, 1991, 81: 473–78.
7 Davis, R H, Leitner, M G, Russo, J M, Byrne, M E, 'Anti-inflammatory activity of aloe vera against a spectrum of irritants', *Journal of American Podiatrists' Medical Association*, 1989, 79: 263–66.

References, anti-microbial

1 Robson, M C, Heggers, J P, Hagstron, W J, 'Myth, magic, witchcraft or fact? Aloe vera revisited', *Journal of Burn Care Rehabilitation*, 1982, 3: 157–62.
2 Fly, L B, Keim, I, 'Tests of aloe vera for antibiotic activity', *Economic Botany*, 1963, 17: 46–48.
3 Lorenzetti, L J, Salisburg, R, Beal, J, et al, 'Bacteriostatic property of aloe vera', *Journal of Pharmaceutical Science*, 1964, 53: 1287.
4 Heggers, J P, Pineless, G R, Robson, M C, 'Dermaide aloe/aloe vera gel: comparison of anti-microbial effects, *Journal of American Medical Technology*, 1979, 41: 293–94.

We also suggest that you read Chapter 64, pp579–88, of the book *Pharmacology of Natural Medicines* by Michael T Murray, ND, and Joseph E Pizzorno Jr, ND.

References, bioavailability

Special thanks to Gene Hale of the IASC for granting us permission to refer to this paper and the accompanying tables. All references (1–36) in this section are detailed in the paper 'Effect of aloe vera preparations on the human bio-availability of vitamins C and E', by Joe A Vinson, Hassan Al Kharrat and Lori Andreolli.

Copies of the study paper and full details of all the references in this section (1–36) are available from the IASC (see Appendix 1.4).

3

Choosing aloe vera products

SINCE 1997 when my first book on aloe vera was published, the demand and the market for aloe vera products and 'products with aloe vera' and other natural products has increased dramatically and the number of companies connected to the aloe vera industry has burgeoned. Like most industries that experience phenomenal growth in a short period, one often finds that demand can outstrip supply and this can lead to a proliferation of products of lower quality being introduced to particular markets, as the less scrupulous suppliers attempt to cash in and make quick returns.

This is when the need for nationally and internationally accepted standards is paramount. I believe that the time has come (certainly in the UK) for companies with products of unquestionable purity, quality and efficacy (and with unconditional customer money-back guarantees) to take positive action to curtail the activities of those manufacturers and suppliers who do not meet the highest quality standards. Such action may help ensure that the market they have worked so hard to develop is not tainted by the less reputable companies with dubious marketing tactics. These companies are just there for the 'quick buck' and can undoubtedly hoodwink enough people to make money for several years before disappearing into the proverbial sunset – leaving the reputable companies to clear up the mess left behind.

Back in the mid-nineties, there were probably no more than ten to twenty different brands of aloe vera products (both drinks and topical preparations) available in the UK market. That figure has increased to well over 100 brands now and that does not include what I call the 'with aloe vera' products that I refer to in the opening paragraph of this chapter. By this I mean products that contain only a small percentage of aloe vera and have little or no therapeutic benefit at all. This is simply a marketing ploy to help sell the product. If you walk into any health food shop or pharmacist now, you will find several brands of aloe vera juices, drinks, topical products, capsules and so on, arranged on the shelves. Some are in clear glass or plastic bottles that may not provide enough protection from possible damage from the light. Many will have labels that suggest the products contain anything between 95 and 100 per cent pure aloe vera juice.

Very often the capsules and the drinks claim to contain concentrated aloe vera, many times the strength of normal aloe vera (whatever normal is!). Phrases such as 'cold-pressed', 'whole-leaf', 'double-concentrated' and even '20–50 times more concentrated than the standard' may be used but what is the standard and what does it all mean to the uninitiated buyer of aloe vera products? Much of this is marketing hype, designed to make the consumer think that they are getting something out of the ordinary in terms of quality and potency. This may be the case with some but a word of caution to those who are unaware of the massive differences in quality, efficacy, purity and potency of the aloe vera products now available in the UK, the USA, Europe, Asia, Australasia, and now Africa.

Obviously the aloe vera marketplace, like any other, will have companies that may adopt misleading labelling, others may use quotations and refer to research that is not just totally out of context but was never meant to be used in association with that particular brand of aloe vera. To get to the root (no pun intended) of the issue, we have to go right back to the beginning.

KEY TIP

When assessing the quality of an aloe vera product remember to consider these six key points:

1. the quality and maturity of aloe vera plants used
2. the soil they are grown in
3. the way they are grown and where they are grown
4. the age at which they are harvested
5. the harvesting methods used
6. whether there is a stringent adherence to quality assurance at every stage of the stabilisation, processing and manufacturing processes.

It is essential that 100 per cent pure, stabilised aloe vera gel is used and that it is the primary ingredient in all aloe vera products.

KEY TIP
It must also be the most significant part, by volume, of any product (the debate of inner gel versus whole leaf is outlined in more detail in Chapter 3), especially if people are wanting to use the products to help treat and manage a particular disorder or ailment.

I have personally tried numerous aloe vera products here in the UK, in Europe and in the USA. Many of them were so watery (and this applies as much to the topical products as to the drinking juices) that in some cases it has been almost impossible to differentiate the aloe vera drink from water. My view of such products is that water is good for you but not if it costs £10 or $10 per litre or more. Similarly, some of the topical creams, gels and shampoos have been found to contain very little active ingredient – i.e. stabilised aloe vera gel.

The stabilisation process must not involve synthetic chemicals and the purity of the product must be guaranteed from the time the raw aloe vera gel is extracted and processed to the time it is bottled and then delivered to the customer. Products must also carry an accredited seal of approval and at the present time the only organisation that has internationally accepted standards is the IASC. See Appendix 1.4 and 1.5. Most products now carry the IASC seal of approval because the respective manufacturers quite rightly conclude that without it they would have difficulty selling their products to a general public that is slowly but surely becoming more discerning, more knowledgeable and more aware of the quality issue.

These days the words 'aloe vera' seem to appear everywhere as manufacturers of everything from shampoos, deodorants, razors and creams to tissues, toilet paper, recreational drinks, face sprays, washing powder, baby wipes and more exploit the 'healing properties' of aloe vera and the boom in demand for products with aloe vera. With all these products around now, how can you – the customer – choose one brand rather than another, and is the cost indicative of purity and quality?

KEY POINT
Unfortunately with many products there is simply not enough aloe vera content to do anything other than provide some form of psychological reassurance to the customers – they are unlikely to derive any physical or therapeutic benefit!

Growing aloe vera

This is obviously the first critical stage in the process of 'plant-to-product-to-customer'. So let's look at what happens – let's follow the plant from the nursery bed through harvesting to stabilisation and processing, and let's keep it simple. Aloe vera must be grown organically, i.e. without the use of or need for synthetic chemicals, i.e. chemical sprays, herbicides, fertilisers, insecticides and pesticides at any time in the cultivation process and growing cycle. Currently, there are thousands of acres of commercial aloe vera plantations in Texas, Mexico, the Caribbean, Australia and South Africa, and other countries enjoying similar climates. There are also plans to further expand plantations to cope with the increasing demand for aloe vera products in places like Latin America, Japan, Taiwan, Thailand, Malaysia, the Philippines and last but by no means least, China and India – arguably the biggest potential markets in the world.

Growing, cultivation and all aspects of crop husbandry are highly labour intensive, as most jobs require manual labour rather than machines. All the weeding and harvesting is done by hand to prevent any damage to the mature aloe vera leaves. In the nursery area, the 'pups' – the small offshoots from the adult plant (rather like the common household spider plants) – are carefully removed and planted out in dedicated areas. These are nurtured until they are robust enough to be transferred and planted out in larger fields. They will remain there for up to four years, being carefully tended until they reach maturity, with their optimum complement of vitamins, minerals, amino acids, enzymes, other nutrients and, of course, the unique polysaccharides. At harvesting, all the outer, mature leaves are cut by hand (not machine), in order to avoid damaging either the harvested leaves or the younger, less developed leaves in the middle of the plant. As the leaves grow and mature at different rates and grow closely together in a rosette pattern, resembling a clump of celery, harvesting is an ongoing process that requires considerable care and attention to ensure the remaining leaves are not damaged in any way.

On arrival at the processing plant, the leaves are transported (on rubberised conveyor belts for added protection) to an area where they are washed, topped and tailed and then filleted. Again much of this is done by hand to avoid bruising or in any way damaging the delicate structure of the leaf.

The leaves are then cut lengthways and the clear inner gel extracted. The rind (outer leaf) is removed and retained for use as an organic mulch and soil conditioner that is integrated back into the fields. This provides a natural, organic, vegetable-based fertiliser for the next growing cycle. The economically important inner gel is collected and piped into vast stainless steel vats, each holding thousands of gallons. It is here that the collected inner gel is stabilised using a unique, patented stabilisation process, with natural stabilisers.

Stabilisation and processing

KEY POINT
The producers of the best quality aloe vera products manufacture them in accordance with the highest pharmaceutical standards and within the parameters laid down by any regulatory or other relevant bodies.

The most stringent quality assurance procedures are adhered to at all times to ensure that there is no physical or bacterial contamination. Regular batch testing ensures that the presence of the anthraquinone fraction is within the 'beneficial' limits for aloe vera products for both internal consumption and external use. No artificial chemicals are added during the manufacturing process and all products are made from the highest grade (food grade) raw aloe vera gel and not from powdered concentrates or other similarly altered raw materials.

KEY TIP
Lots of people don't like the taste of aloe vera (can't think why!). So, they take tablets or capsules instead. Due to the small amount of aloe vera in them, we believe it is doubtful whether they have anything like the same benefits as drinking the 'fresh' gel. Instead, either mix your aloe vera with a strong tasting fruit juice (mango is good) – or give in to the joys of drinking it pure (the taste does improve when you get used to it – honest!).

The world's largest grower, manufacturer and distributor of aloe vera products uses a stabilisation process that preserves the inner leaf gel, which ensures it is 'essentially identical' and has the same freshness and potency as the gel from a fresh, newly harvested, mature aloe vera leaf. This process has allowed this particular company to promote the concept of 'fresh' aloe vera. This compares to most of its competitors that may use a whole leaf process, during which time the raw material must be passed through carbon filtration to ensure that all impurities and bacteria from the outer leaf are removed. The inner leaf gel process took years to perfect and is protected by two worldwide patents. This complex process guarantees the freshness of the processed aloe vera and is known not to interfere with the naturally synergistic workings of all the gel's nutritional components.

KEY TIP
Another benefit of the stabilisation process seems to be that the healing properties of the stabilised gel are not only enhanced, but that they also become more consistent.

Over the centuries, households and peoples from all over the world have benefited enormously from the 'potent' and sometimes 'miraculous' properties of aloe vera as a natural remedy for a wide range of both internal and external disorders. Hence the reason for the large amount of anecdotal evidence that has been gathered over the years relating to aloe vera's healing benefits.

KEY TIP
By simply slicing the leaf lengthways to expose the gel and then rubbing it on the affected area, its cooling and healing properties could be experienced almost instantaneously, as could its benefits when consumed for internal use.

However, until recently, such benefits could be enjoyed only by those fortunate enough to live in warmer climates near fresh aloe vera plants or those with the knowledge to grow aloe vera as a houseplant (though the potency of indoor grown plants is recognised as being considerably less than those grown outside in hot climates exposed to natural sunshine). In the last two and a half decades one company, which now has operations in over ninety countries, has effectively changed the face of the aloe vera industry worldwide. Now everyone, literally from South Africa to Finland and Australasia to California and all points in between, can enjoy the benefits of the highest quality aloe vera products, throughout the year.

Inner gel versus whole leaf

The debate continues with arguments being put forward by both camps as to which type is best. My view is based not just on my experiences of having seen thousands of people benefiting from taking the products made with the inner gel but also on my appreciation of the level of processing that is involved in the whole leaf products.

Nature gave us aloe vera and short of applying or using a fresh, mature leaf every time we wish to take aloe vera (it's not very practical for someone living in a country where aloe vera does not grow), the next best thing arguably is to use the plant in as natural a state as possible. Excessive filtration and/or concentration can materially affect the make-up and balance of the naturally occurring nutrients. The natural salts in aloe vera could be concentrated in such a way as to have a detrimental effect on the natural long-chain sugars or polysaccharides, thus reducing their potency.

KEY POINT
The two activities most likely to damage or destroy polysaccharides early in the manufacturing process are, firstly, exposure to the natural enzyme, cellulase and/or, secondly, the activity of bacteria. Interestingly, both are present in aloe vera just under the rind or on the outer green leaf.

The companies that discard the rind and whose products are based on the inner gel are effectively negating a source of potential economic damage (in their opinion). Whole leaf manufacturers use carbon filtration or other techniques to filter out the bacteria and other impurities found on the rind after the whole leaf has been effectively liquidised. These manufacturers maintain that more of the active ingredients and healing agents are found in the outer leaf area (i.e. the material that is discarded by the 'inner gel' manufacturers). My view is firstly that aloe vera is a living plant and materials and nutrients are transported throughout the plant, and the inner gel contains enough to have significant and wide ranging beneficial effects. Witness the case histories in Chapter 5. Secondly, the filtration process may also expel some materials/nutrients that are highly beneficial. Thirdly, and this is a matter of pure commercial logic, if there was a real and defined difference in relation to the percentage of healing nutrients in the finished whole leaf products compared to the inner gel products, there would be recognised commercial and health benefits.

> KEY TIP
> If whole leaf was better, then why would the largest grower and processor of aloe vera in the world (they would have more leaves to use than all the other manufacturers) not develop and sell products based on the whole leaf production process instead of the inner leaf gel?

To me the jury is still out and until an independent body can categorically prove that whole leaf is better, I am sticking with what I know works and works well. I have seen too many life-changing experiences to be easily swayed by marketing hype, bias or unsubstantiated 'facts'! One always has to recognise that different manufacturers obviously have a vested interest in selling their particular products and in promoting their particular extraction and processing procedures as being better than that of their competitors.

> KEY TIP
> In the end the decision is yours as to what you believe and which product you want to purchase. Never forget that the 'proof of the pudding is in the eating' – just make sure that you've got a cast iron, unconditional sixty-day money-back guarantee on the products you decide to purchase.

Quality – the essential component!

Aloe vera must be 'biologically alive' and must be in a bio-available form if customers around the world are to experience the full scope and range of benefits from this 'wonder plant'. The only way that aloe vera can reach the customer in a 'fresh' state and still be of the highest quality is if the raw inner gel is stabilised immediately. This stabilisation process must also preserve and retain all the active ingredients without the use of any damaging chemicals or exposing the gel to excessive heat.

KEY POINT
Aloe vera, like all living matter, decomposes and if the inner gel undergoes prolonged exposure to the air, it will oxidise and rapidly deteriorate, thus losing its medicinal properties and hence its health, healing and therapeutic benefits.

Aloe vera must be harvested and handled carefully to ensure that the leaves are not damaged prior to the gel being extracted at the stabilisation plant. The world's largest grower and processor of aloe vera owns thousands of acres of aloe vera plantations, in several different countries, where the plants are nurtured using the highest standards of crop husbandry. The plants are carefully tended from the nursery beds right through to the time when the inner gel is extracted from the mature, harvested leaves to be stabilised (using a unique and patented system) and later processed into a wide range of drinks and topical skin care and daily care products. It is important to note that some of the less scrupulous growers, suppliers and manufacturers of aloe vera products may often be tempted to harvest leaves prior to their reaching optimum maturity (i.e. three to four years).

KEY TIP
Normally it takes three to four years before an aloe vera plant is ready to be harvested and sometimes this timescale is reduced to generate quicker income for the companies involved. The real losers in this scenario are the customers or buyers of the finished products because they are not getting the most potent aloe vera available.

The highest standards of production are essential, as is the need to use only fresh, mature aloe leaves from the Aloe Barbadensis Miller plant. The resultant extracted gel must be properly treated, stabilised and preserved to ensure that the highest purity, efficacy and quality standards are met and maintained at all times. Some companies may subcontract the growing of the aloe vera plants to established independent growers who grow plants to strict specifications and crop husbandry guidelines, using organic farming techniques. This should ensure that no synthetic chemicals are ever used that may be detrimental to the purity of the gel in the plant and the finished product and thus its healing properties.

However, smaller suppliers of aloe vera may have to buy their raw material or even the finished product on the open market, with no guarantees that the plants have been grown organically or that they were mature prior to harvesting. Similarly, the inner leaf gel may not have been in the same fresh state as when it was harvested. It may also have lost some of its potency, either through oxidation and decomposition or as a result of an inadequate stabilisation/preserving process, using chemical rather than natural additives and stabilisers. Its potency can also be compromised as a result of overheating the aloe vera during the production process, so destroying many of its valuable nutrients (enzymes, amino acids, vitamins, minerals, polysaccharides, etc.) and healing properties.

KEY TIP

The widely accepted view that it is the presence of the unique polysaccharides and the synergism between all the nutritional constituents that gives aloe vera its 'magical' properties, means that the method of processing is critical to preserving the integrity of its health-giving and healing benefits.

Any processing that involves exposure to excessive heat, high salt concentrations or enzyme actions or extreme filtration or concentration can have a detrimental effect on the polysaccharide content and thus reduce their actions and hence their benefits.

The damaging effects of such processing could result in the aloe vera losing its 'biologically active' properties and associated benefits and would make any such products almost worthless. The largest growers and producers and those with the established business track records recognise that their manufacturing processes must take all these factors into account and therefore manufacture their products to the most exacting standards, in so-called 'clean room' conditions to ensure that quality is consistent. Every batch is rigorously tested in accordance with strict and well established procedures.

What to look for when buying aloe vera

Track Record

When purchasing any item, whether it's a car, a TV, a camera or even just an ice cream, the likelihood is that you would purchase a brand manufactured by a well established company that had some sort of track record and one that had either been heavily advertised or had been personally recommended by someone that you know.

I believe this should also be one of the most important criteria when it comes to buying health and skin care products such as those made from aloe vera. However, in reality, because the unit cost is not that high, people don't seem to care that much and, in general, spend far too little money and effort on their health and health products compared to items like junk food, tobacco, alcohol and so on.

Being healthy and taking decisions about better health and prevention is all about attitude and you have to 'invest' in that process. If your goal is better health, it will require some form of financial commitment. However, prior to spending any money, do some research and make sure that the treatment or the products you want to buy are the best available and are price-competitive. When it comes to aloe vera, the likelihood is that products purchased on a direct basis from companies that have long established trading records stretching back decades are likely to be superior. Very often, these companies are totally vertically integrated and are therefore in control of every aspect of production – from plant to product to you. Generally, aloe vera products from such companies will be far superior in quality, efficacy, purity and potency than those brands that have 'recently arrived' to exploit market awareness and consumer demand. The reason is obvious. The more established brands have stood the test of time and as companies they have invested very heavily in infrastructure and are totally committed to quality assurance and ongoing research and development programmes. Additionally, they have scientists, technicians and specialists monitoring all aspects of the growing, processing, manufacturing, marketing and distribution cycles. This is especially true if the company is accredited by independent organisations or other relevant bodies, for example the kosher rating.

In the UK, the USA and now throughout Europe, there are many companies involved in the direct sales of aloe vera (and other nutritional products) but very few – to our knowledge – are totally vertically integrated.

KEY TIP

Few have any meaningful track record or the necessary financial strength or stability to develop efficient distribution systems that will last and, to our knowledge, only one offers an unconditional sixty-day money-back guarantee for customers on all its products.

If you have any doubts about the aloe vera products you are thinking of buying, stop and ask yourself the question – why do I want to take aloe vera? If the answer is that you want to help treat or manage a particular ailment or disorder, or even that you want to take it as a health tonic and you want your skin to look better and feel better (and yes, maybe even younger!), make sure that the aloe vera you buy is always of the highest quality.

KEY TIP
Never compromise on quality – we have found the most potent aloe vera is still undoubtedly the most cost effective.

Never accept second best – you simply don't have to, anymore!!

KEY TIP
Always look for the guarantee.

The largest manufacturer of aloe vera offers an unconditional sixty-day money-back guarantee. Others may also do the same but, at the time of writing, we are not aware of anything more than the normal thirty-day money-back guarantee.

To have the opportunity to try products for this period is a good way for you to determine their benefits.

Personal recommendation/Third party/Independent endorsement

This is perhaps the most important aspect of any purchasing decision, whether it's a book, a car, a film, a restaurant or yes, even aloe vera and other natural health products! If you are interested in taking aloe vera and you have read something in the media about the benefits of aloe vera and you also know someone who is taking aloe vera and finding it beneficial, the likelihood is that you will purchase the product as much on the basis of that person's recommendation as on the information you have read in the media. It is most important however that you also do your own 'due diligence'. Research the products as much as you want to and ensure that you obtain the best products available. Unfortunately, I have seen many people put off taking aloe vera on an ongoing basis because the particular brand they tried was simply not capable of providing the improvements and healing benefits that they had either read about or heard about or that they were looking for or even caused some form of allergic reaction.

KEY TIP
Very often this is because they have read a case history in the media that may have featured one particular brand of aloe vera. They have then purchased a totally different brand that is subsequently found to have a fraction of the active ingredient or healing properties of the brand originally featured or even other 'less pure ingredients'. It's hardly surprising that they may be disappointed – but do not blame aloe vera – blame that particular brand/product!

This is why it is so important to ensure that if you read an article in the media and you want to buy aloe vera (or any other product featured), you should always contact the company concerned to obtain the relevant information and then make an informed choice. Remember that there is still a vast disparity in the quality, purity, efficacy and potency between the brands of aloe vera available in whichever country you live or visit.

So, in summary

- ➢ talk with people whom you know are taking aloe vera
- ➢ do your research and look around for a brand of aloe vera that offers an unconditional sixty-day money-back guarantee
- ➢ buy a product from a company with an established track record and the IASC seal of approval
- ➢ buy a product where 100 per cent stabilised aloe vera gel is the main ingredient
- ➢ This means that you have sixty days to try the products and if, for whatever reason, you do not like them or you do not feel that it/they have worked, you can get your money back.

Using a product in this way is the best approach to using aloe vera. Try it and see if it works for you. Good luck, I am confident that you'll soon experience the benefits.

Polysaccharides

Often referred to as the 'magic bullet' of aloe vera, these particular long-chain sugars are unique to aloe vera and they seem to work synergistically with the other key constituents. As long ago as 1977, polysaccharides were identified as being a key element in aloe vera's potent healing mechanisms. Dr Albert Leung, in a report in the *Drugs and Cosmetics Journal* (June 1977) noted:

> During the past three years, there has been a considerably revived interest in Aloe Vera as a cosmetic ingredient. Several major cosmetic and consumer product companies have incorporated it into their products and others currently are at the development or pilot stage with their own lines of Aloe Vera cosmetics… .
>
> All take advantage of the age-old reputation of Aloe Vera as a skin healer, skin softener and moisturiser… .
>
> It is commonly believed that the moisturising emollient and healing properties of aloe gel are due to the polysaccharides present. The major polysaccharide present has been determined to be a gluco-mannan. Other polysaccharides containing galactose and uronic acids as well as pentoses are also present.
>
> It is probable that the gel's beneficial properties are not due to the polysaccharides alone but rather as a result of a synergistic effect of these compounds with other substances present in the gel.

If all this seems a little complicated, it is hardly surprising because even after nearly five decades of intensive scientific research, scientists are still only now partially able to explain the almost miraculous, non-toxic and highly potent healing powers of aloe vera.

KEY POINT
These result from a powerful combination of anti-inflammatory, antiseptic, analgesic, antibiotic, astringent, coagulating, anti-pruritic and other agents, as well as pain and scar inhibitors and growth or biogenic stimulators. A well known German research pharmacist named Freytag called the latter a 'wound hormone'.

Dr Danhof is quite forthright in his views on polysaccharides. He believes they are probably the single most important constituents of aloe vera because of the health benefits they seem to impart to both humans and animals.

It is reported that the optimum polysaccharide content in aloe vera should be between 1,200 and 2,000-plus milligrams per litre (that is in the naturally occurring plant). The processing of aloe vera should not compromise that concentration and no simple sugars or starches should be added to try and boost that level during the production process.

KEY POINT
Artificial methods of concentrating aloe vera could cause damage to the polysaccharides through certain processing techniques that may expose the polysaccharides to excessive bacteria or cellulase levels.

Also any increase in the concentration of the natural salts and any changes in the natural ratio of liquids to solids (99.5 per cent: 0.5 per cent) found in the pure aloe vera gel or juice may have a detrimental effect on the properties and benefits.

Although the IASC's standard on polysaccharides content is listed at 1,100 milligrams per litre this should be considered as a minimum level only. For instance the world's best-selling brand of aloe vera, and the one that was the first to gain the IASC's seal of approval, has a polysaccharide content of between 1,900 and 3,500 milligrams per litre – which far exceeds the minimum standard.

KEY TIP
Think of the IASC as a minimum standard (in order to have the right to display the IASC seal of approval) – but also be aware that some quality aloe products can be two to three times richer in essential elements.

International Aloe Science Council (IASC)

Certification – proof of quality

The IASC is an organisation that was set up with the support of the major international aloe vera growers and producers to help develop, monitor and maintain standards (content, quality, purity, efficacy, potency, etc.) in the aloe vera industry worldwide. Its inception came at a time when the industry was almost totally devoid of any regulations or standards and although not strictly 'independent', it is wholly objective and it has overseen significant improvements in standards throughout the aloe vera industry and continues to work towards further improvements. There are some manufacturers who maintain the IASC standards are not rigorous enough and have chosen not to apply to have the IASC seal of approval on their products.

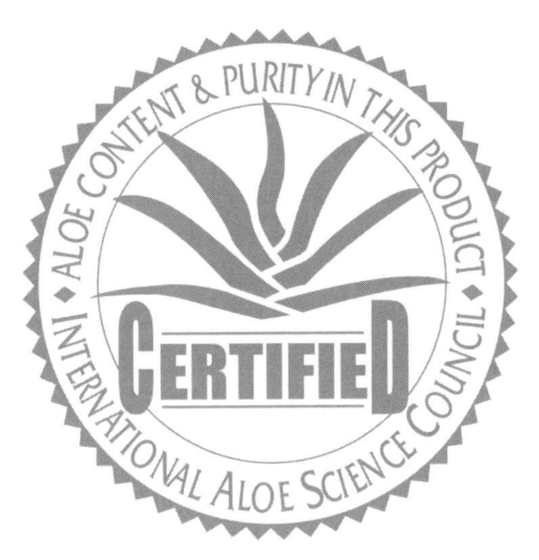

My view is that such a decision is obviously their choice. However, if I was a potential customer wanting to buy an aloe vera product, I would prefer to believe the widely accepted standards of an internationally acclaimed regulatory body over the subjective marketing claims of a commercial producer that has an obvious and direct financial vested interest in selling its own brand of products. The IASC seal of approval has become accepted worldwide as the indicator that those brands that carry the seal meet the minimum standards required. It also means that those particular brands (and individual products) have been inspected and audited and the products and contents analysed. Independent experts use approved procedures developed and laid down by the IASC science and technical committee.

When I wrote my first book in 1997, only one company in the UK (which sells its products direct to the public through a network marketing system and trained independent distributors) had the IASC seal of approval on its products. Since then, many other companies in the UK have now met the minimum standards required to be able to display the seal. Don't forget there is still a wide difference in the potency and in the percentage of stabilised aloe vera gel, between different products and in the methods of stabilisation in products that carry the IASC seal.

I have asked Gene Hale, managing director of the IASC to share his thoughts with you. He states:

> My name is Gene Hale and I am the Managing Director of the International Aloe Science Council – a non-profit industry organization serving its

members and the aloe industry, worldwide. Twenty-two years ago, a group of visionaries from the aloe vera industry met to form a working association that could help mould the future of the aloe industry. These people were driven by a desire to establish strict standards for the industry and not for personal gain. Their work helped forge the framework for an organization known as the National Aloe Science Council, now known as the International Aloe Science Council. This organization is at the forefront of quality control and assurance standards and the development of new research programmes in the aloe vera industry.

The aloe vera plant is a member of the lily family, a succulent, even though its appearance is more like a cactus. Aloe grows in the hot, dry areas of the world and a hard freeze will destroy the plant. While the origin of the aloe family is in Africa, we can now identify over 400 species of aloe. These range from small plants that never grow much more than a few inches high to tree-like aloe plants and a myriad of variances in between. Some have large heavy leaves filled with its precious inner material while others have slim leaves extending from spiny stalks.

There are two totally different products that are extracted and processed from the harvested leaves. One is called the drug aloe or an anthraquinone called aloin. This material is found clinging to the inner walls of the aloe leaf. It can be extracted from the outer leaf then processed and sold to pharmaceutical companies as a natural ingredient in a laxative product. The virtually toxic free balance or remainder of the aloe vera leaf is processed with only small traces of aloin for use in numerous products that are marketed to aid those who demand the fabulous benefits aloe vera offers. It is available in two basic forms. One is the inner material extracted from the aloe leaf and the other the entire leaf. The whole leaf is disinfected, chopped into smaller chunks and ground up leaving everything in it. Next, you must filter out the green outer rind material called chlorophyll and the drug aloe, aloin, that is now in this thick green mixture. Regular filters are used followed by charcoal filtration to remove these two unwanted agents from the aloe liquid. These two very different products are referred to as the inner fillet gel or juice and the whole leaf aloe – this is called the aloe raw material. Experts continue to disagree as to which is best, but we know that products derived from both processes are widely promoted for their benefits. Continued processing can also produce concentrates and powders of both types of aloe.

The primary function of the International Aloe Science Council is to work toward growing its membership and currently we have member representation in over 60 countries. The Council publishes a magazine called 'Inside Aloe' six to eight times a year. This magazine reflects changes in the industry, regulatory alterations, IASC functions and certification of company products and facilities. We also conduct an annual scientific seminar bringing scientific studies to the forefront by inviting the scientists and researchers to deliver their latest findings as to what aloe can do according to their scientific studies. The IASC also works closely with regulatory agencies, responds to actions that are required and works with members to meet industry needs.

The certification of products is probably the most important function of the Council. When companies make application for products to be certified, the Council uses an outside qualified, independent certifier to visit the location to be certified and to review the product work order or formula to assure that the proper and stated amount of aloe is incorporated into the product. They examine both the aloe raw material and the finished products (to ensure both comply with the certification standards laid down) as well as a selection of labels and literature and any related statements that must include the correct information about the specific aloe used. The labels and laboratory analysis of the samples are blinded and then sent to the certification chairman for approval prior to the Aloe Council formerly approving them for certification. The product(s) can only display the official IASC Certification Seal when formal approval is gained.

Recertification is done annually and random sampling is performed periodically. Currently, the certification tests are to have an L-Malic acid test done by HPLC. A total solids analysis, a test to determine the Calcium and Magnesium by A/A and the NMR (Nuclear Magnetic Resonance) Spectroscopy that analyzes 13 areas such as polysaccharides, adulterants, acids, acetyl groups and more. The product to be certified, recertified or random sampled must pass these stringent tests to carry the round IASC Certification Seal that states 'Aloe Content & Purity in this product – Certified – International Aloe Science Council'. This seal is very important for companies to use since it announces to the buying public that the purity and quality of their product has met the stringent standards laid down by the IASC. Unfortunately, many products are still sold to an unsuspecting public that have adulterated aloe, improperly processed aloe or have such a small amount of aloe that it is impossible for benefits to be

> derived from it. The International Aloe Science Council will not grant its 'Seal of Approval' to any product with an aloe content of less than 15% by volume.
>
> Some call IASC the industry watchdog and the steps taken by our organization certainly bring us into the mainstream of informing aloe vera users what they should look for. All labels are certainly not correct and over processing can render some aloe products virtually worthless. We are there to establish, develop and yes, even police, standards of purity, efficacy, quality, aloe vera content, etc., and to maintain those standards that are not only accepted by the aloe vera industry worldwide but are now increasingly being demanded by a much more knowledgeable and 'savvy' buying public. We are unique in what we do and what we stand for and we believe that by maintaining such rigorous standards and ethics, we are helping both the industry and the buying public to enjoy the rewards of this amazing plant.
>
> You can never tell what you are buying just by looking at an attractive label or some fancy packaging. Look beyond the disguise to the real marker – the IASC Certification Seal.

For further information on the IASC, see Appendix 1.4 and 1.5.

Patent

Although this information would not necessarily be displayed on any products, it is nevertheless an important fact that establishes the credibility both of a manufacturing process or a part of that process and the parent company that owns the patent(s). A patent is granted only on a product or method (as in the stabilisation process used by the world's largest aloe vera grower and manufacturer) that can be proved scientifically to be unique and actually to work. The company referred to in this section has two such international patents on its stabilisation process.

Kosher rating

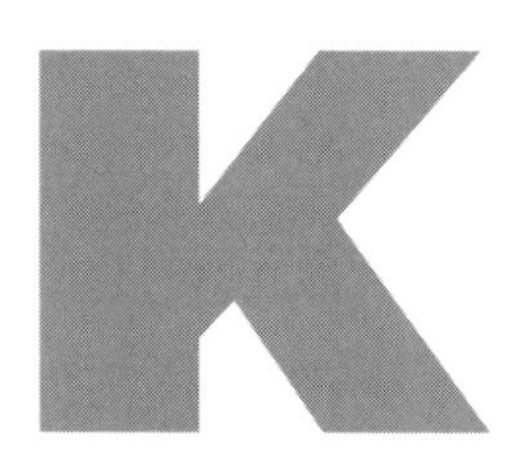

One indicator of quality that is unique to the world's largest aloe vera company is the K mark (see symbol) or kosher rating. This is an internationally accepted symbol of purity and quality that is both recognised and respected throughout the world. To achieve this quality mark, a rabbi from a certified laboratory is required to inspect the processing facilities, the formula of the stabilisation method (in the case of aloe vera), the manufacturing process, the facilities and all the ingredients in the products. The standards set are high and rigidly adhered to and many religious groups throughout the world, not just the Jewish faith, perceive the kosher mark as an accepted measure of high quality and a guide to safer and purer products.

Islamic seal of approval

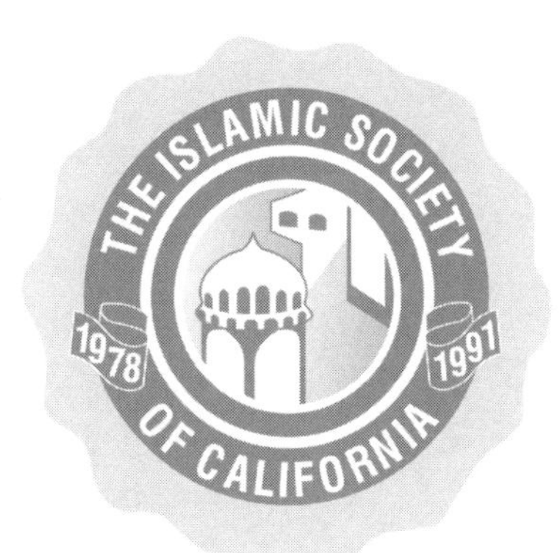

This is also a measure of quality and purity and shows that products conform to the highest standards laid down by this particular religious faith.

Not tested on animals

This is an important factor for many people. To my knowledge, none of the large aloe vera manufacturers uses animals in the testing of their products. There is however no question that aloe vera can be used to help treat and manage and in some cases even cure a wide range of ailments, disorders and diseases in animals. This subject is covered in Chapter 7.

Price is NOT a true indicator of quality

There is still a huge disparity in terms of quality, purity, efficacy and potency, as we have already mentioned, and the same is true of prices. Some aloe vera products are very cheap and if you want 'cheap', the chances are there will be very little aloe vera in the product and certainly not enough to have the sort of healing properties and therapeutic benefits that are now so often mentioned in the media. So beware of products being advertised at ridiculously low prices for a year's supply or more!! However, there are also many aloe vera products that are quite expensive and also have comparatively little aloe vera content as a percentage by volume.

KEY TIP
The most important considerations are to make sure you are getting value for money and that the brand or products you buy have some form of quality certification and money-back guarantee. You, as the customer, must be happy that you have got value for money and that the product(s) you have purchased will provide the benefits that you are looking for.

This is where professional advice (and here I am talking about someone who knows about aloe vera and its properties, potential uses and benefits – and not necessarily a doctor) is not only relevant but I believe is absolutely essential. If you do not feel that the initial advice you receive is adequate, make sure that you find someone who is able to provide objective advice on dosage, usage and product type.

> KEY POINT
> The remit of the Aloe Vera Centre, a retail mail order business and advice organisation, based in London (see Appendix 1.1), is not only to market the finest quality aloe vera and other nutritional and skin-care products, it is also to provide advice and information to anyone interested in aloe vera and its properties, uses and benefits.

Labelling can be misleading

When I wrote my first book on aloe vera there was no requirement to state percentage content by volume of 'stabilised aloe vera gel'. Currently, there is still no requirement to state the percentage by volume of stabilised aloe vera gel on any product containers, be they drinks or topical products. So I make no apology for repeating what I said in my first book. What some companies do is to use product labelling descriptions that can sometimes be misinterpreted by the customer. In the UK, for example, if a label states that a particular product contains a certain percentage of aloe vera (let us say it has on the label 'this product contains 99.5 per cent pure aloe vera juice'), anyone could be forgiven for expecting the contents of the bottle, tub or pot to contain 99.5 per cent by volume of aloe vera.

Well, sorry, you'd be wrong!

Unfortunately that's not the case! In fact it may mean that there is as little as 10 per cent (or sometimes even less) of the stabilised aloe vera gel (or active ingredient) by volume but that the 10 per cent aloe vera content is actually 99.5 per cent pure. Confused? You have every right to be! In other words, I could state that my container contains 99.5 per cent pure aloe vera juice, when in reality I may have added only a small amount of 99.5 per cent pure aloe vera juice to a container that was mostly water. Now, you can perhaps understand why some people who say that they have tried an aloe vera product, and that they did not see or feel any difference or benefit, could or would be disappointed. You cannot always rely on a label to tell you the whole story.

However, what the label may tell you is whether aloe vera is the principal ingredient in the product.

> KEY TIP
> In every case, aloe vera should be at the top of the list of ingredients, i.e. the number one ingredient – if it isn't buy another brand.

Manufacturing processes, conditions and temperatures will obviously vary from company to company but in order to ensure that the biologically active ingredients and all their healing properties are fully retained, temperatures must be strictly controlled and kept below certain levels, and synthetic chemicals should not be added.

> KEY TIP
> For example, when buying a natural product like honey, you should always ensure that it is 'cold-pressed'. This ensures that all the nutrients and other active, immune-boosting and health-giving ingredients will have been retained.
>
> The same is true of aloe vera – it is a 'biologically active' or 'living' food.

To many people, 'whole-leaf' aloe vera may sound like a desirable product but it really depends what has happened during the processing.

The filtration methods used must remove all bacteria and other possible detrimental contaminants and the vast majority of the aloin fraction. During this process, it is quite possible that some beneficial nutrients may also be removed. That is why one could argue that 'the jury is very much – still out' where the 'inner gel versus whole leaf' aloe vera debate is concerned.

> KEY POINT
> The pure aloe vera inner leaf gel, when properly stabilised and processed into drinks, has all the gentle healing and other beneficial properties needed to stimulate the digestive system in a safe, non-toxic and harmless way. It is also highly beneficial nutritionally, boosts the immune system, helps to detoxify the body, helps to increase energy levels and aids absorption of nutrients.

KEY TIP

Make sure that the aloe vera product you purchase has a safety seal (to ensure the quality and purity has not been compromised). Also, there should be no reason why the aloe vera products you purchase (drinks, creams, lotions, shampoos, deodorants, toothgels, etc.) should not have a sixty-day money-back guarantee.

What should aloe vera juice (drinking gels) look like?

I would maintain that aloe vera drinking gel really is the 'original amber nectar!' It is a slightly thick liquid containing natural pulp (much the same as if you peeled an orange and put it in a liquidiser and took out the pips of course!), which is a slightly yellowish colour. The colour can vary, naturally, from batch to batch. Where it's grown and the time of harvest may also have some affect on both the colour, consistency and taste. Unfortunately, there have been manufacturers that have adulterated the product in ways that are not beneficial to the buying public.

Some brands have allegedly been found to contain substances like bleaches and artificial colourings to ensure that the colour is uniform in every bottle. The old adage about aloe vera, 'that if it looks like water and tastes like water, there is a good chance that it will be mostly water', is probably true and if you're not 100 per cent happy, make sure that you choose another brand. I find that the simplest way to describe this is to imagine the difference between the juice from a freshly squeezed or liquidised (the inner flesh only!) orange and much of the orange juice you can buy in cartons from the average supermarket. The latter can just be orange liquid (where the original fruit has probably gone through so many pressings there's almost nothing left of the original orange) where the percentage of actual fresh orange is probably very low but it is still sold as orange juice. If manufacturers and supermarkets had to state in large writing how much pure orange juice there was present in the carton as a percentage by volume, I seriously doubt whether anyone would buy it. But, because both manufacturers and supermarkets make enormous profits from such products they would never willingly declare such information. It is the same in the aloe vera business. There are products being sold that purport to be aloe vera and are sold as such but are, in my opinion, mostly water (not the naturally occurring liquid).

KEY TIP
These products are simply riding on the back of the huge growth in demand for aloe vera products and they are, of course, exploiting the consumers' lack of knowledge and awareness of the vast quality disparity between different products.

Personally, I would never buy a product that looked like water because the naturally occurring pulp has obviously been filtered out (along with what else?!).

If you are unfortunate enough to have had this experience, try and get your money back and if you have no luck, just make sure that you never buy that particular brand again.

Remember, water is good for you but not that good for you when it's sold as 'aloe vera' at around £10 or $10 per litre!

What should aloe vera gel or juice taste like?

High quality aloe vera is not sold for its taste, it is sold for its wide ranging uses and benefits. The taste is slightly unusual and very 'vegetably' and most people think it's an acquired one. Although my wife, Mary, has benefited enormously over the years (she has taken it for IBS and diverticulitis) from drinking aloe vera gel (a potent, unflavoured drinking juice), she is still not overly enamoured of the taste! I however now regard it as my essential 'amber nectar' – I love it! I would strongly recommend that you just get used to it. The real benefits far outweigh any issues about taste and, to be honest, once your taste buds adapt, it really does improve and you hardly notice it. Above all, please remember the 'looks like water, tastes like water' advice and choose a high quality product.

KEY TIP
If you have read this book and have still not found such a product, please call us at the Aloe Vera Centre (020 8875-9915/0870-7555800) or visit the website at www.aloeveracentre.com

Design of the bottle or container

The design and physical construction of the bottle or container should always ensure that the integrity of the contents is not in any way affected by air, light or any other potentially detrimental factor. The container should always be made from a light-deflecting material. Clear glass or plastic will simply not prevent a deterioration in the product. The world's largest manufacturer and marketer of aloe vera uses specially developed containers which do not degrade and have a triple membrane skin that prevents both oxygen and light penetrating the container. The combination of the unique container and the stabilisation process keeps the drink 'fresh' for over three years. Once opened the container must be kept in the fridge and should be consumed within three months. Most aloe vera manufacturers will endeavour to ensure that the containers they use are impervious to both air and light but they must also ensure that whatever stabilisation process they use guarantees the integrity of the drinking juice throughout the duration of its shelf life.

Should you have any doubts about any aloe vera product(s) you are thinking of buying, whether it's a drink or a topical product, you can either decide not to purchase that particular item or you can call us or email us at the Aloe Vera Centre (alasdairaloevera@aol.com) for advice and guidance (see Appendix 1.1).

Four key tests of quality

- the official IASC seal of approval (no imitations!) should appear on the container
- check that stabilised aloe vera gel is the first ingredient on the contents list (with some aloe vera products I have seen, both drinks and topical products, the first ingredient is 'aqua'). That's just the European (Brussels diktat) way of saying 'water' – if that's the case do not buy it
- look for the K (kosher) mark if you are buying an aloe vera drink and you want an additional guarantee of purity
- make sure any aloe vera product you intend purchasing also has a safety seal – this helps not only to preserve the integrity of the contents but also ensures that the product cannot be tampered with

4

The professionals have their say

IN THE last few years, there has been a significant increase in the number of doctors, dentists, vets, other health professionals and therapists who have come to regard aloe vera not only in a more positive light but who are also using aloe vera products as an integral part of their various practices, clinics and treatments. This 'revolution' has been slow to come about but one has to realise that this is probably due to the decades of entrenched thinking and the belief that pharmaceuticals and antibiotics, in particular, seemed to be the answer to all ailments and diseases.

Recently I read an interesting comment about the money now spent on pharmaceutical research and development on the introduction of new 'ground-breaking treatments' compared to when penicillin was discovered. The latter cost 'nothing' to discover and with regard to the former, estimated research and development budgets are currently running at a figure in excess of $31 billion (!). One could ask the question, where is the next generation of so-called 'ground-breaking' pharmaceutical medicines?

While I am not a doctor, Audun Myskja *is*, and I hope that we both have sufficient objectivity to see both sides of the coin. I now believe that slowly but surely the 'allopathic professionals' (i.e. doctors, dentists, vets, etc.) are beginning to realise that some high quality, natural (plant, animal, mineral or insect derived) products may have a significant role to play in the prevention, the treatment and the management of certain conditions, ailments and yes, even diseases.

KEY TIP

As I am writing this book, new research at the University of Wales in Cardiff in the UK has revealed that irradiated, high quality, pure natural honey may be able to kill off mutant bacteria including the deadly antibiotic-resistant superbug methicillin-resistant staphylococcus aureus (MRSA), which is said to be linked to about 20,000 deaths a year in Britain alone and costs the UK's NHS in excess of £1 billion per annum in extra treatment!

This is another example of a natural product, present and available for thousands of years, being found to be effective where 'man-made' drugs have been seen to be seriously wanting or in some cases totally ineffective.

There is now an increasing level of interest being shown in the potential uses and benefits of natural products and plants like aloe vera. An increasing amount of research is being done on the uses of products made from plants such as aloe vera and these projects are conducted by people with conventional medical backgrounds (see Chapter 8). This can only be described as a highly positive step forward that I am sure will result in more and more 'professionals' beginning to understand the potential role of aloe vera (and other natural products such as pure honey) in the prevention of ill health and disease and the promotion of improved general health and overall well-being.

Aloe vera has been used by complementary therapists for many years but it is really only in the past twenty years in the USA, and the last seven or so in the UK and Europe, that therapists have been able to purchase products where the quality, purity, efficacy, potency and consistency of supply was guaranteed. Because of this comparatively recent development, aloe vera is now increasingly being recognised by therapists as a natural and effective way to cleanse and detoxify the body gently. When taken internally as a drink, aloe vera is absorbed by the body thus promoting healthier cells and hence healthier tissue. Given that our bodies are replacing over two and a half million cells every day, it is vital that those cells receive the maximum possible nutrition and aloe vera can play an important role in that process, as many doctors and therapists are now realising.

In the USA, many therapists, including chiropractic physicians, have been using aloe vera, both orally and topically, for over twenty years. They believe it helps the body heal itself. Although in the UK aloe vera as a health tonic and drinking juice is still comparatively new, it is making a significant impact on the way many therapists treat their patients. Even doctors (on both sides of the Atlantic Ocean!) are now beginning to wake up to the fact that aloe vera may be able to play a complementary role in the prevention, treatment and management of certain conditions, disorders and diseases.

This chapter records some of their comments, their opinions, their experiences and examples of certain cases they have treated with aloe vera.

Dr Audun Myskja

Dr Myskja is director of the Centre for Integrated Medicine, Integrated Medical and Health Centre, Norway. See Appendix 1.2 for full contact details.

Dr Audun Myskja is one of that rare breed of 'traditional' doctor who not only had an interest in complementary therapies many years before it became 'fashionable' or 'trendy' but has also studied herbal medicine, energy medicine and flower remedy treatments. He is a teacher of medical music therapy, as well as herbal and flower remedies. He is also a qualified Tomatis therapist and his integrated medical and health centre, which he runs with his wife, Reidun – a reflexologist and homeopath – is one of Norway's leading Tomatis teaching centres. He is a prolific author and has had many papers published and is also the author of several books. His book on music therapy was published in 1999 and his book on flower remedies was published in 2000. He has also written a book on aloe vera in Norwegian – *Aloe Vera – naturens skattkammer*. He is also a consultant to the Norwegian Cancer Association on complementary therapies and terminal cancer care and was, until recently, the head of staff at a hospice in Oslo, Norway. His interest in aloe vera and its potential role in the 'healing' process dates back over two decades and he outlines some of his own experiences and views below.

> One of the most mysterious capacities of the body is its ability for self-repair and self-healing, and we very often take this self-healing capacity for granted until it is lost. One example of a disease that reduces the body's capacity for self-healing is diabetes. It leads to a reduction in the capacity for wound-healing and reduces the body's resistance to infections and inflammations. The word infection refers to an agent-like bacterium, virus or fungus. Inflammation refers to the effect on a tissue. If we use the word inflammation there is no certain infectious agent.
>
> Professor Robert Davis at the Pennsylvania College of Podiatric Medicine conducted a study on mice, published in the *Journal of the American Podiatric*

Medical Association. He made a group of mice diabetic by giving them streptozotocin injections. A control group was given normal feeding, whereas one treatment group was fed with aloe vera. He also extracted gibberellins, glycosides found in aloe vera and injected another treatment group similarly. At the onset of the experiment, all the diabetic mice were exhibiting signs of inflammation, and there was no difference in signs between three groups. After the observation period, the following was found:

> In the control group, there was no change in the degree of inflammation shown. In the two treatment groups, the inflammation decreased exponentially, following the exact dose response rate with higher doses. The mice in both treatment groups receiving the highest doses were completely free from inflammation at the end of the investigation.

What conclusions can we draw from these studies? We may infer that the substances in aloe vera have anti-inflammatory activity – this includes plant hormones like gibberellins. The study showed that there is no difference between giving this substance as a concentrate and injecting aloe vera gel. This is important, given that treatment with a single component of aloe vera, like acemannan, can lead to side effects. So it is then safe to say that injecting aloe vera gel is safer and will give the same effect to support anti-inflammatory activity. Tissue samples showed that aloe vera decreased leukocyte infiltration in normal tissue and increased the growth of normal collagen tissue.

Dioscorides, one of the fathers of the healing arts, mentioned aloe vera in his writings. He stated that aloe vera may increase hair growth, reduce the growth of tumours, lessen stomach pains, help to combat ulcers, help stop bleeding in wounds, reduce boils and aid in the healing of eye infections. This is strikingly in accord with research findings over the last twenty years and shows that the indications for using aloe vera have been evident for centuries – even millennia. Traditional use of aloe vera gives some indication of the belief in its general health powers. In Russia aloe vera was called 'the plant of immortality', in Japan the name for aloe vera means 'no doctor is necessary.' The Chinese traditionally call aloe vera the 'wand of heaven'. These traditional phrases may support our belief in aloe vera as a general tonic and stimulant that may influence health, well-being and vitality.

Anti-ageing properties

As a boy brought up in a relatively poor post-war Norway, it impressed me greatly to hear, in history classes, that Cleopatra, the queen in ancient Egypt, took baths in milk, in order to keep her skin beautiful. We do not know for sure if this milk was actually aloe vera, as many books have claimed, but we do know that aloe vera grew in ancient Egypt and was used for both its internal and topical benefits.

We also know that there is a better chance of rejuvenating the skin with aloe vera than with ordinary milk. Aloe vera penetrates deeper into the skin than milk, and has an affect on the skin layers where rejuvenation actually occurs. One of the reasons for the penetrative powers of aloe vera is the presence of lignin, a relatively inert cellulose-like substance that helps other ingredients to penetrate to the deeper layers of the skin. When we state that 'beauty is only skin deep' we must remember that the texture and youthfulness of the skin is influenced by many deeper layers of tissue. One of the principal qualities of aloe vera is that it is a potent growth stimulator. For example, when used on a cut or a burn, it penetrates below the wound and promotes healing from the inside out. Because it replaces the fluids without stopping oxygen from getting to the wound, it helps both to speed up the healing process and reduce the scarring. Some of the hospitals that are using aloe vera are reporting an increased rate of wound healing, both faster and more efficient than normal.

Synergistic effect

It is presumed that in aloe vera, the whole is more than the sum of its parts, i.e. a synergistic effect. Over the years, many companies have tried to extract individual ingredients of aloe vera. The therapeutic benefits of this is uncertain and there have been reports of serious side-effects in patients using large doses of acemannan extracted from aloe vera.[2]

Although we currently lack proper medical documentation as to the existence of any synergistic effect of aloe vera's 200-plus ingredients, it is safe to say that the ingredients work together and mutually complement one another and have no harmful interactions. In our clinic, we have also had many experiences of synergy between aloe vera and other natural remedies, like garlic, ginger and marine oils. Many cancer patients have reported that they have tolerated the cancer treatment better with aloe vera as a supplement. So we cannot exclude an additional synergism between aloe vera and certain forms of regular medical treatment. To focus too strongly on the single therapeutic agents in aloe vera would probably miss the mark. We have every reason to presume that it is precisely the exact balance between the many groups of biologically active compounds that gives aloe vera its unique and versatile effectiveness.

Although many of the staples of modern medicine are single substances extracted from herbs, modern research has raised objections to the basic assumptions that you can improve on nature by extracting single ingredients from herbs, plants, fruits and obtain an enhanced effect. In plants used as folk remedies, like aloe vera, garlic, onion, cabbage and ginger, vitamins are contained in proportions that are surprisingly harmonious, relating to the body's needs and especially which trace elements the body requires.

The difference between aloe vera and garlic, onion and ginger is that the former has been used primarily as a remedy, with defined medicinal actions and a spectrum of indications for use that has remained surprisingly constant through the centuries. Conversely garlic, onion and ginger have primarily been foodstuffs, though it has been known that, in addition to their respective nutritional values, they may also have a significant therapeutic benefit.

So it is safe to say that we do not know of any other single traditional plant remedy with such a wide and versatile content of essential vitamins, trace elements and substances with as broad a range of therapeutic effects as aloe vera. Although we cannot prove, in the scientific sense, that this is a synergistic effect in that all the elements have a mutually supportive effect on each other, we do know that they work well together.

Many of the reports on the actions of aloe vera (see Chapter 5) can hardly be explained in any other way than through a synergistic effect. Based on the reports of aloe vera users, the synergistic effect may also partly explain the increase in sensation of vitality and well-being. We also know, for instance, that the anti-inflammatory effect of aloe vera is due to the combined actions of several ingredients, including acemannan, glycosides like gibberellins and several anthraquinones. These work on different areas of the anti-inflammatory response in the body and seem mutually to aid each other. When we look at the anti-inflammatory effects of aloe vera, it is safe to say that there is a synergistic effect on different elements. The whole is indeed more than the sum of its parts.

Increased well-being

Judging from the reports of a number of patients and aloe vera users, this is the single most frequently reported effect of using aloe vera over time. General fatigue is becoming an increasing problem not only among patients but also among stressed modern-day employees. Often it can have well defined causes, such as in cancer or in chronic post-viral fatigue. In many cases the cause may also be psychological or an effect of modern lifestyle with stress and sensory overload. Poor diet and a lack of essential nutrients can also contribute to a feeling of general lassitude.

Can aloe vera help humans thrive in the same way as veterinary surgeon David Urch claims? He believes that when animals are given aloe vera, they often become 'bright eyed and bushy tailed'.[3]

Well-being is a complex but important area for future research. Overall health and well-being is difficult to measure, but we come across some interesting paradoxes in the debate between modern medicine and natural therapies. Medical science is reluctant to admit any positive effect of natural remedies, and the main argument is almost always due to the lack of scientific documentation.

However, an investigation of the treatment given by doctors for low back pain and shoulder pain in Norway has shown that only eleven per cent of treatment modalities used in low back pain and nineteen per cent of treatment modalities used by doctors for shoulder pain have been scientifically documented. Researcher Vigdis Moe Christie did a thorough investigation and compared a representative sample of patients' views of both alternative treatment and conventional medical treatment. When Christie looked at the patients' perceived results of visits with the two types of practitioners, ninety-one per cent of patients answered that they were well or better after consulting an alternative practitioner, whereas only twenty-seven per cent felt well or better after a visit to the doctor. Interestingly, only eight per cent were unchanged after alternative treatment whereas forty-seven per cent were unchanged after consultation with a doctor. A further one per cent felt worse after alternative treatment but this figure was twenty-one per cent after medical treatment. The sample included 118 patients, 109 of whom had received alternative treatment and 92 regular medical treatment. This is only one of several investigations that question the basic criticism levelled by the medical establishment at alternative treatments, namely that they do not result in a real change in a patient's condition, thus implying that the difference between medical and alternative treatment is that the former works while the latter doesn't.[4] This view contrasts with investigations like Christie's, which show that the public may actually perceive the results of alternative treatment as being better than the results of conventional medical treatment. There are many possible reasons for this, one being that the groups of patients that have acute medical ailments, like acute appendicitis and other conditions requiring surgery, normally only visit for that specific medical treatment and not for ongoing therapy.

The groups of patients that try both forms of treatments are often patients with chronic degenerative diseases or vague illnesses and ailments. Could this be an indication that increased well-being is a specific area for complementary treatment? There is little doubt that orthodox medicine will remain the chosen treatment for most diseases and serious acute conditions. However, the symptoms of illness and 'unwell-being' may be an area where complementary treatments may take over as a primary approach to better health and well-being. We have reason to believe that aloe vera will prove to be one of the most effective agents in aiding our quest for perceived and improved health and well-being.

Increased energy

'Energy' is a subjective sensation, linked to our degree of vitality – how alive we feel. In many other traditions, like the Indian, Tibetan, Japanese and Chinese cultures, energy is viewed as the main determinant of health and well-being. In these traditions, energy is viewed as giving body and mind life force. It enters body and mind through points of heightened activity and flows in channels, supplying the body with this life force. The most well known health system based on energy is acupuncture. In medical terms this is a controversial subject, but I, since childhood, have had the ability to see and perceive these streams and centres of energy activity.

One of the main reasons for my growing interest in aloe vera is that I have seen many patients with problems around the abdomen who seem to have a pronounced lack of energy in that area, as if the normal protective filter has broken down. After starting on aloe vera, they have become visibly strengthened, as if the filter between their body and the environment has somehow been restored and the energy levels in that area increased. This corresponds with the person's own feeling – often after taking daily doses of aloe vera drinking juice for only two to three months. Talking about energy can often be quite subjective but for those who suffer sudden or prolonged ailments, energy levels are very much a reality.

Dr Gregg Henderson has used aloe vera systematically for many years at his clinic, and finds that many of his patients become visibly energised by using aloe vera. He believes that:

> '...aloe vera is a great energiser and if you drink it on a daily basis, you probably won't need as much sleep. Not only is it a high quality nutritional product but its healing properties benefit both human and animal tissues.
>
> 'However, aloe vera does not in itself heal anyone or anything! The body does its own healing – it just needs to have the right "healing environment", free of any infections. Aloe vera is known as "the healing plant" because it provides the body with the necessary "agents" to take care of itself, i.e. to restore and repair and activate or re-activate normal body functions and the body's own healing process.'

I have been a medical doctor for over twenty years and, in that time, I have always integrated complementary therapies within my practice. I have worked with herbs and plants – as remedies – since the early seventies and have been fully aware of the role of aloe vera in the treatment of burns and the rejuvenation of tissue and skin for many years. I was not fully aware of the real penetrative power of aloe vera skin products until I was lent a spray formulated for use in sports and other similar injuries. Once recently, while on vacation, I played in a football match – on a very hard surface – and unfortunately suffered a complicated and extremely painful knee injury, which left me unable to walk. I used an aloe vera spray (with herbal extracts) soon after and applied it regularly over the next few hours. Amazingly, the pain vanished within a few hours, and much to my amazement I was able to walk the following day! Three days later, I could barely feel any effect of the injury and was able to move my leg quite freely. I then remembered a similar injury I had suffered six months previously when, unfortunately, I did not know about this spray. I had suffered pain for several days after the injury and did not recover fully for over three weeks.

I decided, after this very positive personal experience, that I would use the aloe vera spray and other products on any patients of mine who had similar painful injuries. I quickly found that the effect was better than the combination of anti-inflammatory and painkilling drugs (with physiotherapy) – the traditional treatment. There appeared to be no side effects, the cost of treatment was lower and the days off sick were reduced. Having both experienced and seen these very visual benefits personally, I decided to look closely at the research that had been done on aloe vera and was surprised to find that the benefits of using aloe vera internally were perhaps even greater than the topical benefits.

Immune deficiencies, intestinal diseases, cancer

Immune deficiencies, intestinal diseases and even cancer have been positively affected by the use of aloe vera and one could also document which components in the plant seemed to produce these effects. I found it incredible that the areas where aloe vera seems to act so powerfully are on those functions where conventional medications or drugs have shown little benefit. They are in the areas of immune deficiency, post-viral fatigue, general debility and weakness, exhaustion and lack of energy. I have many patients who are benefiting from using aloe vera products, both internally and topically, but one in particular comes to mind. This young patient had rheumatoid arthritis and we managed not only to reduce his pain but also cut down on his use of medication or drugs by using an aloe vera gel drinking juice internally [see 'Erik', Chapter 5].

After over twenty-five years' experience with healing plants and herbs, I am in no doubt that I have found no other plant that is quite so versatile or so potent as aloe vera, when presented in a pure, quality controlled state, i.e. high quality products produced by research based, quality conscious companies.

Further details of Dr Myskja's experiences with using aloe vera are included in the sections on case histories – Chapter 5.

Alan Watson, chartered physiotherapist

Founder of the Bimal Clinic, London (see Appendix 1.3 for full contact details), Alan Watson is a state registered and chartered physiotherapist who specialises in the management of chronic injuries of both a sporting and non-sporting nature. He established the Bimal Clinic in London and has since developed the clinic's formidable reputation as a centre of excellence in injury management. Alan has treated some of the UK's most prominent sportsmen and women and is often asked to help treat complex cases.

Muscular lesions, spinal conditions, arthritic joints

Alan has been using aloe vera products for the last six years and he believes it has had a profound affect on his treatments of soft tissue, and in particular muscular lesions and spinal conditions. It has also proved particularly effective in the treatment and management of arthritic joint conditions. He highlights his own personal experience with aloe vera:

> I have found that by using the aloe heat lotion in particular [a proprietary brand of heat cream], the pain in my own finger and wrist disappeared within a couple of months of using it. It was something I had been plagued with for many years and was mainly due to the manual nature of my occupation. For years, it had given me considerable discomfort whenever I was treating my patients.
>
> All the clinicians in the practice have found that the combination of the aloe heat lotion and arnica work extremely effectively together to alleviate muscular spasm, pain and inflammation. This combination of creams, with deep tissue therapy, facilitate the reduction in muscle hypertonicity and enable the clinician to progress with manipulative and mobilisation therapy with fewer post-therapy symptoms. The aloe heat lotion is much more effective as a massage medium than massage oil, as the constitution of the cream is smooth and easily absorbed and has longer lasting effects than other heat related creams. Compared to most other heat creams (which are ostensibly skin irritants) that may draw blood away from the injury, the effect of the aloe heat lotion is that it seems to penetrate deep into the tissue, promoting the healing process. Our patients describe a feeling of sustained and comforting heat sensations, which ease stiffness and pain in both muscles and joints.

Dr Gregg Henderson

Doctor of Chiropractic Medicine
Director of the Fallbrook Chiropractic Center in California

Dr Gregg Henderson, DC, FCTS, is a doctor of chiropractic medicine, a multi-disciplinary nutritionist and director of the Fallbrook Chiropractic Center in California. He has been using aloe vera as an integral and essential part of his patient care for over twenty years. In the following subsections, he details his experiences with aloe vera and his views on its role in the promotion of overall healing, good health and nutrition.

Burns and pain inhibitor

Aloe vera is mainly known for its ability to inhibit pain with injuries such as burns, and it is very easy to explain why it has this particular quality. It contains several analgesics and it can also penetrate the layers of the skin, moisturising the skin, soothing the nerves and reducing inflammation.

Anti-inflammatory

As an anti-inflammatory, it has a particular property that we do not fully understand, causing it to penetrate quickly and deeply into the skin and fight inflammation. This is probably why so many people seem to experience positive results with inflammatory diseases such as rheumatoid arthritis. Aloe vera moves in and competes with the enzyme that causes inflammation, so that it does not spread or become any larger. Research has shown that aloe vera enhances blood flow, stimulates the immune system, speeds repair and reduces scarring.

Cleansing and purifying

Aloe vera also contains an ingredient that actually emulsifies cholesterol, thus enabling the body to eliminate it. It stimulates the cleansing and purifying of the blood in the liver and acts as coagulator in cases of bleeding. Because it is a natural product that is recognised by the body and absorbed easily, good results can often be achieved in a comparatively short period of time, depending of course on the ailment. It also helps to speed up the replacement of body tissue and improves or replenishes the tissue through healthier cell production. Additionally, it contains uronic acids that actually strip away harmful materials from the body, and aloe vera also has an antibiotic effect that is well proven and well documented.

Over the last two or three decades we, in the so-called Western world, have developed and are routinely using 'superdrugs' and, not surprisingly, as a result have created 'superbugs' that are almost totally resistant to these drugs. The current situation in UK hospitals with the superbug – MRSA – is a good example of this situation. This has been referred to earlier in this book.

Salmonella, streptococci and staphlyococci

What I find most interesting – and I come across this virtually every day in my practice – is that the high quality aloe vera products that I use in my clinic are still effective against such organisms as salmonella, streptococci and staphlyococci.

Growth stimulator

One of the principal qualities of aloe vera is that it is a potent growth stimulator. For example, when used on a cut or a burn, it penetrates below the wound and promotes healing from the inside out. Because it replaces the fluids without stopping oxygen from getting to the wound, it helps both to speed up the healing process and reduce the scarring. Some of the hospitals in the USA that are using aloe vera are having an increased rate of healing, which can be fifty per cent faster than normal.

In our own practice we use aloe vera frequently with cancer therapies, such as chemotherapy and radiation therapy, because it reduces the negative reaction of patients to the effects of both the chemicals and the radiation. Our patients who use aloe vera do not normally lose their hair, they do not get sick during the therapy courses and they tend to respond much faster to the treatments.

Aloe vera is also a great energiser, and if you drink it on a daily basis, you probably won't need as much sleep. Not only is it a high quality nutritional product, but its healing properties benefit both human and animal tissues.

Colitis and diverticulitis

In the intestines, we can have many disorders, such as colitis and diverticulitis (to mention but two), and aloe vera has proved to be an excellent healing aid for all these.

> KEY POINT
> Basically, aloe vera will work in any situation where there is an '-itis' or inflammation, so that is why it can help with such problems as arthritis, colitis, diverticulitis and so on. It has the ability to soothe, protect, heal and cleanse the intestine, to detoxify the body and thus help to eliminate chemicals and other toxins (and free radicals) that we absorb from the atmosphere and processed foods, etc.

Aloe vera does not in itself heal anyone! In all my years of practice and in all my discussions with doctors, I have not met one yet who has healed anyone! The body does its own healing – it just needs to have the right 'vehicle' at the right time. Aloe vera is known as the 'healing plant' because it provides the body with the necessary 'agents' to take care of itself, i.e. to restore and repair and activate or re-activate normal body functions and the overall healing process. For example, it can destroy the bacteria that cause peptic ulcers – up to ninety per cent of the time.

Accelerated healing

Still, after all these years, one of the most remarkable and visual examples that I have ever seen (and I have seen a lot) is the way in which aloe vera can accelerate the healing process. This particular example relates to a plastic surgeon I know who uses what is effectively a chemical peel when performing face lifts.

He uses a product called aloe activator (a pure aloe vera liquid for topical use) to help accelerate the healing process and hence the healing and recovery time of his patients. This 'time period' has now been reduced from six weeks to just over one week. The use of just this one product resulted in a reduction by a factor of six in the duration of the 'healing process', and it is undeniable proof of what can be achieved using the incredible healing powers of high quality aloe vera products.

Dr Gary Fischbach, MD

Dr Fischbach is a private practice doctor in south eastern USA, who is a founding member of the Fairborne Institute and has pioneered the use of various natural compounds, including aloe vera, over the last few years. His book, *Nature's Miracles*

– *An MD's Experiences*, provides a revealing insight into the views of someone who was trained at one of the top medical schools in the USA and subsequently became a conventional medical practitioner. However, his realisation that the health care profession, of which he was a member, was ignoring some key factors that could have a profound effect on improved health and well-being, led him to consider 'complementary' or 'alternative' ways of treating patients. He, like many other doctors and therapists, soon identified that the origin of many of the ailments and diseases that afflict the so-called developed world are the 'free radicals'. These oxidants, or as he puts it 'unstable oxygen molecules', are released by pollutants, stress, the chemicals in our food and drink, the metabolic process itself and the sun.

Free radicals

Most people now accept that these 'free radicals' are responsible for so much of the degenerative process and are the single largest contributor to diseases like cancer (the scourge of the twentieth and twenty-first centuries). It would seem that 'free radicals' wear down our immune system, thus reducing the body's ability to defend itself. It is then that the diseases, infections and so on can take hold and wreak havoc with people's health and general well-being. There is no question that changes in lifestyle and diet (see Chapter 6) can help, as can improvements in the quality of the air we breathe and the water we drink, and how much regular exercise we take.

We can help ourselves mainly through diet (and using water and air filtration wherever and whenever practicable), and the increased intake of more anti-oxidants, to include higher intakes of the so-called ACE vitamins, i.e. vitamins A, C and E.

According to Dr Emanuel Cheraskin (*Journal of Orthomolecular Medicine*, 10: 2, pp89–96, 1995), free radicals have been implicated in over sixty different diseases and disorders, including Alzheimer's, cancers, cataracts, heart disease and high blood pressure, infertility, macular degeneration, mental illness, immunity and infections, rheumatoid arthritis, etc.

Conventional and complementary medicine

Conventional medicine has often fallen woefully short of the need to adopt a more proactive and preventative approach to healthcare. Dr Fischbach maintains that conventional medicines, as remarkable as they can be, have been no match for some of the most devastating and life-threatening diseases – those that carry with them the highest concentration of free radicals. The result has been a huge increase in the numbers of people dying from or ill with arthritis, cancer, strokes, diabetes, high blood pressure and numerous other disorders and diseases. Dr Fischbach is concerned that many conventional physicians are still trained to focus on the treatment of conditions only once they have arisen. The concept of 'preventative' care and the role of improved nutrition and the real health benefits of taking natural supplements has been almost totally ignored. He believes that changes to such set attitudes are being driven more by individuals rather than by the establishment, i.e. the medical and health profession.

No treatment ever has a 100 per cent success rate

He also advocates that his colleagues in the medical profession should not necessarily 'throw in the towel' when conventional treatment does not always work (no treatment ever has a 100 per cent success rate). He believes that they should consider the use of complementary therapies and some high quality natural supplements – many of which have a long history of healing. In his book, Dr Fischbach discusses such natural compounds and products as maritime pine, colloidal silver and aloe vera (and their properties, uses and benefits), and it his views on aloe vera particularly that I will refer to in this section. Dr Fischbach confirms that the legendary healing powers of aloe vera have been well documented through the ages and that many people are now very familiar with its healing, moisturising and soothing properties.

> KEY POINT
> Aloe vera has been proven to help in the healing of burns, wounds (surgical and others) and in chronic skin conditions like dermatitis, psoriasis and eczema, as well as helping to treat cancerous and pre-cancerous lesions.

However what is not so well known is aloe vera's wide ranging benefits when taken internally. He believes that in order to lock in all of the beneficial ingredients, it is essential that 'cold-processing' techniques are used to stabilise aloe vera. Dr Fischbach also confirms that it is the presence of the unique polysaccharides and one in particular, acemannan, that gives aloe vera its potent healing and immuno-modulating properties. He believes acemannan has a significant health benefit on both the gastrointestinal and immune systems.

The Western world now suffers from increased chemical pollution, infection, stress and nutrient deficient food (the 'well fed and badly nourished syndrome'!!), the combination of which can destroy people's immune systems. That makes the presence of an immune-building plant like aloe vera all the more valuable.

Dr Fischbach is convinced that the resultant diseases of the immune system, such as Epstein-Barr syndrome, systemic candidasis, ME and AIDS all have a common feature in their symptoms, and that is a dysfunctional digestive system.

KEY POINT
He believes that the inability of the stomach and intestines to break down food properly causes retention and subsequent absorption of too many toxic substances through an irritated, permeable bowel wall, allowing them easy access to the rest of the body. The result is a breakdown in the absorption of nutrients, cellular depletion, toxic build-up to levels the body cannot cope with and a degeneration of the immune system.

Added complications are that poorly digested food provides an excellent medium for the onset of fungal disorders such as candida that further deplete the body's immune system and inevitably lead to a downward health spiral and possible further infectious attack.

The acemannan component

What he found with aloe vera and its acemannan component is something that all medical practitioners should note. Acemannan can have a positive impact on each of these areas in the following ways:

- by inserting itself into the body's cell membranes, it can normalise cell function by regulating the transport of both nutrients and waste in and out of the cells (this was also confirmed by Dr Danhof). This enhances both cellular function and general metabolism
- it acts as a powerful anti-inflammatory agent, neutralising many toxic substances and restoring bowel impermeability
- immune cells are stimulated
- it helps eliminate bacteria, viruses, fungi and parasites, and with AIDS patients it seems to help protect the immune system from the toxic side effects of AZT (a prescribed medication for AIDS)

He lists other key substances and properties of aloe vera:

Anti-viral substance

Acemannan is a potent anti-viral substance found in aloe vera that is effective against herpes, measles and HIV.

Anti-inflammatory and analgesic properties

Salicylates have anti-inflammatory and analgesic properties. Other substances found in aloe vera have been found to relieve pain, reduce itching and lower blood sugar levels. Dr Fischbach advocates the daily intake or use of a high quality aloe vera drinking juice, whether you are ill or healthy, and suggests that aloe vera can be used to help with a number of conditions. He has listed the following conditions, ailments and diseases where he believes either aloe vera drinking juice or a topical aloe vera gel can be of benefit.

Dr Fischbach's uses for aloe vera drinking juice

KEY POINT

Acne, AIDS, allergies, asthma, bronchitis, bursitis, cancer (internal and skin), candida, carpal tunnel syndrome, high cholesterol, ME, colds, colic, constipation, contusion, Crohn's disease, diabetes, diabetic retinopathy, diarrhoea, diverticulitis, eczema, Epstein-Barr virus, fibromyalgia, gastritis, genital herpes, gingivitis, gout, haemorrhoids, hepatitis, indigestion, infections, inflammation, influenza, joint pains, leukaemia, lupus, osteoarthritis, phlebitis, PMS, psoriasis, rashes, rheumatoid arthritis, seborrhea, systemic candidasis, ulcerative colitis, ulcers, vaginitis, viral infection, yeast infections.

Dr Fischbach's uses for aloe vera topical gel/gelly

KEY POINT

Abrasions, acne, athlete's foot, boils, burns, cancer (skin), carbuncles, cradle cap, cuts, nappy rash, frostbite, haemorrhoids, Herpes zoster (shingles), infections, insect bites and stings, measles, rashes, sunburn, warts.

Dr Fischbach is the author of the book *Nature's Miracles – An MD's Experiences*. (See Appendix 2.)

Dr Peter Atherton

Author of The Essential Aloe Vera – *see Appendix 2.*

Eczema

Dr Atherton was a GP for over twenty-five years prior to being introduced to aloe vera by the mother of one of his patients. She had decided to treat her own son's eczema because the conventional medication that been prescribed had failed to solve the problem and she was reluctant to use any more medications. The little boy's eczema cleared up after using a topical aloe vera cream with bee propolis (a natural antibiotic from the beehive).

Although initially sceptical, Dr Atherton, who readily admits he was a 'strictly conventional' doctor, was open minded enough to read some literature on the range of aloe vera products and to study some research papers on aloe vera.

What convinced him to try using aloe vera was a paper from the Acne Research Institute of California that was published in the *Journal of Dermatological Surgery*. The paper focused on 'post-dermabrasion wound healing' and highlighted the use of this particular surgical technique to treat skin scarred by facial acne. The technique involves the effective removal of the scarred epidermis layer of the skin to leave the underlying dermal layer to produce a smoother and, hopefully, unblemished epidermis. Post-surgery, the trial used a topical aloe vera gel on one side of the various patients' faces and the normal treatment on the other.

The results were highly significant – the aloe vera patients had a twenty-five to thirty per cent faster healing time than the patients using normal treatment. This persuaded Dr Atherton, who had a keen interest in dermatology, that this strange, so-called 'cactus-like' plant merited further research. Some time later he was awarded a fellowship at Green College, Oxford, where he was able to pursue his work on the use of aloe vera, both topically and internally as a drinking juice. He worked in the department of dermatology and with the Oxford Institute of Wound Healing. It was this experience that led him to a fundamental change in his career path, from that of a senior partner in a successful GP practice in Buckinghamshire to the director of Tyringham, all in the space of five short years. So aloe vera can be life-changing in many different ways! Dr Atherton has become one of the UK's leading authorities on aloe vera. His work underpins its uses, properties and benefits and its role in improved healing, health and general well-being.

Chronic venous leg ulcers

Dr Atherton is involved in ongoing research work on aloe vera and has written many papers on the subject. The most significant to date is, I believe, the result of his work on how topically and orally administered aloe vera may aid healing in patients with chronic venous leg ulcers. Dr Atherton's paper, which was also published in the *Nursing Standard* in July 1998, is summarised in Chapter 8 (reprints of the *Nursing Standard* article are available from the Aloe Vera Centre. See Appendix 1.1).

My hope, like so many others involved in the aloe vera industry, is that people like Dr Atherton and others (and there is a growing number!!) will, through their ongoing work, create an environment in which their 'conventional' medical colleagues will throw off the shackles of pharmaceutical-only medications and treatments and adopt a more holistic approach to health care. They could start by looking more positively at how high quality aloe vera products can play a complementary role in their various treatments and practices.

Dr Atherton, like Drs Danhof, Myskja, Henderson et al, has described in detail the properties, benefits and potential uses of aloe vera, as well as describing the key role of those seemingly 'magical' polysaccharides.

David Urch, BSc, MA, VetMB, MRCVS – veterinary surgeon

David Urch had been in clinical veterinary practice for nearly twenty years before he became aware of aloe vera and its vast potential as a healer. It was purely by chance that he was introduced to this efficacious plant. He had been involved in a serious accident and was introduced to aloe vera for its general healing and therapeutic properties. He was astounded by the way it contributed to the improvement in his overall health. His positive experience regarding his own improved health led him to start using the same range of aloe vera products within his veterinary practice and soon he was witnessing similar healing benefits on a wide range of both domestic pets and large commercial animals. Some details of his work with aloe vera and his ground-breaking book, *Aloe Vera – Nature's Gift. Aloe Vera in Veterinary Practice* (see Appendix 2), are in Chapter 7.

David has also been kind enough to share some of his unique library of pictures with us – we thank him for this.

We would also suggest that anyone wishing to know more about the use of aloe vera in veterinary practice orders this book – the most comprehensive and informative book on aloe vera and its use in the animal world. See Appendix 1.6 for further details of how to order David Urch's book.

Richard Sudworth, BDS, LDS, RCS (Eng) – dental surgeon

In his paper that was published in *Positive Health* magazine in 1997, Richard Sudworth considered the dental uses of aloe vera and found that there were numerous opportunities to utilise aloe vera products in general dental treatment.

Use of aloe vera in general dental treatment

Aloe acts in many ways. It is particularly known for its penetrating capacity to reach deeper layers of the dermis when applied topically. It has strong antiseptic properties, being bactericidal, fungicidal and virucidal. It promotes cell growth. It is neurologically calming and also acts as a detoxifying agent.

Gingivitis

There are many potential applications for aloe vera in dentistry. It is extremely useful in the treatment of gum disease – gingivitis and periodontitis. It reduces swelling of the soft tissues and consequently this reduces the bleeding of the gums. It is powerfully antiseptic in gum pockets where normal cleaning is difficult, and its anti-fungal properties help considerably in treating Denture stomatitis, i.e. red and sore mucous membranes that are permanently covered by a denture. This is a form of thrush, against which aloe vera is very effective.

Herpes, shingles and viral complaints

Cracked and split corners of the mouth are also subject to fungal infection, and this can also be cured by using a topical aloe vera product. Its anti-viral properties help in the treatment of cold sores (Herpes simplex) and shingles (Herpes zoster).

Use in root canal treatment

It is a powerful healing promoter and when inserted into extraction sockets is highly beneficial. It can also be used in any surgical wound and has a use in root canal treatment as a sedative dressing, healing promoter and file lubricant.

Forms of aloe vera for dental treatment

The various forms of aloe vera that can be used in dentistry are:

- aloe toothgel
- aloe vera gelly for healing promotion
- aloe propolis cream for use on hands to counteract frequent hand washing and the wearing of latex gloves
- aloe activator spray which is excellent for throat infections, painful erupting wisdom teeth and joint pains

Lastly, aloe vera gel drinking juice can be used in conjunction with any topical treatment for skin lesions, joint lesions and for problems such as IBS. The drinking juice is also a powerful detoxifying agent and, if used in conjunction with the planned removal of mercury amalgams, acts as a scavenging agent for mercury and a neuro-sedative and an immune enhancer.

Most of the work on the use of aloe vera in dentistry has been conducted in the USA and at the moment the only additional information we have is that listed in Chapter 4 (Dr Timothy Moore), and Chapter 8.

Fluoride – good or bad?

When talking to many dentists there seems to be a fixation on the need for all toothgels and toothpastes to contain fluoride. Many experts believe that there is already enough fluoride available in what we eat and drink without having to put extra amounts into toothcare products. The British Dental Association has apparently urged toothpaste manufacturers to specify levels of fluoride on their packaging. There are fears that fluoride may have harmful as well as beneficial effects and there is a growing body of opinion, and not just within the 'complementary' or 'alternative' fraternity, that fluoride is a toxic material, with potentially serious health implications.

It would seem that there are two totally contradictory opinions about the presence of fluoride in our toothpaste products and additional fluoride in our drinking water. The 'pro' lobby argues that it is essential for good dental health while the 'anti' lobby maintains that there is little documented or substantive evidence to show that the presence of fluoride reduces cavities. Much of the fluoride debate revolves round whether it is natural fluoride or artificial fluoride, i.e. the type the authorities add to our drinking water. It is the latter type that has the apparent health risks. They also argue that there is growing evidence to suggest that fluoride can cause damage to teeth, bones and soft tissue and can be linked to other health disorders. They also maintain that the 'pro' lobby never mentions that much of the fluoride absorbed by the body is not orally but through the skin when immersed in water.

Since 1997, in the USA, the FDA has apparently required that all toothpastes containing fluoride carry a poison label! In the same year, over 1,000 scientists at the US Environmental Protection Agency (EPA) declared that,

> Our review of the evidence including animal and human studies, indicates a causal link between fluoridation and cancer, genetic damage and neurological impairment.

Check out the study on the information and scientific evidence available on the National Pure Water Association (NPWA) website, http://www.npwa.freeserve.co.uk/.

Other information can be obtained from the Fluoride Exposure Group in the UK: tel +44 (0) 1455-828778.

Also, an internet search for 'fluoride' on any of the major search engines will show up the huge number of reports on the subject of fluoride in public drinking water. Try this out on one my favourite search engines, http://www.google.com.

I was staggered when I read some of the information – there is no question in my mind that we should all be very concerned at the prospect of any further pollution of our water sources and especially so when it is approved by government departments. There is also an increasing number of studies, from different parts of the world, that question the decisions of public health authorities throughout the world to continue to introduce fluoride into public drinking water. One should really ask the question – is good dental healthcare dependent on the presence of fluoride in toothpastes and other dental products, and if not is it necessary to have fluoride in any toothgel or toothpaste or additional fluoride in our drinking water? If it can be categorically proven that the presence of fluoride in toothcare products is critical to good dental hygiene and healthy teeth, then obviously we must have it in 'safe' levels. If it is not, then we have to rethink the whole fluoride policy.

The reason that I have included this reference to fluoride is to give readers an example of a potential toxin that we may all be consuming on a daily basis (at what levels we simply do not know). To maintain good health and well-being, we must ensure that we maintain a regular intake of natural detoxifiers, such as aloe vera. Aloe vera juice taken daily helps to detoxify the body and boost the immune system – countering the harmful actions of toxins and free radicals.

Anoosh Liddell, MISPA, ITEC – reflexologist and aromatherapist

Anoosh is a reflexologist and aromatherapist who has used aloe vera to help in the treatment of a number of ailments, disorders and diseases. Here she outlines four of her more interesting cases.

Fatigue and menopause

Fay was in her late forties when I first saw her and was experiencing the early stages of menopause. She had unbearable sweats accompanied by hot flushes that were so bad she had taken to going out into the garden at night in her nightgown and walking barefoot on the cold wet grass to cool off. Her GP had advised her to take hormone replacement therapy (HRT), which she did for a period of two months, but she was unhappy about taking HRT tablets as they raised her blood pressure and made her body bloated. She came to see me to find a natural way of alleviating her symptoms. I observed that she was overweight and had very dry body skin but oily face skin. Assessing her internal metabolism using reflexology techniques, I found that she suffered from an incomplete emptying of the bowel and kidneys. Her general state of health was good but her body felt 'clogged', hence she was fatigued and lethargic. I advised Fay to cut out drinking all tea and coffee and instead to drink two litres of still water per day and also four cups of dandelion herbal tea. This would start to flush out the kidneys and purify the blood and liver generally, and would also moisturise the body skin. Next I advised her to take aloe vera juice (fifty millilitres three times a day) and slippery elm powder (one teaspoon three times a day, mashed into half a banana) and also to take acidophilus and bifidus to enhance the friendly bacteria in her digestive system. This she had to do for three to ten days, eating nothing else except three portions of boiled rice (as little as possible).

The objective of the treatment was for her to have three soft bowel movements per day before introducing a normal healthy diet very slowly over a period of three weeks or so. I tested her on her first visit with a full body massage and used clary sage, geranium, lemon and sage pure essential oils. I prescribed a lotion of the same oils to apply to her lower back and abdomen each morning, and a blend of the same oils to use in the bath each night. One week later, when I saw her again, she said she had suffered all week with extreme headaches. This is a normal reaction of the body when it is going through a detoxification process. We continued working together and by the fourth week she felt wonderful. She has now been off HRT (her own choice and decision) for three weeks and has had only one mild hot flush. Her treatments are continuing and the progress she is making is extremely good. I have treated about six clients in this way and each one of them has shown wonderful results.

AIDS and HIV

Working with people with AIDS is a very hard thing to do as we in complementary health care always struggle to help alleviate the awful side effects of the powerful drugs that have to be used to keep opportunistic infection at bay. The main body systems that are affected by these drugs are the digestive system (which includes the whole alimentary canal, from the mouth to the stomach, liver, pancreas, intestines and bowel) and the urinary system (kidneys and bladder). Aloe vera juice taken each day (sixty millilitres three times a day or more) soothes and repairs the damage done to these internal organs, giving the person less constipation, stomach cramps and burning urination, and promoting healthier skin. Although by no means a cure, aloe vera, combined with total holistic aromatherapy, has proved to be extremely helpful in improving the quality of life for many of those suffering with HIV and AIDS.

Psoriasis

The first case of psoriasis I treated was a young child aged seven. Her psoriasis was mainly confined to severe scalp infliction and also bad itchy scabbing behind the ears.

Her mother had visited the doctor regularly for three months asking for help, as the child was scratching her scalp so often, causing bleeding, and she was scared of infection.

The usual shampoos and steroid creams were applied but there was little or no relief. I recommended a gentle change in the child's diet – slowly eliminating all dairy produce, convenience foods, white flour products, all fizzy drinks and pickled foods and all oranges and tomatoes. As psoriasis is related to the nutritional integrity of the skin, and as the health of the skin as a whole is dependent on the nutrients that reach it from the blood vessels in the body's connective tissue, aloe vera juice was the main ingredient I used to relieve the psoriasis. The nutritional value of aloe vera would in this case correct any increased body needs for certain nutrients that were not being supplied and possibly creating a deficiency, so resulting in psoriasis symptoms. I also prepared an oil blend containing jojoba, sweet almond, evening primrose, sesame seed and borage oils, together with essential oils of benzoin, bergamot, cajuput, neroli, birch and rose otto. These were to be massaged into the scalp and behind the ears each night, and then washed out with a mild vegetable-based shampoo the following morning. As a tonic after washing, I prescribed a few drops of a blend of essential oils (bergamot, carrot seed, german chamomile, eucalyptus and lavender) mixed in 100 millilitres of water in a plant sprayer, to be applied to the damp hair, making sure the scalp was well moistened. The child's hair tonic and aloe vera were continued for one week. Within two days all the scabs had lifted and come away, leaving behind soft new pink skin and no itching whatsoever. As the weeks passed the child continued to take aloe vera each day, but the need for the hair oiling and spraying grew less until it was done only once a week. After a year, the child was still totally free of psoriasis.

Eczema

I had been regularly treating older children and adults who had minor attacks of eczema from time to time, but had never seen such a bad case of eczema as that of a four-year-old child I treated. Almost her entire body was covered, and her arms and legs needed constant covering up to stop her scratching them, causing bleeding and the added risk of infection. Her mother was very concerned, as each time she went back to her doctor another stronger dose of cortisone cream was prescribed. I suggested that she bathe the child each day in spring water to which Dead Sea salt had been added, and thereafter she should apply pure aloe vera juice with a soft pastry brush all over her daughter's limbs and anywhere else where the eczema was apparent. Small sips of aloe vera juice were also given throughout the day, as well as wild blue-green algae. At first the eczema got worse and I recommended that she persevere as I felt confident that the condition would improve. It took six months before changes were noticed and, during this period, I also recommended a slow but drastic change of diet. The child's diet was particularly high in cow's milk, dairy products, sweet, sugary foods and drinks, and highly refined white flour products (all mentioned in Chapter 6), as being sources of allergies or intolerances and being nutritionally 'bankrupt'. Both the child and her mother suffered a great deal during this transitional period, but the results were, in the end, worth all the effort and pain.

Once the eczema had settled down and was only very mild, I made up a liquid blend of aloe vera juice and some key essential oils including geranium, german chamomile, juniper, sandalwood, lavender and myrrh, which was to be applied all over the body each night, after a bath. The change in the child's eczema was significant and I estimated it to be at least ninety per cent improved.

Patrick Holford – nutritionist

Nutritional broadcaster, author and the founder of the Institute for Optimum Nutrition, Patrick Holford is one of the UK's most prolific authors, speakers and broadcasters on the subject of health and nutrition and a tireless advocate of the need to emphasise the links between inadequate diet or poor nutrition and illnesses and diseases. One of his books entitled *Say No To Cancer* has had a significant and profound impact on me both because of my father's death and the fact that some close friends have also been afflicted by this 'scourge'.

Say No To Cancer (see Appendix 2) pulls no punches as to where Patrick Holford believes the blame lies:

> ...the single greatest cause of cancer – even greater than smoking – ...is the modern diet.

However he also believes that most people can reduce their risk of cancer by up to fifty per cent by improving their diet and taking the correct intake of nutritional supplements. The book, while obviously giving no health guarantees, is a simple and easy-to-read guide to adopting a more healthy regime, and parents should also take note for their children and read Chapter 6 very carefully.

Patrick's book details:

- ➢ How to assess and reduce your risk
- ➢ Which foods and what type of foods decrease risk and which foods increase risk
- ➢ How to reduce your exposure to cancer causing chemicals
- ➢ Why hormone related cancers are on the increase
- ➢ How to beat prostate and breast cancer
- ➢ How to fight cancer with nutritional medicine
- ➢ A prevention programme and nutritional support for each type of cancer

His views and opinions are those of someone who has witnessed significant changes over the last twenty years as to what constitutes the average diet in the UK and many other so-called developed countries. My personal view is that we need to remain open minded enough to listen to the arguments and observations of those who, like Patrick, fully understand both the positive and negative ways in which diet can impact on our health. We would also begin to reject the 'stranglehold' that large food conglomerates, manufacturers, retailers and fast food outlets have exerted on the national diet, nutritional levels and ultimately our own health, that of our children and the health of the nation as a whole. I believe if more of us exerted more pressure through 'voting with our wallets', we would soon be a much healthier nation.

Let me pose some questions for you:

- what if through improved diet and nutrition, the incidence of cancers and other serious and often fatal diseases was significantly decreased and the requirement and demand for expensive medications and treatments was reduced as a result?
- what if natural products like aloe vera, honey, etc. were found to have such significant healing properties and benefits that people's health, life expectancy and quality of life could be significantly improved, and what if these natural products could even replace many common medications?
- do you think that the large global pharmaceutical conglomerates would be prepared to accept this reduction in their business, profits, influence and control?

Venetia Armitage, DTH, nutritionist

Venetia is a registered nutritionist who has been taking aloe vera herself and recommending it to her patients, mostly as a general health drink tonic, for about eight years. Several years ago, she was introduced to a more potent aloe vera gel drinking juice and very quickly realised the significant difference in the quality and content of its active ingredient. She soon recognised the positive impact that the new product could have on her patients and she began giving it to them in a more potent yet natural form.

She describes here how she uses it:

> For their initial consultation I usually suggest that my patients take aloe vera along with a cleansing, high-vitality diet. The aloe vera drinking juice

soothes and heals the gut, encouraging good bacteria and rehydrating the system. Although the body will always try to heal itself, without good tissue and sufficient fluid it is difficult and, in some cases well nigh impossible, to achieve any significant results. With its powerful moisturising abilities, aloe vera is able to keep the body well moisturised so that healing can begin. Once the body is cleansed and re-hydrated it can better utilise vitamins and minerals from food and nutritional supplements.

As the majority of my patients have digestive problems and some are very debilitated, aloe vera is invaluable for relieving pain and discomfort and easing the painful spasms caused by problems like IBS, a debilitating condition that is becoming increasingly common in today's stressful society. Many IBS sufferers swear by their daily dose of aloe vera and in some cases they are eventually able to dispense with their medication. I use aloe vera with the utmost confidence, having seen it change the lives of many of my patients who have benefited so much.

Medical herbalism

It is really only in the last twenty-five years that there has been something of a European 'renaissance' in herbal medicine and practice. However, there still seem to be numerous, influential, vested interest lobbies who are determined to ensure that legislation will make it either very expensive or illegal to practice without formal certification or the payment of expensive licences for each so-called herbal medicine. I will leave it to the reader to determine what sort of companies could be behind the ongoing lobbying – especially in Europe – for such legislation.

Could it be those companies who are involved in the manufacture of expensive pharmaceuticals and the financial institutions that back them who view the growth of herbal medicine as a possible long-term erosion of both their monopolistic positions and the huge financial returns they enjoy?

Herbal medicines cannot be patented and are making a comeback for two main reasons. Firstly, more and more people around the world, both therapists and the general public alike (especially those in the more affluent, developed countries), are realising that pharmaceuticals and synthetic medications do not hold all the answers to diseases and illness. Secondly, herbal medicines and natural healing plants and products, e.g. honey, which have long track records of healing (in some cases like aloe vera – dating back thousands of years) can have a significant role to play in both the prevention and management of numerous disorders and diseases. Again aloe vera and honey cannot be patented.

Andrew Chevalier, MNIMH – medical herbalist

Andrew Chevalier is an experienced medical herbalist and a leading figure in the field of herbal medicine. He is both a leading author and a commentator on herbal medicine. He is a past president of the National Institute of Medical Herbalists and chair of the Council of Complementary and Alternative Medicine. He was also responsible for pioneering the development of the first ever degree course in herbal medicine at Middlesex University. His book, *The Encyclopaedia of Medicinal Plants* (see Appendix 2) is the most fully illustrated, comprehensive and practical reference guide to over 500 key herbs and their medicinal uses available today.

One of the most interesting general points he makes relates to how conventional medicine established an almost monopolistic control of medical practice throughout Europe by the end of the nineteenth century. This led to herbal medicine becoming illegal in many major European countries and herbal practitioners being persecuted and even imprisoned if they did not have official medical certification.

KEY POINT
His book is an essential item of reading for anyone who wants to know about the history of herbal medicine, its role, continuing development and influence in the different countries of the world.

He also explains how and why it is now experiencing such a huge 'renaissance' (in Europe and the USA) and, most importantly, he lists details of the 550-plus different herbal medicines featured and how best they can be used and for what sorts of ailments, illnesses and disorders.

KEY POINT
In particular, the references in the book to aloe vera and its properties, uses and benefits help define the important role that this plant has had in herbal medicine over the centuries.

The development of Ayurvedic medicine in India dates back over 5,000 years and comes from two words – 'ayur' meaning 'life' and 'veda' meaning 'knowledge' or 'science'.

KEY POINT
Aloe vera has been an integral part of the herbal remedies associated with the ancient practice of ayurveda, which, to this day, remains one of the most widely practised and accepted systems of healing in and around India (where one fifth of the world's current population lives!). It is also gaining broader acceptance in the so-called developed world.

Aloe vera also figures prominently in Chinese herbal medicine, so its importance as a healer and restorative tonic cannot really be questioned.

KEY TIP
'Extensive research in the USA and Russia, since the 1930s, has shown that the inner gel of an aloe vera leaf has a dramatic and effective ability to heal wounds, ulcers and burns, putting a natural protective coating on the area and speeding up the rate of healing and reducing the risk of infection. This action being due in part to the presence of aloectin B, which stimulates the immune system.'

In the 1950s, further research confirmed its ability to heal burns and it was also found to be a highly effective treatment for radiation burns. Chevalier quotes:

KEY TIP
'The aloe vera gel is an excellent first-aid remedy to keep in the home for such skin disorders such as eczema, minor burns and wounds, grazes, scalds, sunburn, rashes, minor bites, stings and swellings.'

KEY TIP
'Internally, it has been found to ease the discomfort and pain of internal disorders such as IBS and peptic ulcers.'

Aloe vera gel can even assist in the treatment and eradication of viral infections like warts.

KEY TIP
'Pregnant women who suffer with stretch marks have found that the elasticity of the skin can be improved by rubbing in a topical aloe vera gel.'

KEY TIP
'Also people suffering from varicose veins have found the application of a topical aloe vera gel to be helpful.'

Penelope Ody, NIMH – medical herbalist

Penelope Ody is another author, commentator and lecturer on herbal medicine who has had several books published, including *100 Great Natural Remedies* (see Appendix 2). In this book she mentions aloe vera's wide ranging properties and benefits, specifically those related to digestion, skin disorders and wounds.

KEY POINT
She also refers to its place in Ayurvedic medicine as a restorative tonic when taken internally and as an increasingly popular ingredient in skin creams and cosmetics. Aloe vera can also be used to help with disorders like eczema and fungal infections such as thrush and ringworm.

She also confirms its usefulness as a convenient household first-aid 'tool' for minor burns, wounds, insect stings and bites and inflammation.

KEY POINT
Other disorders for which she mentions the use of aloe vera include: circulatory problems and chilblains; skin problems such as eczema, acne and psoriasis and nappy rash in babies.

Rosemary Titterington, MIHort

Rosemary Titterington is the founder and owner of Iden Croft Herbs in Kent, an internationally renowned centre for aromatic and medicinal herbs. She comments on the benefits she has found from using various products containing aloe vera below.

> For many years I have used, and recommended to others, the natural juice of the aloe vera plant. It has proved invaluable when used in the home, as a leaf can be removed and the juice used for first-aid on burns, blisters, skin irritations and insect bites. However, it is not the most convenient plant to take in your luggage when travelling!
>
> I was thus delighted to find a source of the highest quality aloe vera, with the added convenience of being packaged to protect the integrity of the product. Pure 'aloe vera juice in a tub' was a huge improvement in terms of no longer having to cut and prepare the leaf.

Burns

KEY TIP
'From my own experience and from verbal reports from our customers I have found that topical aloe vera gelly is good for burns, providing good, quick first-aid on clean, cooled skin (I apply running cold water first to reduce the heat), and for treating blisters from burns.'

My daughter burned her foot on a hot water bottle, and a dressing of aloe vera beneath a 'ring pad', for protection, prevented the huge blister from bursting, reduced the swelling and the wound healed without a scar.

KEY TIP
'I have used or recommended aloe vera for eczema, dry skin (particularly for older ladies), sunburn, insect bites, heat rash, nettle rash, and so on. It is extremely soothing and also reduces itching.'

Itchy scalp

KEY TIP
'Some customers have found aloe vera jojoba shampoo very useful for dry, itchy scalp conditions, psoriasis and so on, and generally useful with sensitive skin and dry hair. Aloe vera lip balm is also very good for dry lips caused by wind and weather.'

I have also recommended to a group of people with Parkinson's disease that they tried drinking the aloe vera juice, and the feedback has been very promising. I know that some of the Parkinsonians are still using it, and some of the carers have also found it beneficial for them – it seems to help to reduce the problems caused by tension.

Cystitis and acne

One of my clients was having a bad attack of cystitis. She was under a lot of stress and was drinking lots of coffee to keep her going. After a week of drinking aloe vera gel twice a day her symptoms had gone. She also applied aloe vera gelly topically whenever she visited the bathroom, which she said gave immediate relief locally. However, she noticed that the tube wasn't going to last very long and remarked on it to her sixteen-year-old daughter, who admitted that she was using it on her acne, which covered her face, upper chest, upper back and shoulders. More tubes were acquired and they too were used quickly. It transpired that her brother was using it for his acne, too! The good news was that within a matter of only six weeks they didn't have a spot between them!

Dr Timothy E Moore, DDS/MS, PC

The following information relating to Dr Moore was extracted from the IASC website at www.iasc.org, email iasc1@email.msn.com. See Appendix 1.4 and 1.5 for full details on the IASC. In his paper entitled 'Aloe vera: its potential use in wound healing and disease control in oral conditions',

Dr Moore describes his experience using aloe vera over the last fourteen years. He states that aloe vera has been shown to enhance defence mechanisms and it has a variety of components to help combat periodontal disease and other oral conditions. As a periodontist utilising aloe vera in various consistencies and with over 6,000 documented patients who have been treated with applications, he has observed remarkable healing, reduced edema and pain control.

There are seven main uses of aloe vera in dental practice:

- applications directly to the sites of periodontal surgery
- applications to the gum tissues when they have been traumatised or scratched by toothbrush-dentifrice abrasion, sharp foods, dental floss or toothpick injuries

- extraction sites respond more comfortably and dry sockets do not develop when aloe vera is applied
- acute mouth lesions are improved by direct application on herpetic viral lesions, aphthous ulcers, canker sores and cracks occurring at the corners of the lips. Gum abscesses are soothed by the applications as well
- other oral diseases that are chronic in nature respond. Gum problems experienced by sufferers of AIDS and leukaemia can be relieved
- denture patients with sore ridges and ill-fitting dentures and partials can benefit as fungal and bacterial contamination are reduced, as are the inflammatory irritations
- aloe vera can also be used around dental implants to control inflammation from bacterial infection

Other oral disorders such as candidiasis, desquamative gingivitis, vesiculobullous diseases, acute monocytic leukaemia, haematological disorders and nutritional problems all respond to the use of aloe vera. There is a gathering momentum for products like aloe vera across the USA as researchers become more interested in alternative therapy utilising natural products versus synthetic agents. Aloe vera research is currently being undertaken at Oklahoma University and Baylor University. Dr Moore also refers to the use of aloe vera in the tragic bomb disaster in Oklahoma City in 1995. Many bomb victims were treated with aloe vera and the attendants, the doctors and especially the injured themselves learned that the healing capabilities of aloe vera far exceeded their expectations in terms of pain control and healing-time reduction. He concludes by saying that he believes that aloe vera has an unlimited future in new applications and that he feels that in dentistry, the profession is just on the cutting edge of 'promising utilisation for anti-inflammatory procedure, antiviral and immunological benefits for patients'.

Michael Peuser – Aloe – Empress of the Welfare Plants

Michael Peuser is German by birth and has lived in Brazil for over twenty years. He worked with a large European group and was sent to Brazil on assignment in the 1980s. During his time in Brazil, Peuser has become more involved with natural, plant-based medicines, including aloe vera. In his book, *Aloe – Empress of the Welfare Plants*, Michael Peuser talks about the long history of aloe vera (over 4,000 years) and its use in over fifty double-blind studies since the 1930s. He talks of over sixty diseases where aloe vera can be used alongside conventional medication (as what he calls an 'accompaniment') to help the healing process. He focuses particularly on the use of aloe vera in those suffering from certain types of cancer. This is obviously an extremely contentious and emotive subject and we have included reference to him and his book within our publication in order to ensure that our readers are fully aware of what other authors of books on aloe vera are referring to in their writings.

In 2002, Michael Peuser was interviewed on mainstream television in Germany – in a programme called *Fliege die Talkshow* – a popular TV programme that focuses on natural medicines. He mentioned the case of his father-in-law, in Brazil, who had terminal prostate cancer and was at home on his deathbed. The doctors who had operated on and treated him, but to no avail, had prescribed morphine to ease the pain of the cancer in his last few days. Coincidentally, at about this time, his wife had read about a Franciscan monk in Brazil called Romano Zago, who had written about a particular elixir made from aloe vera, pure natural honey and sugar cane spirit. This 'potion' was reputed to have powerful healing and health-giving properties (similar in many ways to the drink that the Knights Templar used to fortify themselves many centuries before, called the 'elixir of Jerusalem'). Zago had also spent some time working with pilgrims at the Church of the Holy Sepulchre in the Holy Land, so it is quite possible that he came across information on the uses of aloe vera in the treatment of illnesses, diseases and disorders when he was in the Middle East. She felt that they had nothing to lose and so decided to prepare the recipe and gave it to her husband four times per day. Within a few days the lesions on his body from the bedsores started to heal and the pain from the cancer subsided. He started putting on weight and his bowel movements improved. He did however die four months later – not from cancer but from influenza – there was a flu epidemic in Brazil.

On the face of it this would seem to be something of a miracle, and let us not forget miracles can and do happen and that the medical fraternity does not always have an answer for such phenomena! I can just hear the 'guffaws' and 'laughter' from all the sceptics out there. I would however err on the side of caution and consider whether this particular 'elixir' could have significant healing properties. Just think about it: aloe vera has a track record of healing dating back over 4,000 years, pure honey also has potent healing and curative properties and pure cane alcohol also has therapeutic properties.

Peuser, who himself has a scientific background, was understandably slightly bewildered by and a little sceptical of what he saw as something of a miracle. He decided to do some research for himself. He read many books and accessed countless research papers and scientific trials and also advertised in Brazil for anyone who had themselves experienced the healing benefits of aloe vera. He was excited by the response and on closer examination of all the respondents, and from his own research, he concluded that most of the illnesses where aloe vera, whether taken internally or topically on the skin, seems to be most effective in its action is where there is capillary constriction (he stated on the TV programme that the human body has about 150,000 kilometres of capillaries), which can often cause serious medical problems. Aloe vera helps to open the capillaries and thus increase blood flow around the body, transporting all the healing nutrients, vitamins and other substances to the required areas.

Peuser is convinced of the 'curative' and therapeutic properties of orally administered aloe vera juice in relation to various cancers and many other serious diseases and illnesses.

Details of the recipe for the 'elixir' to which Michael Peuser refers and copies of the videotape of the interview with Michael Peuser on the German television programme (with English language dubbing) are available from the Aloe Vera Centre (see Appendix 1.1).

Adrian Blake – complementary therapist

Adrian Blake has been involved in complementary medicine for many years, and in the following subsections describes two of his most interesting cases involving aloe vera and its benefits.

Stomach pains

> Jenny was a housewife in her late forties who came to us for homoeopathic counselling. For twelve years she had been going to see her GP, complaining of pains in her stomach, but although numerous tests were done, nothing could be found. She was admitted to hospital for further investigation. On opening up the abdomen and examining the internal organs there appeared to be haemorrhaging from various sites but no cause could be found, so as a routine precaution, the appendix was removed. Unfortunately, two months later, the pains in her stomach recurred and she went back to her GP who again referred her to the hospital. This time it was decided to remove her spleen. For the next eighteen months she made various trips to her GP and back into theatre for exploratory operations, and also had her gall bladder removed. Each time the haemorrhaging improved temporarily and then returned six to eight weeks later. It was therefore as a last resort that she came to us for help. We looked at Jenny's case history and decided that there had been so much shock and trauma that she needed a remedy to

restore the balance. She seemed to be quite poorly nourished, had trouble absorbing and digesting many foods and her appetite was poor.

We decided to use aloe vera juice as a way of healing the internal organs in her body as much as possible with the micro-nutrients that are contained in aloe vera. The juice would also increase the life force and energy of her internal organs. Initially we started her off with as much aloe vera as she could tolerate without causing a loose bowel. On some days she would consume over 200 millilitres of stabilised aloe vera gel, taking small amounts throughout the day. After a few days she reported that her bowel movements were much more regular and over the next couple of weeks her appetite improved. Within a month she seemed to be a much brighter, stronger and an altogether more centred person. She continued with the treatment for the next three months, during which time neither the pains nor the haemorrhaging recurred. We can only assume that she was able to absorb the nutrients and take the healing from the aloe vera and therefore restore her body to normal. She is now capable of absorbing and digesting nutrients from everyday foods and is naturally very pleased not to have return to her GP or to hospital for further exploratory operations.

Ulcerated colon and other problems

The second case concerns Gerry, a fitness fanatic aged thirty-eight, who used to weight-train several times a week. Unfortunately his problem appeared to be the result of over-exercise! He had exercised his abdomen so much that it seemed to have gone into spasm. This had left him bedridden for a couple of weeks and unable to do any exercise. Unfortunately, while this was happening – while his abdomen was in spasm – the colon became underactive. So normal viruses, parasites and bacteria that would routinely be eliminated by daily bowel movements began to build up and he experienced extreme pain and discomfort every time he tried to have a bowel movement. This situation continued and it soon became extremely ulcerated. He also discovered that he could not pass anything that was at all abrasive without experiencing pain. After about a week bleeding ensued and the combination of this, the ulceration and spasms continued for several more weeks. He then went to his GP who gave him some painkillers, told him to rest and indicated it would heal up in a few days. The problem continued for the next month and there was no evidence of any healing. Gerry came to us in desperation for homeopathic counselling. As soon as we saw his condition we knew something needed to be done quickly to alleviate the widespread inflammation and pain in the abdominal area.

KEY TIP
We put him on aloe vera gel drinking juice immediately to reduce both the inflammation and the pain and to help heal the ulceration and thus stop the haemorrhaging. He initially started on a few tablespoons and found that it was very soothing, allowing him to have a bowel movement more freely and without as much pain. Within two weeks the haemorrhaging stopped.

He tried increasing the dosage slightly over the next few weeks and found that he was again able to tolerate the foods that had previously given him so many problems. Gerry had also become slightly anaemic and lethargic because of his experiences. However, over the next few months he found that, apart from healing his abdominal problems, the aloe vera was acting like a tonic on the rest of his system.

KEY TIP
'Aloe vera is what we call a universal healer and acts at a cellular level to help heal and regenerate healthy tissue.'

Gerry was able to resume his gym activities within a few months, stronger and fitter than he had been before the problem began. This is a fine example of the way in which a high quality aloe vera drinking gel or juice can work, not only to heal a specific internal disorder and tissue damage, but also to work right through the body as a health-giving and healing tonic.

Sports-related problems and injuries

Although in the USA aloe vera products have been used extensively for nearly two decades to help with a wide range of sports-related injuries, there has yet to be the same widespread acceptance of these products and their benefits among UK sports therapists. Alan Watson, the founder of the Bimal Clinic in London (see his comments earlier in this chapter), is a staunch advocate of the potent healing powers of a particular proprietary aloe vera heat cream.

Sports injury practitioners, physiotherapists and other specialists, in whatever country they practice, should consider the reasons why he feels aloe vera can make such a powerful contribution to the healing regime at the Bimal Clinic.

Increased professionalism and massive investments in more and more sports and sports stars will mean that therapists in the UK, Europe, the USA and elsewhere will be under increasing pressure to find new ways to accelerate the healing and rehabilitation process and get injured athletes and players back into action more quickly. Any professional sports club's major assets are its players, and if they are not playing regularly because of injury they can quickly become a serious and expensive liability. They are generally a club's most expensive asset and inactivity could have serious financial repercussions for both club and player alike. Even if she or he is an independent sports competitor, inaction through prolonged injury means no competition income. Sports therapists will be facing major challenges to reduce the healing cycle and thus help sports people get back to 'work'.

Edward L Clarry, MFPhys

Edward Clarry specialises in sports injury treatment and exercise physiology. By chance he read an advertisement for aloe vera juice, which recommended its use in sports medicine. He began to use it in his clinic, with some remarkable results. In the following subsections he describes two cases he has treated successfully using aloe vera products.

Bleeding muscle

> Robert was a twenty-seven-year-old American footballer. He had a massive contact haematoma (bleeding within the muscle) of the left thigh that extended to the ankle, an infected astroturf burn over the left knee and inflammation and grazing to the right shin. He came into the clinic supported on two crutches and could not straighten or bend his leg.
>
> The injury was one week old and x-rays had confirmed that there was no fracture. The hospital had advised rest. Normally I would expect this type of injury to take between six and ten weeks to heal. I used ultrasound with aloe vera gel for five minutes, and an aloe compression wrap with intermittent compression for twenty-five minutes, and advised him to take aloe vera juice (thirty millilitres four times per day). I also prescribed some remedial exercise. After the first treatment he was able to straighten his leg and walk without crutches. Three days after the second treatment the bruising was clear over the treated area and the astroturf burn infection was healing. He

played American football in the third week. After just four weeks and the fifth treatment, the injury was completely healed, as was the astroturf burn.

I was particularly pleased with this result. Direct impact injuries of this kind can be complicated. If immediate treatment is inadequate, deep located intra-muscular bleeding may gradually become calcified, which can lead to myositis ossification, a lengthy inflammatory process that normally requires treatment over a long period of time or the surgical removal of the ossification. The aloe vera sports spray healed the astroturf burn in a fraction of the time normally expected. With this type of burn due to secondary infection, it is quite common for the injury to last all season.

KEY TIP
I have never seen a single case of secondary infection when the aloe spray has been used in first-aid treatment, and the burns normally heal within a few days. When the injury has been infected due to lack of adequate first-aid care, it has healed in one or two weeks after treatment with the spray.

Fractured foot and ankle

The second case was Helen, a secretary in her thirties, who had not worked for two years due to a domestic injury. She had fallen from a stepladder and had fractured her foot and ankle. She had undergone surgery, during which a steel plate and steel pins had been inserted, followed by physiotherapy at the hospital. After two years Helen could not move her foot, ankle or toes and was suffering from extreme pain when walking. The foot and ankle were swollen, discoloured and inflamed. She had not worn normal shoes for two years and needed a stick for support. Her foot was very sensitive to the touch, indicating nerve irritation or pressure. I applied an aloe compression wrap with intermittent compression (twenty-five minutes for each treatment), aloe massage lotion and aloe sports spray after the foot became less painful to the touch.

KEY TIP
I also recommended that she drank thirty millilitres of aloe vera juice three times a day as an anti-inflammatory and that she applied the aloe vera compression wraps when she went to bed at night. It was also important that she tried to exercise her foot and ankle as her condition improved, so I gave her a progressive routine to follow.

There was an improvement in the swelling and soreness after the very first treatment, with a progressive improvement after each subsequent treatment. In just three weeks and after six treatments the pain, tenderness and swelling had reduced considerably, with the shape of the ankle reappearing. The dark brown discoloration had changed to pink and I was able to apply pressure in massage. Limited movement returned in her foot, toes and ankle. The limitation was due to calcification – not surprising after two years' lack of treatment. At four weeks she was walking without sticks and has now bought new shoes after two years. She informed me that the orthopaedic consultant had stated that he had not expected her to regain so much movement and advised her to keep on with her treatment. My patients are now recommending aloe vera to their families and friends. They are claiming some incredible improvements in overall well-being, performance, energy, niggling ailments clearing up, improvements in arthritic conditions and skin problems.

KEY TIP
They also report some 'unbelievable' improvements in conditions such as IBS, colitis and ME.

Use of aloe vera on sports injuries and related problems

Aloe wraps are very effective for knee and ankle injuries as part of a compression programme. Aloe ice-block massage after applying heat packs gives good results as part of a hot and cold treatment. Aloe vera products are now an essential part of my changing-room and field first-aid kit.

KEY TIP
I have found that aloe massage lotion, when massaged into the cervical, thoracic and lumbar spine regions, can be very useful in relieving the symptoms of back pain. This is especially so when the aloe sports spray is used as part of the massage programme or as part of ultrasound or interferential treatment and also as a part of a self-treatment programme.

I now believe that many athletes and players of a wide range of different sports in the UK and other countries, as well as an increasing number of therapists, are beginning to realise the incredible healing powers of high quality aloe vera products.

Can all of these health professionals be wrong?

Although traditional medicine does not hold all the answers and solutions to the many disorders listed and described, many doctors may still, I am sure, cast a wary eye over what they have read in this book and in this chapter in particular. They may even be highly sceptical of the opinions of the various health professionals mentioned. However, what I would like to suggest is that all of those involved in allopathic medicine take a more positive view and ask themselves these questions:

What if Dr Myskja is right?
What if Dr Fischbach is right?
What if Dr Danhof is right?
What if Dr Henderson is right?
What if Dr Timothy Moore is right?
What if Dr Atherton is right?
What if David Urch is right?
What if Alan Watson is right?
What if Patrick Holford is right?
What if all the people mentioned in this chapter are right?

All the people mentioned in this chapter are independent health professionals and authors with recognised qualifications, who have one thing in common. That is, they were either already involved in complementary therapies and products or they were open minded enough to consider that there was an alternative or complementary approach to allopathic or conventional and traditional medical practice and medicines.

For those who were already in the herbal-alternative-complementary 'camp', they were also prepared to consider aloe vera as an integral part of their treatment and therapy programme and/or they wrote of its important properties, benefits and uses in their various books and publications.

They all share the same opinion about the role and importance of aloe vera and have now introduced it into the various clinical practices and health regimes they are involved in.

KEY POINT
They all believe aloe vera can play a significant and important role in the treatment, healing and ongoing management, or in some cases the prevention, of numerous ailments, disorders and diseases – even in some chronic cases.

Aloe vera, provided it is administered correctly in the form of a high quality product or products, with guaranteed quality, purity, efficacy and potency, either topically or internally, is an important complementary therapy that does not tend to contra-indicate with medications, and in some cases can actually enhance their effects and benefits. If anyone reading this chapter has any doubts, I would suggest that initially they email me at the Aloe Vera Centre on:

alasdairaloevera@aol.com

5

What aloe vera can do for you

Case histories: the people have their say

THIS CHAPTER more than any other – apart from perhaps the one on animals – is the one that will probably help you decide whether or not aloe vera is something that you feel could help you, someone in your family or someone you know. I have tried to include case histories and examples covering as broad a spectrum of diseases, ailments, disorders and injuries as was practically possible.

This chapter is based on the personal experiences of the many people who have found that aloe vera has played an important role in helping alleviate pain or other symptoms or has helped treat and manage the ailment, disorder or condition from which they have been suffering. We are not suggesting for one moment that anyone with any sort of medical condition or problem should stop taking their prescribed medication. We would, of course, advise against adopting any such course of action. We are simply reporting the experiences, observations and comments of those people who have found aloe vera to be helpful.

> KEY TIP
> In some instances, they have found that by using aloe vera (either internally, topically or both), it has significantly improved their condition so that they no longer suffer to the same degree, and that, because the condition is more under control, their quality of life is dramatically improved.

The positive impact such events can have on families can be life-changing. Just imagine if your wife, husband or child had been suffering for years with Crohn's disease, chronic IBS or arthritis and the use of aloe vera had substantially improved their condition. Just imagine if one of your children had been suffering with chronic eczema or asthma and the use of aloe vera had substantially improved their condition. How would you feel? Elated no doubt and wanting to share your experiences with other people.

We have witnessed scores if not hundreds of examples like these where people (some of whom had suffered for years with little hope of any improvement in their condition) have benefited to such an extent that both their own and their family's quality of life has improved dramatically – as a direct result of taking aloe vera.

It is important to stress before people read this chapter that aloe vera should never be regarded as some form of 'cure all' or universal 'panacea'. The following accounts have been selected from hundreds of letters and other communications we have received here at the Aloe Vera Centre and from people we have met in the last few years. Some of the names have been changed to ensure the privacy of the people concerned.

Bronte: third degree burns

Carrie tells the shocking story of when her young daughter was badly burnt.

> Six years ago, in 1997, our family was devastated when our two-year-old daughter was burnt after her clothes caught fire from an open gas flame. The burns were extensive, covering fourteen per cent of her body, mainly on the insides of both legs, her thighs and stomach. We were ambulanced to Warwick Hospital, where she was assessed and then sent to the special burns unit at Selly Oak Hospital in Birmingham.
>
> At the time, the treatment for full thickness or third degree burns was to prick the large blisters that had quickly formed and give her morphine and antibiotics and place her on a saline drip. The skin was left exposed and she was placed in a high dependency room for several days under a large drying unit that beamed hot air all over her skin. The skin graft process began after several days and once the burns were finally covered and bandaged, the healing process began.
>
> We were a family that ate a wholefood, mainly organic diet, with a strong belief in homeopathic and herbal remedies and were committed to

Aloe Vera – Nature's Silent Healer

The Body Map Index

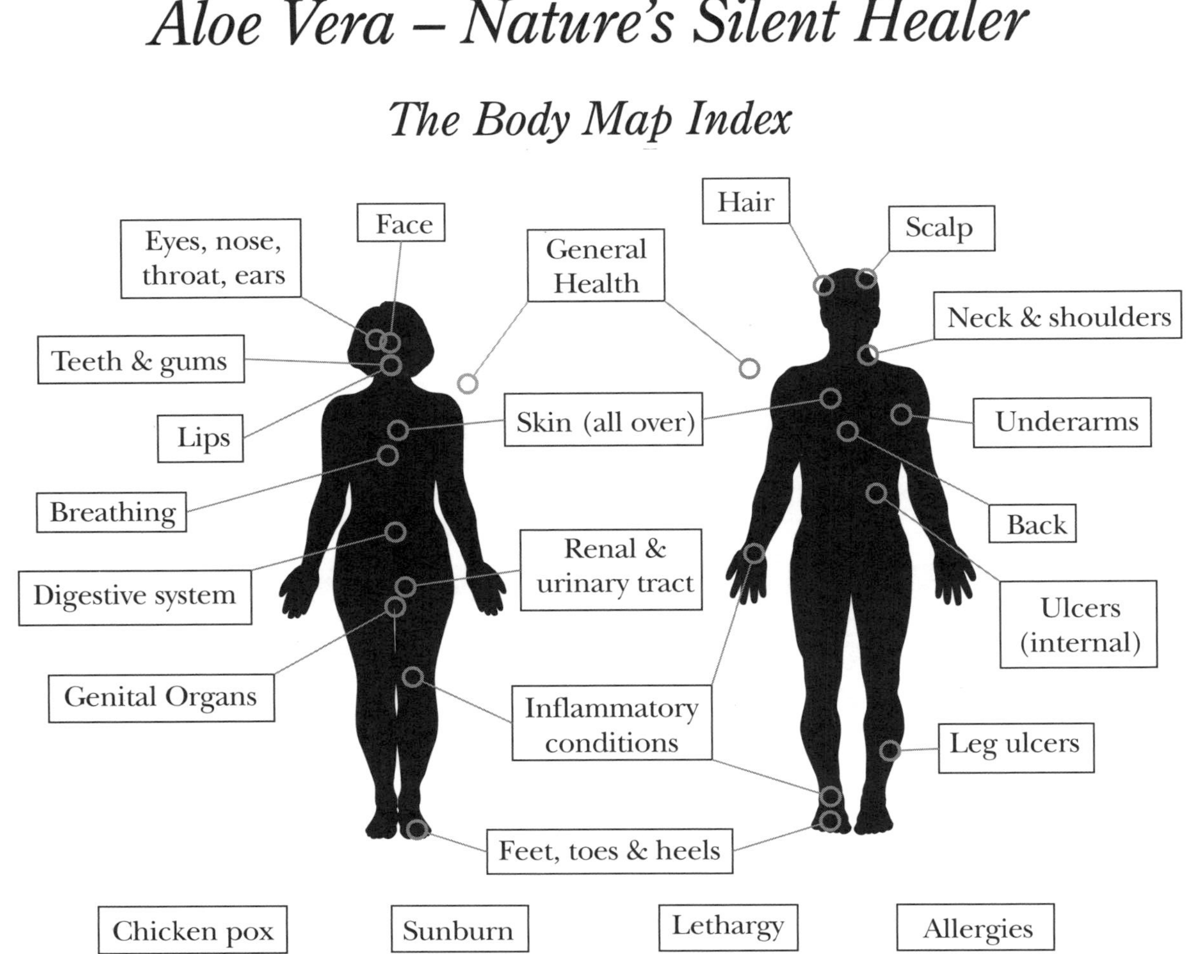

complementary therapies. Even as an ex-nurse, I was horrified to see the amount of drugs that were being used to sedate our tiny daughter and keep her free from infections, to say nothing of the blood packs that she required each time she had a new skin graft (five in all).

The consultants and staff would not let us apply any topical products to aid the healing process, so I decided to take the initiative and contacted friends in the complementary health business. Several of them mentioned an aloe vera gel drinking juice, something she could drink rather than apply. My husband had used this particular product before to help with an inflamed joint problem, so we were able to obtain some immediately, and began to add the gel to our daughter's fruit juice, two or three times a day. We then had a period of some four weeks where the burn sites were dressed and bandaged, the outer bandages being changed every couple of days. We continued with the aloe vera drink.

At the first bandage removal, some thirty-one to forty-five days after the initial incident, we were told that our daughter would probably need to be sedated with ketamine to make removal of the complete dressing feasible. The sites would be very sore, sticky and extremely painful. The innermost dressing would have adhered to the sticky exudate and be very difficult to remove. We prepared ourselves for the worst. As a family who had never even used Calpol before this event, I was loath to allow the doctors to administer ketamine. The outer bandages were removed and as my daughter stood up to back away from this latest intrusion to her body, the inner bandages slipped down her legs revealing dry, pink, smooth scar tissue. There was no pain!

The atmosphere in that room was amazing – you could have cut it with a knife! The registrar was called, followed by the consultant, then another consultant. No one could believe that my daughter's third degree burns followed by numerous skin grafts could have healed so quickly.

'How have you done this?' we were asked incredulously. Of course we were still shocked at the fact that our daughter was scarred.

Being involved with a burns patient is a slow dawning of realisation that this is something that we will live with forever, but I have to say that we were delighted with the reaction from the staff and we knew that something unusual and totally unexpected had occurred.

My answer to their question was: 'An aloe vera gel drinking juice!' The looks that then passed between the nurses spoke volumes. 'No, seriously,' I said. 'We have been giving her two or three fluid ounces every day. Now the bandages are off, can we put it on her skin too?'

Normally at this stage the burn site would be re-dressed and re-bandaged for a further examination in two weeks, but we were able to leave the site uncovered and begin topical application of an aloe vera gelly immediately, followed by early pressure garment fittings. Two weeks later the graft sites had almost completely recovered, with very little pain and virtually no itching. No infections occurred and no drugs were required to help with her recovery. It must be said that we were delighted and the staff bewildered by what had happened. For a patient not to have secondary infections following a burn of such magnitude was almost unheard of.

Six years on, we still apply aloe vera every day. We now use a proprietary aloe vera cream with bee propolis – a natural antibiotic – which has helped give the scar tissue a soft elasticity and has reduced the colour.

Bronte's case history was the subject of a presentation in May 2002 by her mother Carrie, to the thirty-fifth Annual British Burns Conference in Birmingham – attended by over 250 delegates from leading burns centres from all over the world.

We are extremely grateful for the opportunity to share Bronte's story with our readers and wish to thank Bronte, Carrie and Michael for allowing us to do this and to use the photographs (see Colour Plates numbers 5, 6, 7, 8). We hope that Bronte's story will give hope to other burns patients around the world.

Should you wish to contact Carrie Holmes, please refer to Appendix 1.7.

Sarah: Crohn's disease

In the summer of 1989, when Sarah was twenty-nine, she developed eyeritis in both eyes, causing blurred vision and a sensitivity to light. She then suffered with chronic diarrhoea, abdominal pains and had painful ulcerations on her tongue and in her mouth. As a young mother with three children – the youngest was only two – Sarah was physically and emotionally drained by her worsening health. After consulting two GPs, Sarah was finally admitted to hospital for tests. There followed a series of different tests including barium meals, a barium enema, x-rays and an endoscopy. All the tests confirmed that Sarah had ulcerative colitis and Crohn's disease. She was immediately hospitalised for five weeks and tube fed with Pepti 2000 (eight bottles every twenty-four hours). Although her bowel condition improved, she was suffering from chronic anaemia and had to undergo blood top-ups to stabilise her condition.

By March of 1990, her weight had dropped from 112 lbs (51 kgs) to 70 lbs (32 kgs), her haemoglobin had dropped to six (it is now twelve to thirteen), she had thrush and ulcers in her mouth and in her bowel, and she nearly died. When she came out of hospital, she was bedridden and had to have a private nurse for two months. The following year, in August 1991, she had another Crohn's attack and had to have two blood transfusions.

For the next five years she suffered constant flare-ups and was being treated with steroids, and so also developed osteoporosis in her joints and spine as a result of that treatment. She was however determined to avoid having a colostomy bag fitted and continued with her medications, including steroids (at one point she was taking nearly thirty tablets per day, which included forty milligrams of steroids). In 1996, her new consultant suggested that she come off steroids and start on a programme of '6 Mercaptopurine'. She also took salazapyrin as an anti-spasmodic medication and iron tablets.

In 2001 she was introduced to an aloe vera gel drinking juice and since then her life has changed dramatically. Within only one month she started feeling significantly better than she had done for the previous twelve years. Her energy levels increased and the pain she had suffered almost constantly for over a decade was receding. After only fifteen months on aloe vera, she is a completely changed person. The pain and the spasms, the bloating and the diarrhoea and constipation have gone and her latest bone density scan has revealed an improvement in her osteoporosis condition.

Although she still has to have a blood test every three months, because of the medication she is on (immune suppressants), she feels she is now able to lead a more or less normal life, but with a dramatically improved lifestyle. She can now go out without having to worry constantly about where the nearest loo is! She takes her regular medication, alongside aloe vera and calcium tablets. Whereas before she was on seven or eight cartons of Elemental 028 every day, now she doesn't take any. Her daily intake of medication, i.e. tablets, has also been reduced from about twenty-eight to six. Sarah no longer drinks tap water without it being boiled because of the potential for bacterial infection and also uses an aloe vera toothgel (without fluoride because of its potential toxic effects).

Sarah's husband Tim and her three children have been a source of constant support for her throughout her illness, and Tim has become a tireless campaigner over the last fourteen years on matters to do with Crohn's disease.

Tim Page is head of the Chronic Crohn's Campaign and liaises closely with Professor John Hermon-Taylor, who is pioneering research work in the UK into the development of a vaccine to cure Crohn's disease.

If you or anyone you know suffers from this illness and would like to try using aloe vera, please contact us at the Aloe Vera Centre (see Appendix 1.1).

For details of the Chronic Crohn's Campaign, please contact Tim Page, whose details are listed in Appendix 1.9.

Sarah: breast cancer, radiotherapy

On 29th May 2001, Sarah's life was changed forever. She found a lump in her left breast. By 12th June she had been diagnosed as one of the more than 39,000 women in Britain with breast cancer. By 17th June she had had an operation to remove two malignant tumours. Sarah may have been more fortunate than most in that she was able to have the treatment faster because of her husband's private medical insurance.

Everything happened so quickly, as she recounts.

> I was only forty-one, I was a non-smoker and drank very little, and there was no history of cancer in the family (my grandparents had lived into their nineties). We had a healthy lifestyle and I was always careful about maintaining a good nutritious diet. I was in the bath and just felt this lump. I was sure it couldn't be anything serious but it was my husband, Simon, who insisted I arrange a check-up immediately. Within a week I had seen a consultant breast surgeon (he found two lumps, not one) and he felt that at my age although it was unlikely to be serious, he wanted me to have a mammogram and ultrasound examinations. The consultant radiologist saw a solid mass and I thought it must be a cyst. I saw the surgeon again that evening and he confirmed that he wanted to have a biopsy done, but again reiterated that at my age such tumours were in nine cases out of ten usually benign. That Monday night was awful and on Tuesday, when I went back to see the breast surgeon, our worst fears were confirmed: I had not one but two malignant tumours, with some changes to the surrounding tissue. The surgeon was very reassuring and told me that it was curable, it was not a high-grade tumour and that we had caught it early.
>
> He gave me a plan of action that included four key stages. Stage one was surgery – a lumpectomy to remove the lumps and surrounding tissue and removal of the lymph nodes. Stage two was a course of radiotherapy to kill

off any small cancer cells in the area. Stage three was a course of chemotherapy treatment that may not have been necessary providing stages one and two were successful. Stage four was hormone therapy treatment (more on that later). During stages two to four, I would be in the care of a breast care nurse and an oncologist.

After the operation, I was in hospital for over a week. I was in a lot of pain and my left arm was immobilised for five days. I was on morphine and other painkillers and although I had very restricted movement of my left arm, I was able to raise it to shoulder level after about a week. I had the stitches out ten days after the operation and I then had to prepare myself for the radiotherapy treatment that was due to start at the end of July. It was at this stage that the subject of aloe vera was mentioned. Both the breast surgeon and the breast care nurse recommended that I started using aloe vera at least four weeks before the radiotherapy treatment was scheduled to begin. I had also seen a homeopath and I was given the same advice.

Coincidentally, through my daughter's school, I met another parent, Alasdair Barcroft, who runs the Aloe Vera Centre in London and I called him to ask his advice on what to do. He suggested that I use a topical aloe vera gelly to rub all over the area to be treated and also to drink aloe vera juice daily as a way of helping build the immune system, detoxify the body and promote the internal healing process. Aloe vera is rich in many nutrients, including the antioxidant vitamins A, C and E.

I started on the aloe vera regime immediately. My radiotherapy treatment was scheduled to include thirty-two days of treatment over a seven-week period. When I started the treatment I was very aware of pain in my rib area and tightness in the surrounding tissue. I was examined every week by the oncologist to check my lungs and my breathing and the tissue around the treated area. I also saw the breast care nurse every week. I was drinking aloe vera juice every day and using the topical gelly about six times per day. My skin was only slightly pink and much less 'angry-looking' than that of some other patients not using aloe vera – their skin was almost 'lobster red'. The oncologist even remarked on how well my skin was doing. I suppose I was quite fortunate to have a breast surgeon and an oncologist who were both pro-complementary therapy. I used the aloe vera products from July right through to November to ensure that I gave the products time to help with the healing process.

Luckily the pathology tests after my operation had determined a grade two tumour with no lymph node involvement, and that meant I did not need to have any chemotherapy treatment. I finished my radiotherapy treatment but it took from September 2001 to April 2002 to recover. The whole process was very traumatic and what helped me through it was the support of my family and friends and also an organisation called the Haven Trust, which helps people who are undergoing or have had breast cancer treatment.

I started my hormone treatment on 29th September, three weeks after finishing the radiotherapy treatment. I was extremely concerned about the possible side effects of the treatment, though I was told that if I went through with the treatment (eight injections over a two-year period) there was a ninety per cent chance of non-recurrence. Within only three weeks of the first injection, I was experiencing severe headaches and migraines, constipation and heavy bleeding, and my periods stopped. I just felt I was in a state of toxic overload and I was prescribed strong painkillers and anti-depressants. Having just got over the radiotherapy, I felt awful. The oncologist was extremely concerned and arranged for an MRI [magnetic resonance imaging] scan that revealed nothing. The neurologist that I saw recommended that I start on a heart regulator pill. By this time I was fed up feeling ill and I decided to stop taking any more chemicals. In June 2002 I had a mammogram and ultrasound examinations that were clear. So far so good.

I now see the breast surgeon and the oncologist every three months, and I have to do this for the next two years.

As far as the aloe vera is concerned, I felt vitalised when I drank the aloe vera juice, and the topical gelly helped to reduce any skin damage, and I also use an aloe vera deodorant stick. My diet is now totally free of dairy products and I drink a lot of freshly squeezed juices.

It is possible that like so many other people undergoing radiotherapy treatment, Sarah may have suffered from a condition identified as 'radiation fibrosis', where the tissue in the surrounding area is affected and becomes hard. However, the fact that she used aloe vera products (rich in anti-oxidants and other healing nutrients) topically and internally may have minimised the damage. Her oncologist noted how well her skin looked during her treatment.

In October 2002, during Breast Cancer Awareness month, Sarah was one of over a dozen women and one man – all of whom had had breast cancer – who took part in a fashion show at the Hilton Hotel in London, to raise awareness of and money for breast cancer. The show, which was a fun event, sent a very clear message to everyone who was there and all the media who covered it, being, that you can make a full recovery from breast cancer and get your life back and start enjoying yourself again. Sarah was convinced that all the holistic care she received made a significant contribution to her recovery. Sarah has continued her career as a speech and language therapist.

Details of the Haven Trust can be found in Appendix 1.16.

Diana: ME

Diana, who is in her fifties, is someone I met only recently at a business conference, and her story is one of triumph and perseverance over great personal trauma, adversity and illness. She told me that at school she was very fit and was involved in lots of sports, including athletics, hockey and horse-riding. However, she did remember suffering from what was called 'growing pains', more probably glandular fever, in her pre-teenage years, which kept her off school for a year.

In the 1980s, despite needing her sleep, she went on to develop a successful, senior executive career in human resources in fashion retailing, working with one of the UK's foremost retail groups. She was married with three children and enjoyed a very comfortable lifestyle. Little did she know that within a few years everything she had worked for and built – her career, her marriage and her family – would come crashing down. In 1988, after the birth of her third child, she became quite listless and increasingly tired and experienced a lot of stress in her marriage. In 1991 she had three operations in six weeks, each using general anaesthetic, related to the removal of pre-cancerous cells in the cervix. In early 1997 she went on to have a hysterectomy, and at the same time her young son was diagnosed with ME. Although her operation was a success, because of her son's condition and with two active daughters, she was not able to convalesce as much as she perhaps should have, and her own condition deteriorated. She had no in-house help but was recommended to a healer to help with her son's ME, and by September he was able to resume full-time school.

In March 1998 the situation had become so bad at home and her condition had worsened to such an extent that she felt she had no option but to leave and live in a rented flat nearby. For a mum with three kids it was a particularly difficult decision to make, but she knew she had to do something to try and recover her health, and that she couldn't do this in an increasingly stressful home environment with a failing marriage. She lived in rented accommodation for three years with the help of part-time carers, and in January 2001 moved into her own house. In June 2001 she started drinking aloe vera drinking gel – a decision that has totally changed her life. She takes up the story herself.

> As someone who had suffered from severe ME (at its worst I had level three ME, and there are only *four* levels!) for over ten years, I had been on various medications including anti-depressants. I was taking up to fifteen different supplements every day, I had attended a clinic in Harley Street, I was a semi-recluse with no self-esteem, and I was emotionally and physically fragile. I needed a wheelchair for extended trips and struggled up the stairs in my house. Basically nothing that I was doing or taking seemed to have any positive benefit. In 1997, a very old friend of mine, whom I had known for over twenty years, suggested I should try taking aloe vera and bee pollen as it had helped others with ME. For whatever reason I refused and it was only in June 2001 – four years later – that I decided to start drinking this 'wacky cactus juice' and taking bee pollen tablets. It really was life changing! Within four weeks I felt my energy coming back and my muscles responding to exercise. Within a couple of months I was able to do some gardening and to start going out and having a social life. I felt the shackles falling away after over ten years!
>
> I continued to improve and just fifteen months later – in September 2002 – something dramatic happened: I ran in the Flora Five Kilometre Challenge in Hyde Park, in London! This was something I could never have dreamed of in those dark days of ME and family break-up, and I remember how good I felt when I sprinted that last 300 metres. It was as if I had climbed my personal Everest – it gave me a feeling of incredible achievement and has proved to be a 'watershed' in my life. With my friend's help, I have now started to build another career – this time in health and nutrition. Now, I am not only able to work again but more importantly I have regained my self-esteem and my confidence, and I have my health back again. For anyone out there with ME, don't give up, you may find that using aloe vera and bee pollen can improve your life and give you the second chance you deserve.

Diana now has her life under control again and believes that drinking aloe vera was the turning point. For any doctors out there who remain sceptical, you may have to start listening to the patients and look at what they are doing. Allopathic medicine has been of little help to ME sufferers over the years, and it was not that long ago that anyone with ME was dismissed almost out of hand for malingering, or it was just 'yuppie flu'!

Julia: acne

Julia had suffered from acne for many years and had resigned herself to a life on medication. She was extremely unhappy about the situation because of the well documented and potentially serious side effects involved in taking some of the anti-acne prescription drugs. She, like so many other acne sufferers, was aware of the adverse publicity surrounding certain drugs and the possible links between them and conditions like arthritis, hepatitis and depression. Researchers in the UK have apparently found that in a small percentage of cases one particular anti-acne drug may even induce life-threatening diseases. With her options very limited, Julia felt she was 'between a rock and a hard place' and had little choice but to continue with the conventional medication, as she describes.

> It's quite scary when you read newspaper reports about the medication you're taking when the journalism is not only very negative about it, but also claims, in some circumstances, it could have potentially deadly side effects. It's almost like playing Russian roulette. It was quite by chance that I saw another press article that mentioned aloe vera and how it had been used for centuries for a wide range of both internal and external disorders. I was fascinated that something that was plant based and had no toxic or other side effects may help my condition. I wrote off to the company and after receiving the information pack, I spoke to someone who advised me to purchase an aloe vera drinking gel and a topical gelly to put on my skin.

> KEY POINT
> Looking back over the last three years, that was probably the best decision of my life. I am no longer plagued by acne and I no longer feel self-conscious, because my condition has improved so much.

> I still suffer occasionally but I have found that by applying the topical aloe vera gelly more frequently and increasing my intake of the drink (you can't overdose on these products!), the problem soon disappears again.

Catriona: Alopecia areata

Catriona was only seventeen when she was diagnosed as having Alopecia areata. It was a profoundly traumatic time for her and her family, as her mother, Juliana, describes.

One evening when Catriona was getting ready to go out to a party, a friend of hers noticed a small bald patch at the back of her head. After looking at it and realising the patch was completely bald – not even broken hair as a result of some previous hair treatment – we immediately made an appointment to see our GP. To our absolute horror and amazement, she diagnosed ringworm and prescribed a fungicidal cream to treat the problem. Having seen ringworm on a few occasions previously, we suggested to the GP that we didn't think it was ringworm. However, she persisted in her diagnosis, adding that there were many forms of fungal infection and this was one of them. We left the surgery unhappy, dismayed and uncertain. My partner, who had been brought up using natural herbal remedies, suggested we should not use the cream if we didn't believe it was a fungal infection, and we therefore decided to opt for the Chinese herbal route. After a thorough examination, a detailed consultation and a barrage of tests, Catriona embarked on a course of tablets, together with rubbing ginger into her scalp. The patches were expanding but she continued to take the tablets (thirty-eight per day at a cost of £42 per visit – one visit every two weeks: this was quite expensive!). About that time, we also moved surgeries and the new GP suggested, while not wishing to interfere with the treatment, that we should try garlic instead of ginger to rub on the scalp.

Catriona's patches continued to increase and she became more and more depressed. What could I tell my daughter who was a pretty seventeen-year-old – that she was facing up to the possibility that if we couldn't find anything to help, she could end up being completely bald? More patches were appearing and, in desperation, after a few months, her grandmother took her to a trichology clinic in London. The consultant there said she had Alopecia areata and that it was likely to render her bald in due course. They said they could help and suggested a twelve-month course of treatment, with bi-weekly visits for scalp massages and ultraviolet and white light treatments, and gave her some shampoo, conditioner and a lotion – all of which cost over £900! Catriona continued with the course and after about two months and very little improvement, I decided to go with her so that I could talk to the original consultant whom she had not seen since the initial consultation. After her regular treatment and an hour-and-a-half wait, we finally saw another consultant, who was surprised that there had been no reduction in the hair loss. If anything, it was becoming worse.

The consultant then suggested Catriona come in on a weekly basis, and prescribed hormone drops, which she said may lead to increased facial and/ or body hair growth, and said it was up to us to decide if we were to continue using it, if such an effect began. We decided to try this additional treatment but also felt that Catriona could do with a break, so we sent her away on holiday with a friend for a week.

As you can imagine she was in quite a state – seventeen years old, her hair falling out in very large amounts and no hope of a cure. She was almost suicidal. It was while Catriona was away on holiday that a friend rang and suggested we speak to someone called Alasdair Barcroft, who had written a book on aloe vera – a plant with powerful healing properties. In desperation we rang him and spoke at length about our daughter's problem. After listening to us, he suggested Catriona might benefit from using certain aloe vera products and we arranged to meet Alasdair on the day that Catriona returned from holiday, so that he could see the problem for himself. When we showed him the severity of her problem and he saw her state of mind, he fully understood our anxiety and distress. He suggested we try a range of aloe vera products, which included a potent unflavoured aloe vera drinking gel and three topical products – an aloe jojoba shampoo, an aloe jojoba conditioner and an aloe vera gelly, the latter to rub into the bald patches. He advised us how often to take the drink and how to use the other products. What impressed us about him was his depth of knowledge and his patient guidance. We bought all the products – enough for a three-month treatment, and it cost us a lot less than either the Chinese herbs or the trichology clinic.

Catriona started the treatment immediately, and although the aloe vera drink had what had been described as an 'acquired taste' (Catriona thought it tasted awful!), she was able to take it quite freely mixed with a fruit juice (another of his suggestions). Prior to Alasdair's visit, Catriona had became more and more depressed, not wanting to go out or see her friends. She just stayed in her bedroom and cried. We said that if it would help her, we would all shave our heads so she wouldn't feel so isolated. We even enlisted the co-operation of some of her friends who said they would do the same in the name of charity. However, she refused, saying it would do no good and why should everyone else suffer? Eventually we got her friends to cajole her into going out again and bought her an impressive selection of hats and caps so that the bald patches were less noticeable.

She started to use the aloe vera drink and gelly three times a day, having put aside the other treatments, and she also used the shampoo and conditioner every day. Before bed she would always ask us to look at her hair to see if there was any change. That night (this was about seven days after she started the treatment) to our amazement we saw there were some very fine little baby hairs growing in all the patches. I had to pluck one out to show her before she would believe me. I cannot explain the transformation that took place in the days that followed. Every day we checked and the fine hairs became stronger and fuller. Thank God, at last something positive was happening! I contacted Alasdair and he suggested we increase Catriona's intake of the drink slightly and that she should use the gelly more often to rub into her scalp. Within six weeks of starting the aloe vera treatment, Catriona had good hair growth coming through where previously there had been absolutely none. Her state of mind improved dramatically and very soon her self-confidence returned and she was back to her normal happy self. She now tells everyone who knows her and knows about her hair how things have improved. From our point of view, it seems to be a miracle. Her hair has grown back vigorously, where before there was no trace, and she has her old vitality back. She seems to be well on the road to recovery.

KEY TIP

Because of the impact aloe vera had made on Catriona's life, I then started to take the aloe vera gel drink and also started to use the topical gelly. The effects were staggering. It seemed to heal the skin problem I had suffered with for years, it gave me more energy and I now feel better than I have done for a long time.

Aloe vera has given back to our daughter not only her hair but also her spirit and self-confidence, and she is now able to enjoy life to the full again. We feel, from the bottom of our hearts, that everybody, old or young, should try taking this aloe vera for a healthy skin and a healthy body. It seems to make you healthier and more vigorous and it does wonders for your skin. No wonder it is known as the 'silent healer'.

Gina: rheumatoid arthritis

Gina's life had been ruined by arthritis and the side effects of the medication she had been prescribed. It had all started after the birth of her second child, when she was only thirty-three. She recounts the impact it had on her and her family, and how some so-called 'wacky cactus juice' changed her life, forever.

About six months after the birth of my second child, the large toe on my right foot became inflamed and very painful. I didn't recall hitting it against anything but I decided to visit my GP and have it examined. To my surprise he suggested that it might be arthritis and advised me to come back and see him in a few weeks' time, if I developed any pain in my other joints. Within six weeks my right knee had swollen up, and my nursing training made me acutely aware that there was something seriously wrong. The doctor prescribed non-steroidal anti-inflammatory drugs, but within ten days I had to stop taking them because I was developing severe gastric pains. The endoscopy I had soon after revealed severe inflammation and it took two years (on zantac) and three courses of antibiotics before the problems with my stomach were resolved. Over the years, the arthritis became progressively worse and my knees, in particular, were the worst affected. Everyday routines, like climbing the stairs and shopping (which most people do not think twice about), became my worst nightmare – because of the pain. My GP even told me that I had 'better enjoy life as much as I could now' because it could only get much worse. In early 1997, the pain became so unbearable that I was seriously considering moving to a bungalow to avoid having to walk up and down stairs. My GP also suggested that I consider using a stick for walking, and he arranged for me to receive an orange disabled sticker for my car.

Over the years, however, I had steadfastly refused to believe that my condition could only get worse and nothing else could be done. I pestered my GP, remained positive and was always on the lookout for new ideas and alternative therapies. I even persuaded my GP to refer me to the London Homeopathic Hospital and, over the years, I tried all sorts of 'possible cures', including elimination diets, fish oils and even faith healing. Unfortunately none of these gave me any relief or even hope. In March 1997, quite by accident, I was introduced to something called aloe vera gel – a potent, unflavoured aloe vera drinking juice with a long track record of healing success. The person who introduced me to this 'natural vegetable juice' told me how he had cured himself of a chronic sinus infection that had not previously responded to over three years of conventional medication and treatment, including two painful operations.

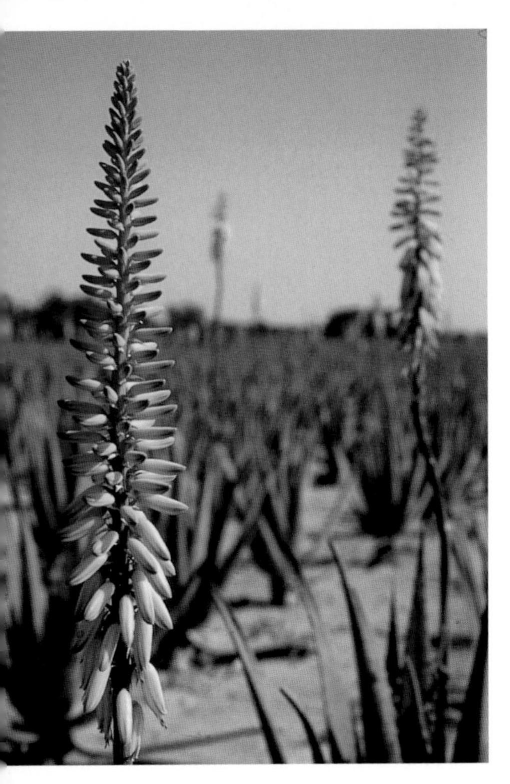

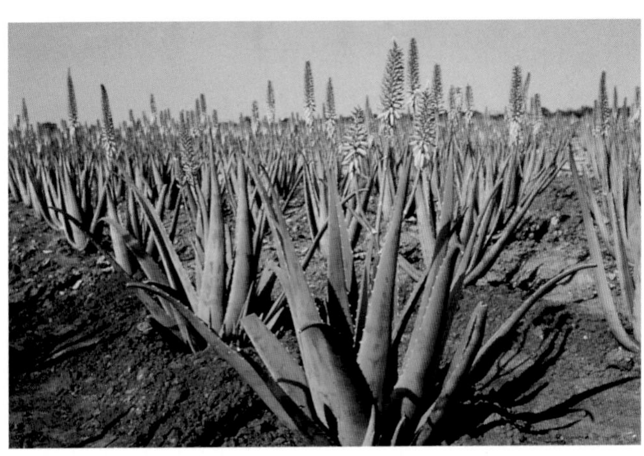

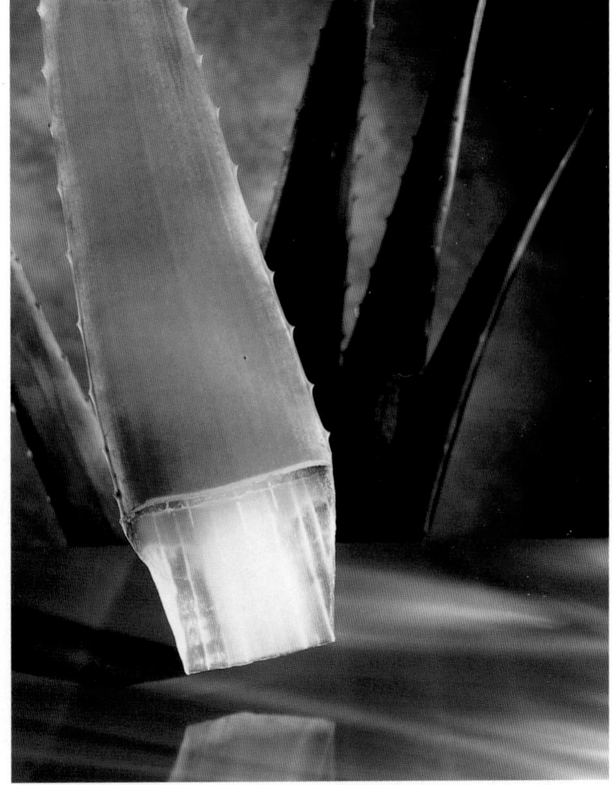

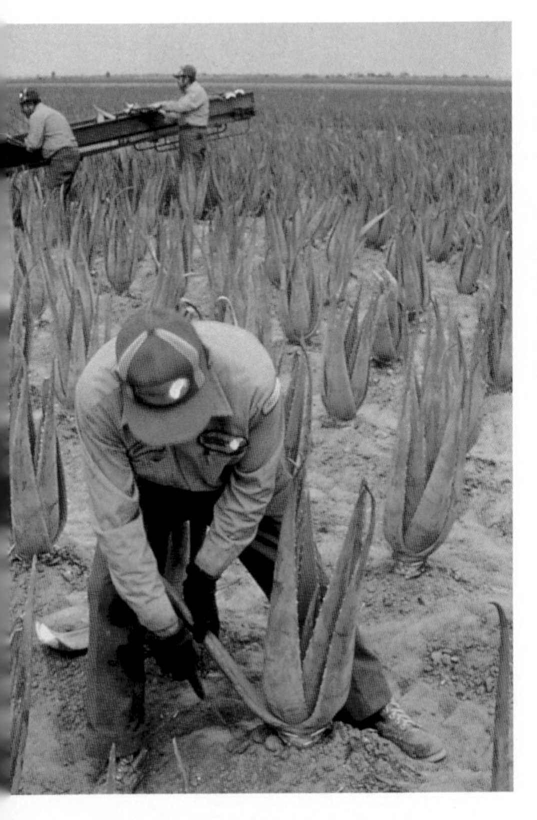

1: Aloe vera plants, showing the central stem with yellow flowers.

2: A plantation of aloe vera plants.

3: Harvesting aloe vera by hand.

4: Cross section of an aloe vera leaf.

Bronte – 3rd degree burns

5 & 6: Shots taken in 1997, showing extensive third-degree burns.

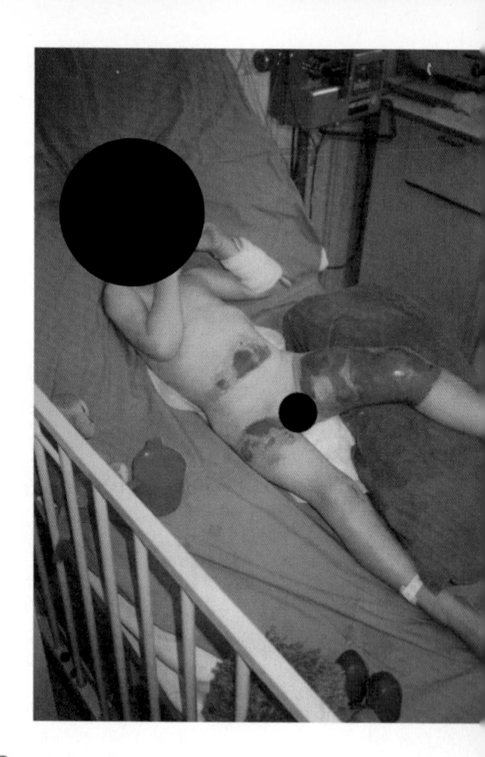

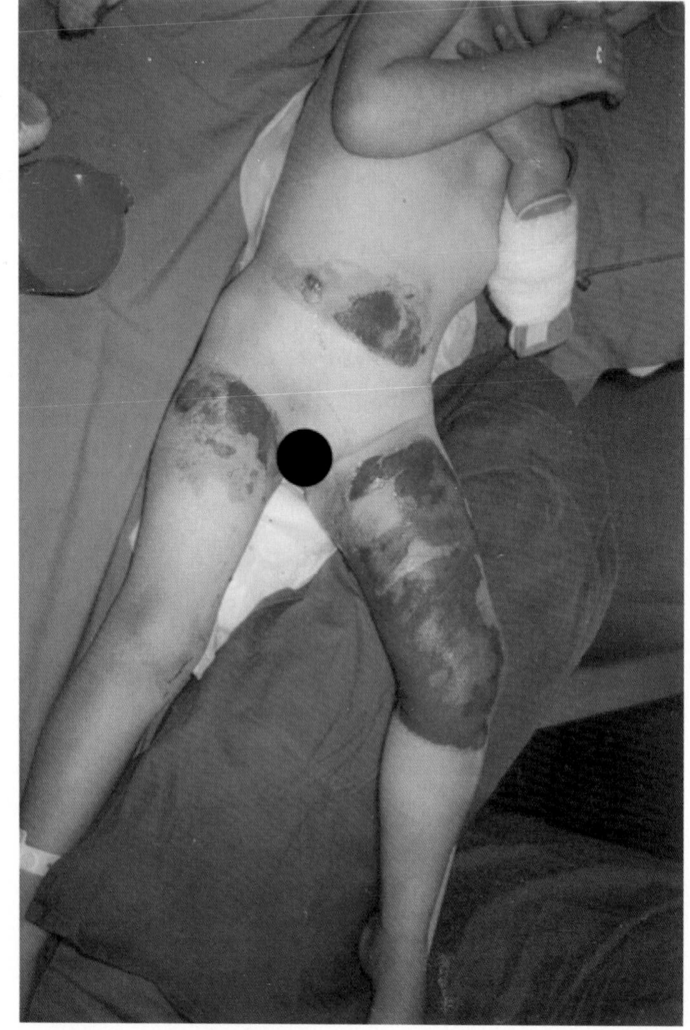

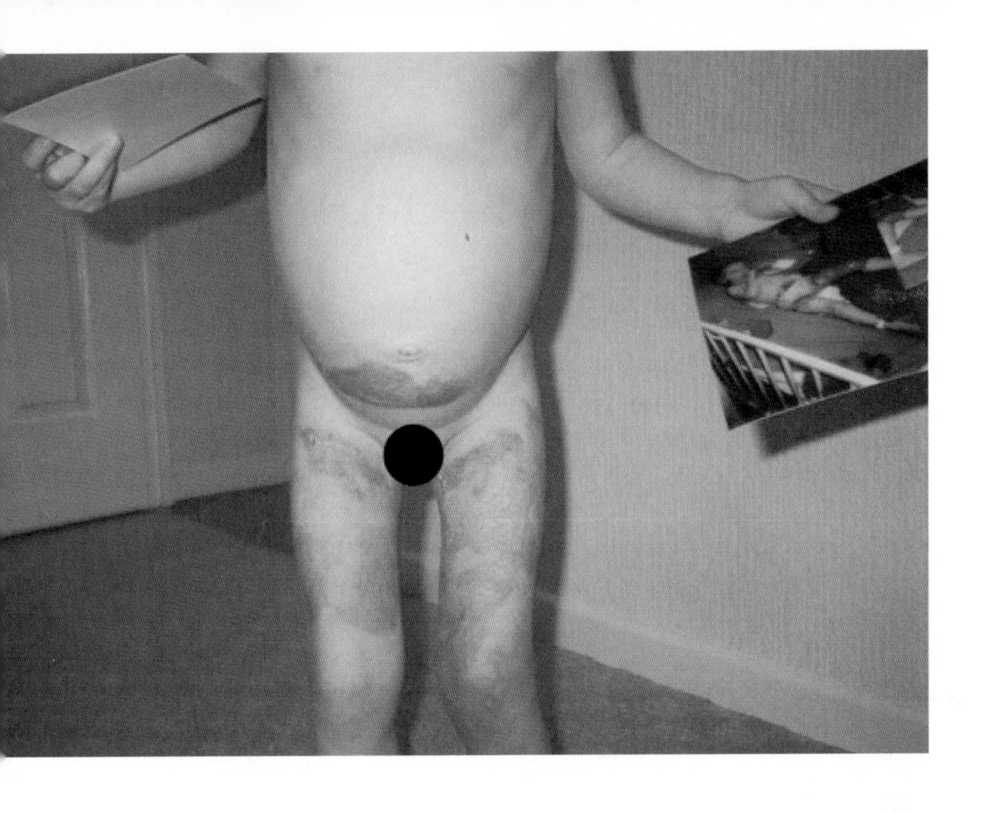

7 & 8: Shots taken two years later, no operations and no infections.

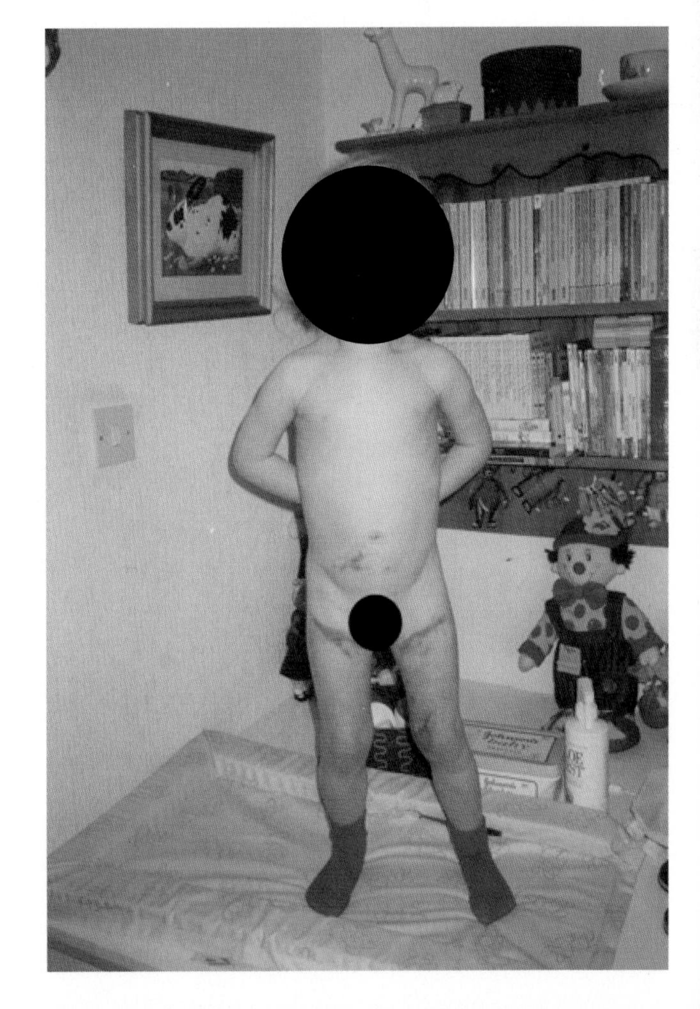

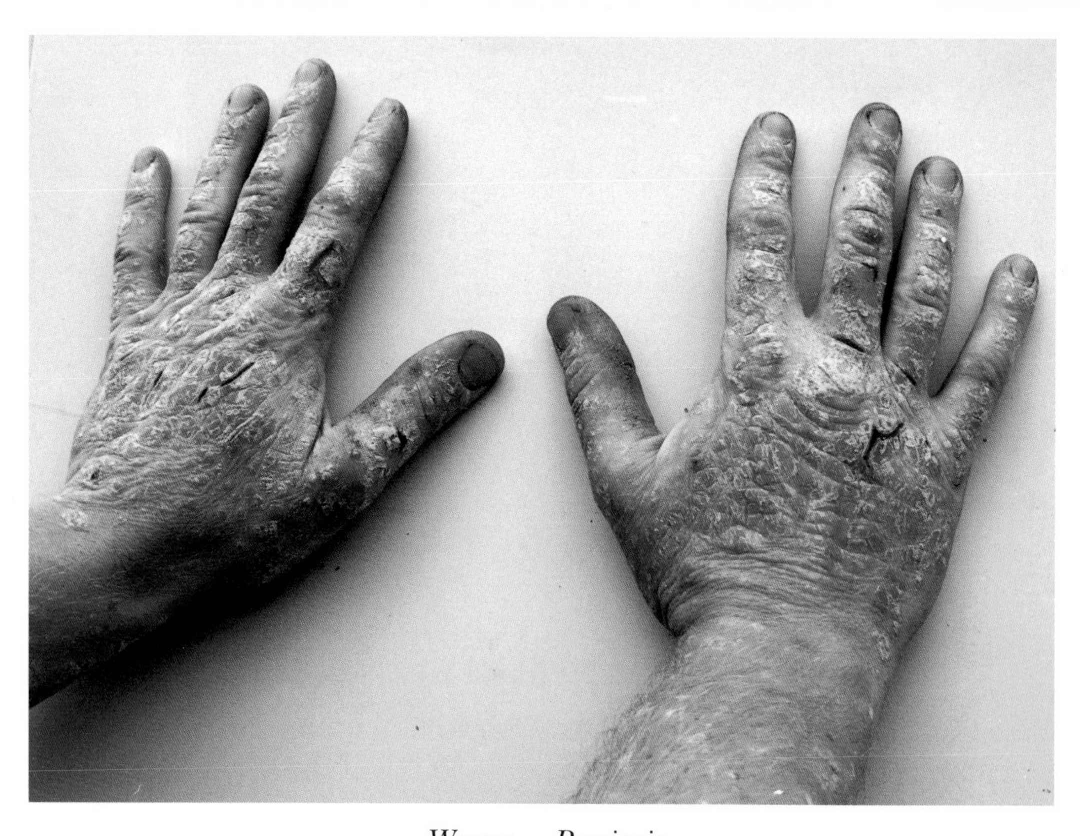

Wayne – Psoriasis
9: Shows hands (with psoriasis) before using aloe vera.
10: Shows the degree of healing on the hands after using aloe vera.

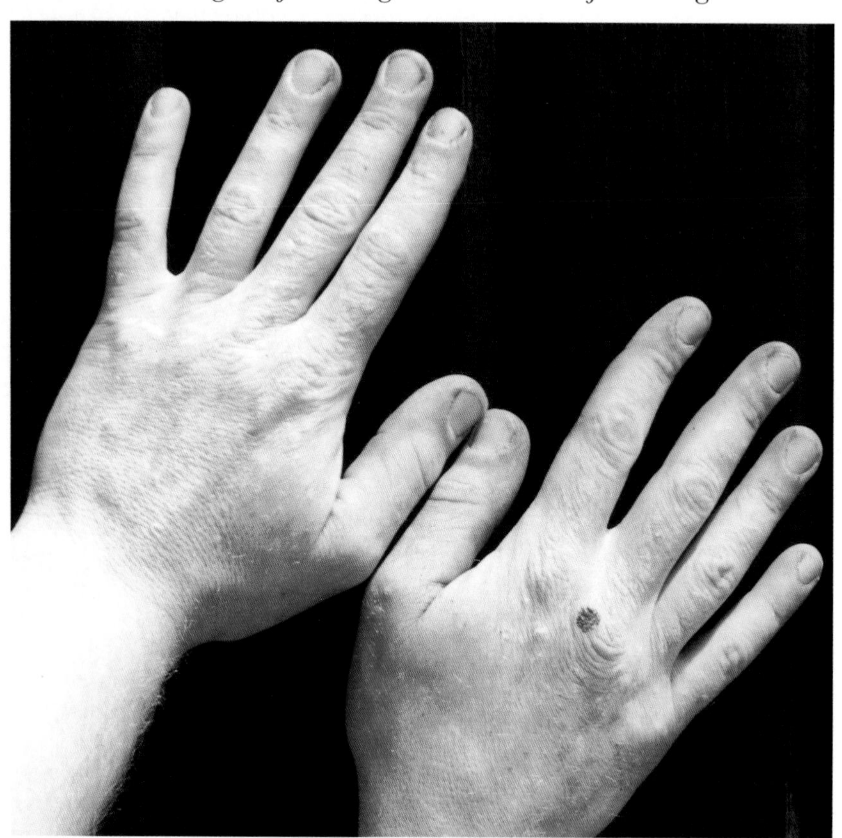

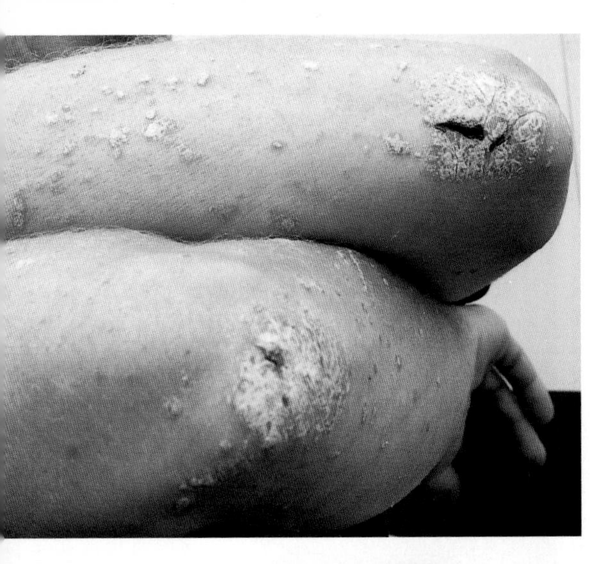

11: Shows elbows (with psoriasis) before using aloe vera.
12: Shows the degree of healing on the elbows after using aloe vera.

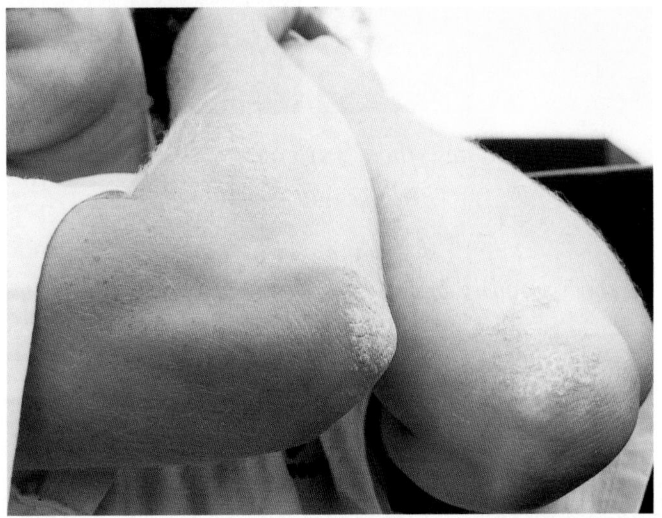

14: Shows the degree of healing on the knees after using aloe vera.

13: Shows knees (with psoriasis) before using aloe vera.

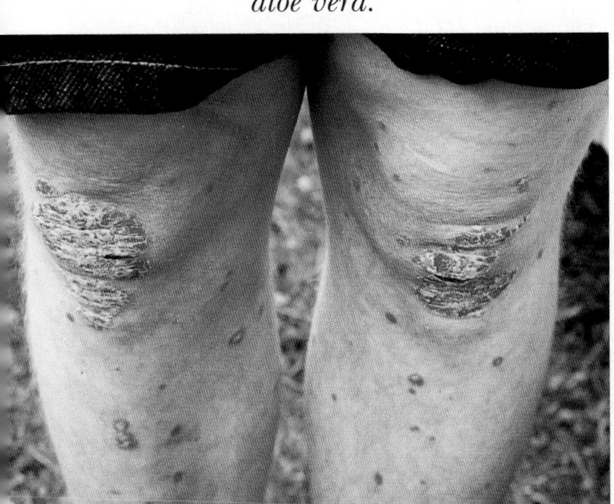

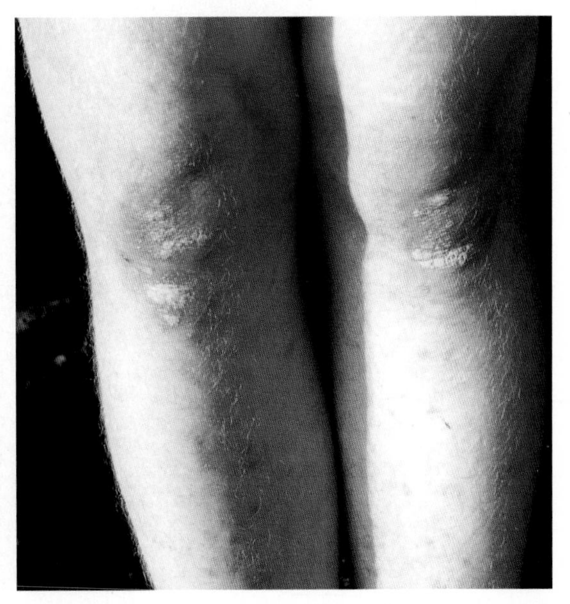

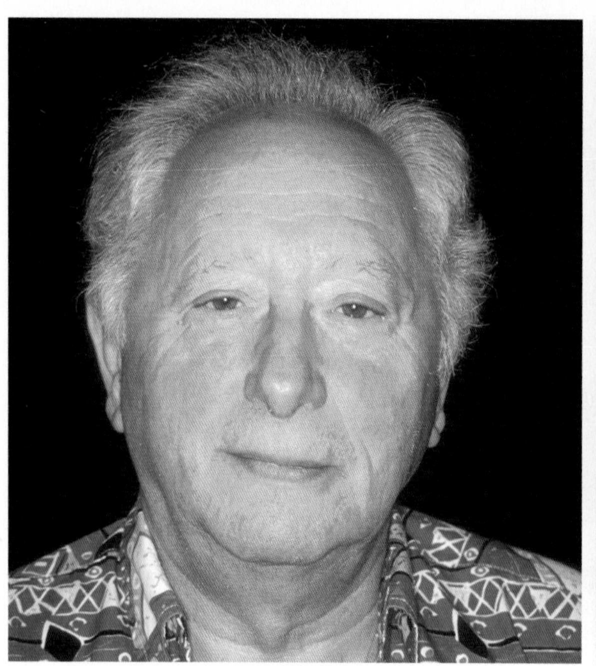

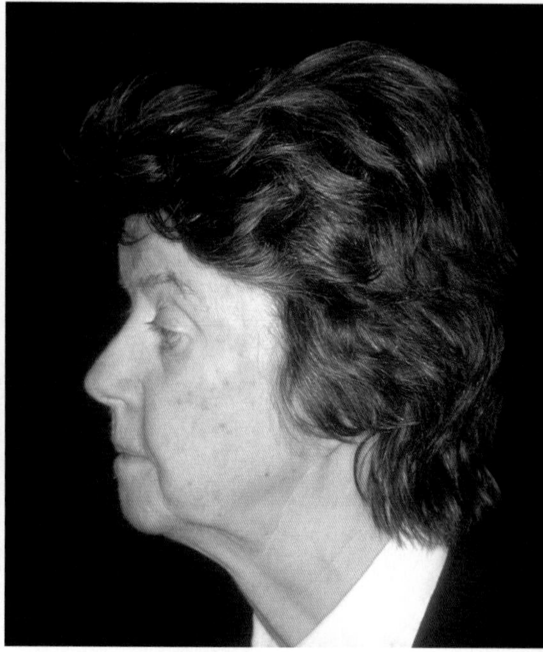

15 & 16: Acne roseaca. Show typical sufferers of this condition with the 'rosacea' markings on the face.

Meadow – Sarcoid
17: Shows Sarcoid growing between forelegs, prior to application of aloe vera.

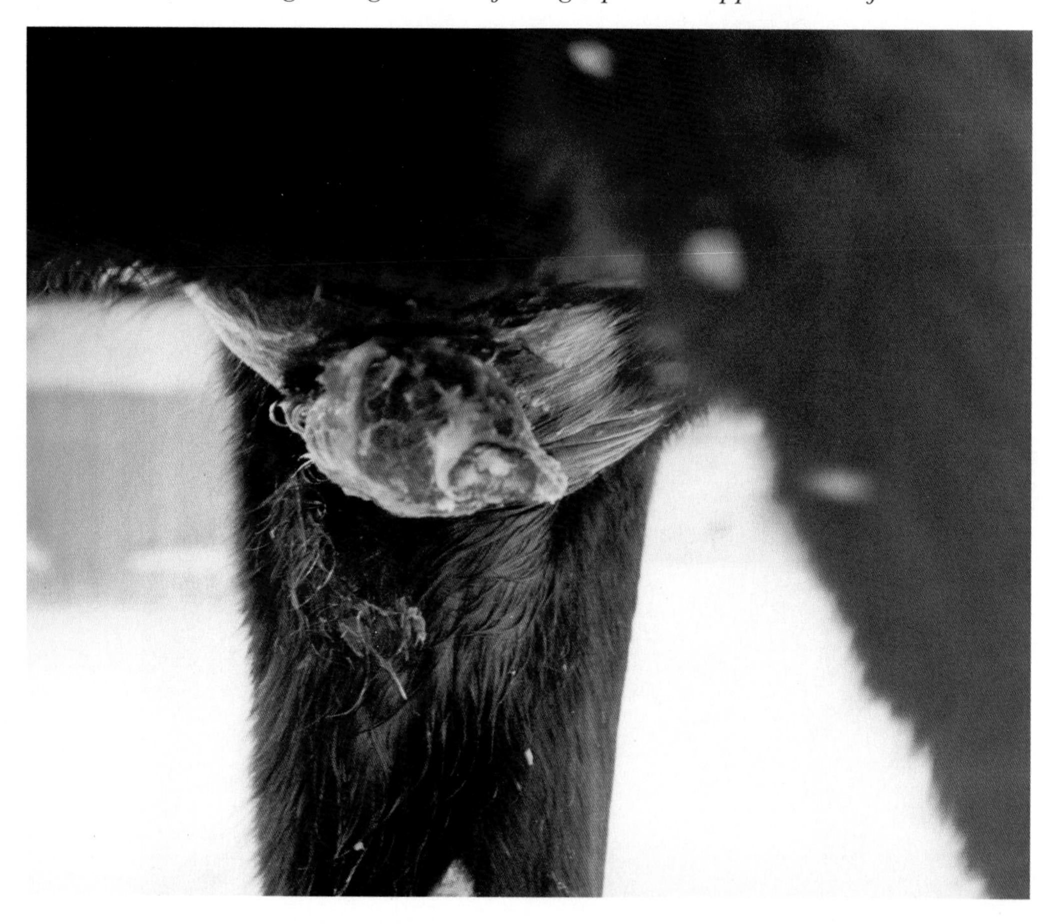

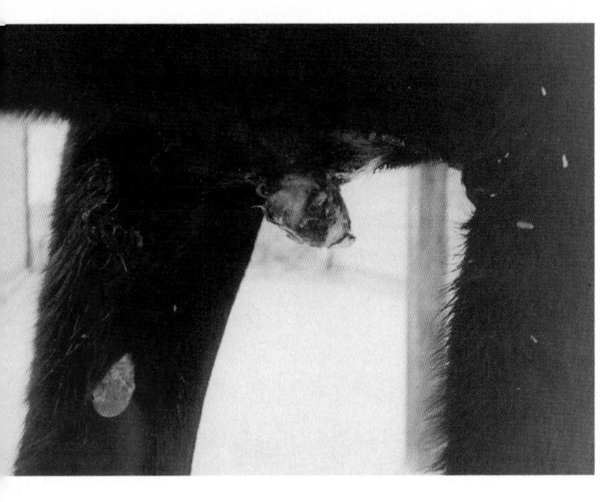

18: (left) Shows Sarcoid – during application of aloe vera.

19: (below) Shows Sarcoid after falling off – tissue healing underneath.

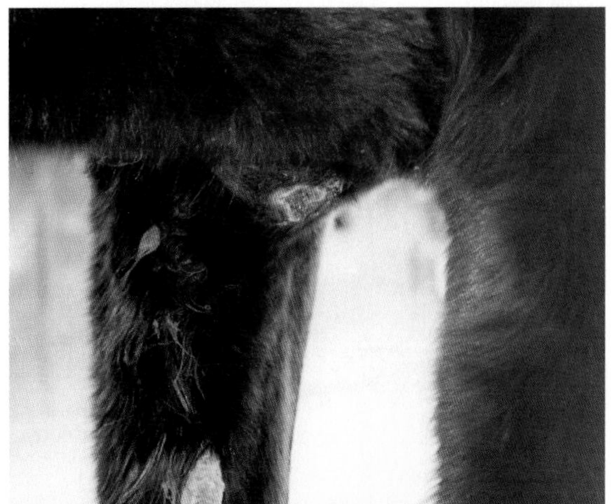

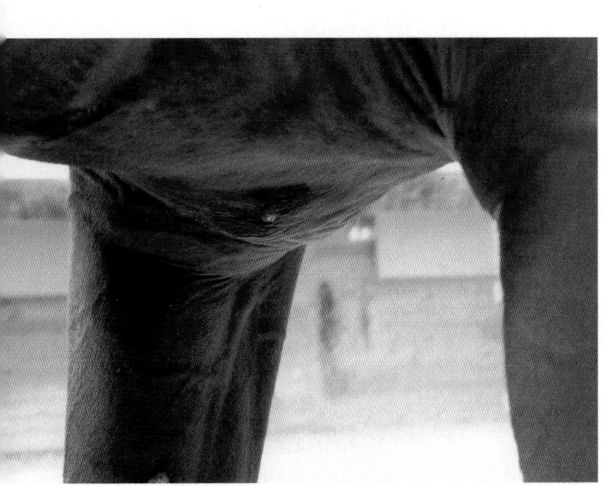

20 & 20a: Meadow – totally healed.

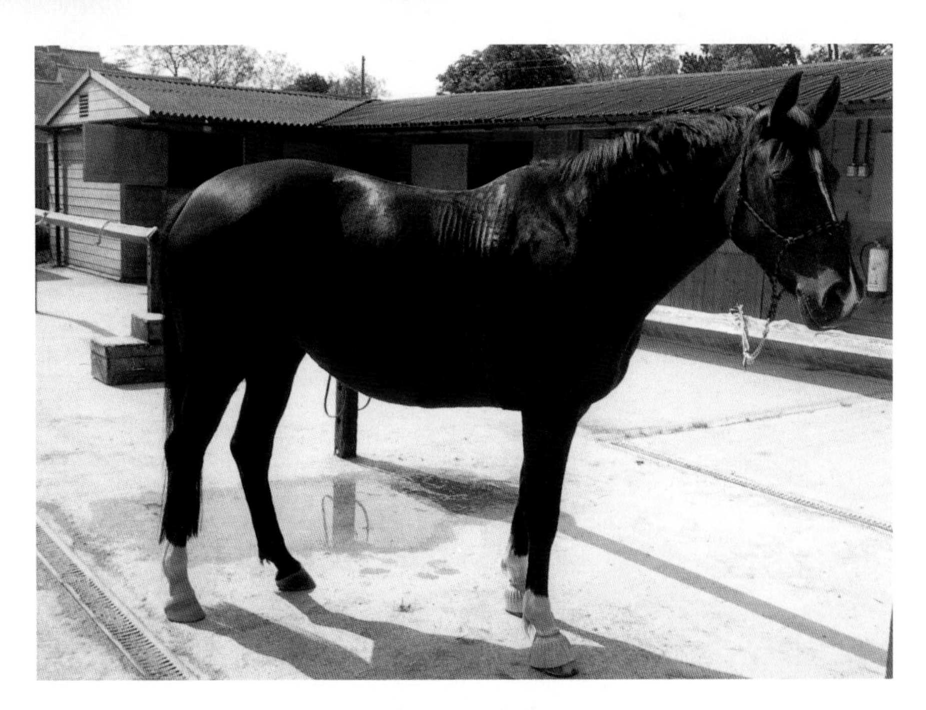

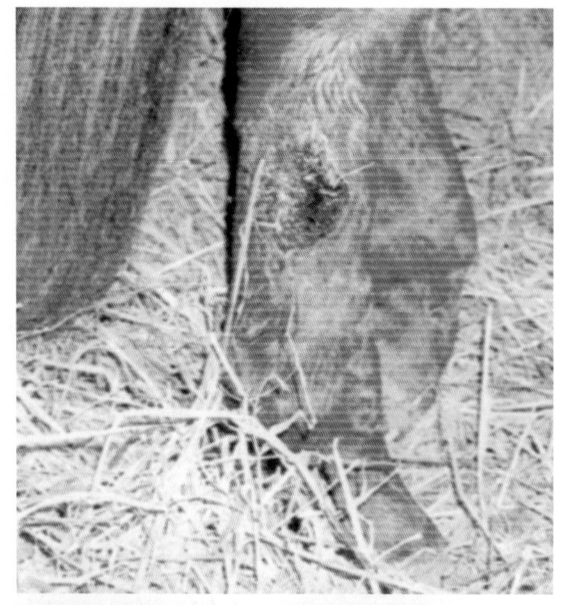

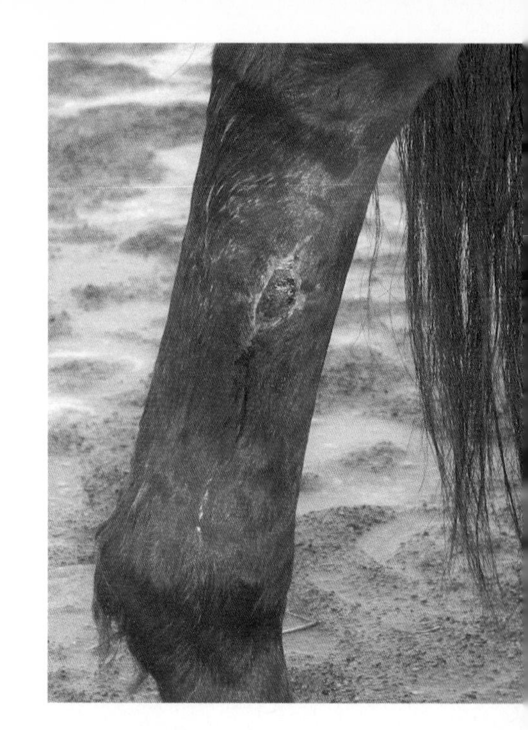

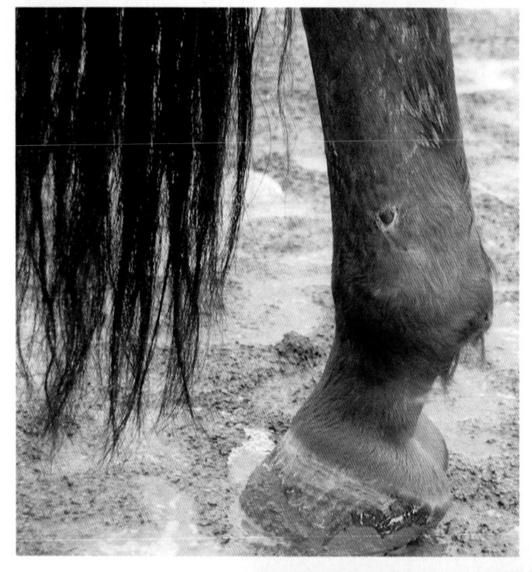

Sevenge – leg injury

21: (top left) Protruding wound with proud flesh– one month after accident.

22: (top right) Two weeks later – wound healing and all proud flesh has gone.

23: (left) Four weeks later – wound area has decreased by fifty per cent.

24: (below) Sevenge – totally recovered.

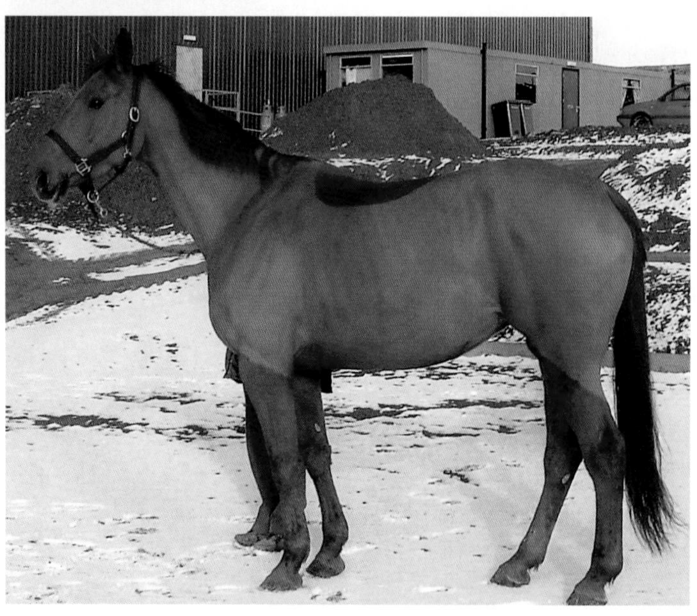

He had used three particular proprietary products to cure himself: an aloe activator nasal spray, an aloe vera gel drink, and bee propolis (a natural antibiotic). As a result of his own personal success, he had set up the Aloe Vera Centre in London, to both market aloe vera products and advise other people on the benefits of what is known in many parts of the world as the 'miracle plant'. He told me that he was not a doctor and that over the years he had been selling this particular brand of aloe vera (and other natural products). He said that there had been some very positive results and measurable benefits for people suffering with a wide range of ailments, both internal and external. He confirmed that aloe vera had a long history of healing and although it had powerful anti-inflammatory properties, there weren't, to his knowledge, any clinical trials relating to its use for arthritis. He also told me that the aloe vera drink was definitely not sold for its taste but that it was the purest and the most potent on the market and that if I saw no benefits within ninety days, I could get my money back.

He mentioned that some people's symptoms could get worse before they started to feel any improvement. I was initially extremely sceptical because I thought I had exhausted all possible alternative routes, but I decided to give it a try – I really had nothing to lose. I was instructed to take two tablespoons, twice a day, and to ensure that I took it consistently morning and night, every day for at least three months. Within only two weeks, I was amazed to notice that there was less stiffness in my joints in the mornings. Within about four weeks, I started to notice an increase in my energy levels and the depression I had felt for so many years started to disappear. Within only two months, I was almost totally pain free – after thirteen years of suffering. It was almost too good to be true – but it was real, it wasn't a dream!

I remembered being told that aloe vera was not in itself a cure for anything. It was the beneficial effects of over 200 different, identified nutritional constituents and the way they acted synergistically, that could help reduce inflammation and pain and promote healing, as well as boosting the immune system and energy levels. Everything I had been told about the benefits of taking aloe vera seemed to be coming to fruition. I was feeling better than I had done at any time in the last thirteen years, and all because of a natural vegetable juice! Six years later, I still make sure I take my aloe vera 'religiously' every day. I am aware that I still have arthritis and that I have not cured it. However, there is no question that my daily doses of aloe vera have kept all

> the painful symptoms at bay and it has none of the chronic or toxic side effects of many of the original drugs I was prescribed. I now feel fantastic. I have lots of energy and no pain! I am able to enjoy life to the full. I have a successful career and I have my life back. Like so many people who take aloe vera to help them with a particular condition, I now believe I am controlling my arthritis – it is no longer controlling me!

Oliver: asthma

Oliver is in his late forties and a director of a UK-based multinational engineering company. As a child he had severe asthma and bronchitis, and he was not expected to survive past the age of eleven. He did and it was subsequently discovered that he was allergic to a wide variety of things, especially grass pollen. He had various treatments over the years, including anti-allergy injections that left him with a lung that is approximately ninety per cent efficient compared to normal.

As he grew older the impact lessened, but in winter particularly he has had to use a combination of inhalers, one to dilate the lungs, and the other to control local infection. Within a few months of first taking a proprietary aloe vera gel drink he realised that he was no longer having to use either of the inhalers, and this has now been the case for more than six years. In the last eighteen years he has never had such a long usage gap. Previously, he was also prone to fairly frequent sore throats in the winter, which he believes were related to his respiratory problem, and these too have now disappeared. He still travels abroad frequently and is in a high-pressure and fairly stressful job – all things that can bring on an asthma attack. Although he still carries the inhalers he has never had the need to use them in the past few years.

Claire: asthma

When Claire was a child she suffered quite badly from asthma. After a while it improved, but in her thirties it came back again, which she found extremely frustrating. Then she was introduced to aloe vera. She was told about a drink called aloe berry nectar and advised to take about three tablespoons per day, every morning as a general tonic and energy booster. She describes how things improved.

> After a couple weeks I realised that I was wheezing less, as well as having increased energy, so I rang my niece to find out whether aloe vera could possibly help asthma. She said, 'Yes, didn't I tell you?' Within six months I had stopped taking my inhaler altogether. The interesting thing about it was that I didn't even know aloe vera could help asthma, so it wasn't a

> question of mind over matter. Having been off the inhaler over a year, and free of asthma, I then went on a two-week sailing holiday without my aloe vera. Within a few days I had a recurrence of my asthma and had to purchase an inhaler locally. However, on returning to the UK and restarting my aloe vera juice, the asthma disappeared again and hasn't returned, and I no longer need to use my inhaler. What an amazing natural drink!

Oliver and Claire's cases are by no means unusual. Many people with asthma report similar effects and benefits and say that by drinking aloe vera gel or aloe berry nectar, they have been able to dispense with their inhalers. It does not happen overnight, however, so anyone considering the use of aloe vera should ensure that it is of the highest quality and should persist with it for several months to see if it can help.

Rowena: burn

One Christmas, Heather's mother, Rowena, accidentally tipped a pan of hot fat over her hand. She was immediately taken to the accident and emergency unit of her local hospital where she was given painkillers, her burn was dressed and she was told to return in three days. When she returned to have the dressing changed she was shocked to see how bad the burn was looking – it covered nearly two thirds of her hand. She could not bend her fingers and there were huge blisters all over it. Again she was told to return in three days. By this time the blisters were gone but the skin was very badly cracked and looked even worse than before. The doctors told her that it would take approximately five months for her hand to heal properly. That was when Heather stepped in, as she recalls.

> I spoke to someone I know who originally recommended aloe vera to me and they suggested I use a natural antibiotic cream with aloe vera and bee propolis.
>
> The next day I put this cream on my mother's hand and told her to apply it at least two or three times a day and occasionally bathe her hand in aloe vera gel (the drink) before applying the aloe propolis cream. Within only five days she had the bandages off and was washing dishes with detergent. The wound was completely healed except for a slight pink tinge to the affected area. My family were so amazed that we wished we had taken 'before and after' pictures to show the difference.

Benjamin: chronic asthma

When he was only two, Benjamin's mother noticed that after any physical exertion or just being out in the cold air he experienced breathing problems. Obviously in someone so young this was a real worry, and not long after, when he caught a cold, it went straight to his lungs. Here she recounts what happened over the next few years and the positive impact that drinking aloe vera had on Benjamin's health.

> For the next two years, Benjamin underwent numerous tests to try and determine what the root cause of his increasingly serious bronchial problems were. He was prescribed both allopathic medicine and herbal remedies. We changed his diet to eliminate various foodstuffs that were thought to be 'triggers', and we focused very much on the homeopathic approach. We discovered that his condition was much better in the drier months and worsened noticeably from September onwards. He sometimes had up to seven asthma attacks each night and that was very worrying. On one occasion his condition became so acute that we had to call in the emergency doctor to administer an injection to help his breathing (it also had horrendous side effects) and other medications, including a strong cortisone pessary. The doctor suggested that Benjamin also took some special capsules (containing something called theophyline) and another spray, which unfortunately also contained cortisone. We had always given Benjamin vitamin supplements and tried literally everything, from special breathing techniques to changing the bedclothes, purchasing a new bed and throwing out all the stuffed toys. About this time, the homeopathic doctor conducted another 'bio-resonance' allergy test and he discovered Benjamin was allergic to milk. We immediately stopped all milk products (this was difficult for Benjamin because he was drinking up to two litres per day). It was incredible how quickly his condition improved.
>
> When he was four, I read an article about aloe vera and its healing properties. I am so glad I did because about that time, Benjamin had reverted to about three asthma attacks during the day and sometimes four at night. These attacks sometimes happened for no apparent reason, even when he was sitting quietly reading a book and not exerting himself running about. We started Benjamin on about two dessert spoons per day of the aloe vera gel drink and the improvement was almost immediate.

Prior to starting on aloe vera, Benjamin would come home from playschool with a cold and then, because the cold went straight to his chest, he would be ill for a week or ten days and would have to miss school. His illness was having a very detrimental effect, not only on his health but also on his development, because he was having to miss so much school and he was not able to do what other children did. I had increased the aloe vera dosage to about three tablespoons per day, which seemed to provide that extra boost his immune system needed, and although he had a few 'near misses', these 'post aloe vera' colds never really developed into anything serious.

Benjamin's condition may well improve as he gets older, but there is no doubt in our minds that the introduction of this strange tasting and very potent aloe vera juice has made an enormous impact on Benjamin's overall health and general well-being. He knows himself that it's helping him and although he doesn't like the taste, he has never refused to take it. He has even said that nothing else so far seems to have helped – it's only his aloe juice that does. The frequency and severity of attacks were considerably reduced, when before we were constantly aware of the dangers from the possible side effects of any cold or other infection. Now we are able to be more relaxed. This aloe vera drinking gel has had a massive, highly positive and life-changing impact on our family and it's something that anyone else with a similar condition or in similar circumstances should consider.

Liza: candida albicans

For over ten years Natalie had been waging war with candida albicans. This left her with constant thrush, fatigue, acne, tissue and joint inflammation, food intolerance and chemical and pollen allergies. A few years ago she started taking aloe vera and has noticed a steady improvement in her health ever since, as she describes.

KEY TIP
I drink aloe vera gel twice daily, which soothes my irritable bowel and bladder, eases my fatigue and improves my energy levels considerably. Aloe vera gelly is excellent for acne, painful joints and gingivitis. The aloe propolis cream and aloe moisturising lotion are excellent for eczema, as well as for sunburn.

I believe, however, that the aloe activator (aloe vera and allantoin) is the most versatile of all the products I have tried. As a mouthwash, it soothes sore and inflamed areas, reduces inflammation and inhibits bacterial and fungal growth. For sinusitis and hay fever, it can be trickled into each nostril and sniffed. It makes your eyes water but it works well. For sore throats, again it can be trickled into the nostrils and allowed to run down the back of the throat or it can be gargled. It stings initially but stops the soreness in its tracks. For earache, trickling some into the affected ear works wonders. It has even made a slight difference to my mother's hearing loss! Either aloe activator or aloe vera gelly can also be used on a tampon to ease vaginal discomfort from thrush, and I imagine would also help dryness if that was a problem. All in all I have found aloe vera products an all-round and very necessary and successful aid to my body's journey in regaining its good health, and I shall be forever grateful.

Holda: chronic fatigue

For many years Holda had been suffering with chronic fatigue, and she was also plagued with splitting headaches, stomach pains and bloating. She was prone to skin allergies and was unable to find any solution to her ongoing problems. She had consulted various doctors and complementary therapists and had tried numerous medications and natural remedies, without any real success. A friend of hers recommended that she start to drink aloe vera as a way of boosting both her immune system and her energy levels and soothing the digestive problems.

Holda takes up the story.

I am from Mexico and I vaguely knew about aloe vera but I was not aware that I could benefit from drinking the juice. After about six weeks, I started to notice that I was less tired and the stomach pain and bloating were eased. Within three months, my skin had improved and my headaches had become less frequent. It seemed as though the aloe vera was helping my body to regain its balance. Because of these improvements, I started to use other topical products on my skin and have found them to help alleviate any skin problems, and I seem to be much less prone to skin allergies than before. Others in my family who have seen the improvement in my general health have now started to use the products and are experiencing the benefits first hand. I would recommend aloe vera as a good all-round tonic, healer and immune-boosting agent to everyone. It just makes you feel good, gives you more energy and improves the skin.

Laura: ulcerative colitis

Laura is in her forties and started suffering from ulcerative colitis in her mid-thirties. At first she was given steroid enemas and sulphasalazine tablets. She was allergic to the sulphasalazine, so she was put on asacol – a medication she has taken ever since.

After a while the steroid enemas could no longer cope as the condition worsened, so she was put on steroid tablets. The amount she took varied, ten milligrams a day being about average, but she had great difficulty getting below five milligrams a day without a flare-up, and then having to increase the dose.

Laura explains.

> My consultant spoke to me several times about surgery, which seemed the only way out, and he agreed I could have some time to try alternative remedies. I had already tried aromatherapy and reflexology and various homoeopathic remedies, but none of these had done much good. I was very depressed, constantly tired and I had also developed a fistula in my colon. I suffered from chronic pain, diarrhoea, bleeding, always rushing to the loo (and scared of not being able to get there in time). I was also terribly fatigued and was very nervous about going out – often I was just simply too tired to make the effort. I had put on about two stones in weight because of the steroids (an increase of some twenty per cent in my normal body weight), and my face had become very puffy – the typical 'moon-face'. I had also developed a fungal infection on my foot and in my groin. I suffered from terrible mood swings and had trouble sleeping, and pernicious anaemia had also been diagnosed. Then I saw a newspaper article about some natural plant extract that you could drink, called aloe vera gel. After contacting the person concerned, I started taking it a month later.
>
> For the first few weeks I felt strange (headaches and so on), but you often get that when your body is detoxifying. After that I started to feel better. Six weeks after starting on the aloe vera gel, I went into hospital to have a colonoscopy, to see when (not if) I would have to have the surgery. My consultant was surprised but pleased to inform me that I was so much improved I no longer needed the operation. I very slowly cut down my steroids until I was off them completely, and I gradually lost the puffiness and excess weight. When I saw my specialist after six months he was amazed at the continued improvement in my condition and asked me to send him information on what I had been taking. I used to have flare-ups at least

> once a week, but since I have been drinking the aloe vera this has been reduced to one or two and only during periods of stress.
>
> I am now feeling considerably better than I have done for nearly ten years, and I am able once again to enjoy things I have not been able to do for years. My incredible recovery and continuing improvement – I call it a miracle – is due to taking aloe vera. I do, however, have a word of caution for any fellow ulcerative colitis sufferers, or anyone with Crohn's who wants to try this remedy. Please make sure that the aloe vera you buy is of the highest purity and quality. There are many brands on the market (I bought some from a health food shop once and it was just like water and had no benefit at all). I have written to the National Association for Colitis and Crohn's Disease to tell them how aloe vera has changed my life, and hopefully my story and positive experience may help the thousands of other fellow sufferers out there. Finally, I would like to say to anyone who has a serious condition like mine, aloe vera is not a cure but it could help improve the quality of your life enormously. Talk to your doctor and/or specialist and tell them that you want to try aloe vera, and keep them updated.

Leanne: conjunctivitis

Leanne woke up one Saturday morning with inflamed eyes and throughout the day the problem gradually became worse. Being a very busy mum, she had little time to think about it during the day, but by that evening it was obvious she had quite a severe bout of conjunctivitis. She was too late to get to a chemist, as she remembers.

> Stupidly I put off going to the chemist, and by the time I thought about it all the shops were closed. I was in a lot of discomfort, and I couldn't see a thing as I had to take my contact lenses out (without them I'm as blind as a bat!), and I never wear glasses. I was very concerned on two counts: firstly it is extremely contagious, and I didn't want to infect the rest of my family; and secondly I was in so much pain that I really needed something to help quickly. I remembered a good friend of mine telling me only the week before that her husband had used an aloe vera product to help cure his conjunctivitis, so I phoned her. Luckily she had some of the 'magical' aloe activator, so my husband went round and picked up the product and I used it immediately, diluted on a one-to-one basis with boiled, filtered water (it had cooled down by the time my husband came back!). Within half an

hour the pain and inflammation had been reduced. I rinsed my eyes again before I went to bed and when I woke up in the morning my eyes were totally clear, no pain, no inflammation and none of that awful yellow 'gunk'. I rinsed my eyes once again for good measure and put my contact lenses back in – without any problems.

Sanjay: diabetes

Sanjay was first diagnosed with diabetes in 1992, and he decided almost immediately that he was not going to take any medication. For five years he was able to control the disease by carefully monitoring his blood sugar levels on a daily basis and adhering to a strict diet regime, which eliminated certain foods like rice and potatoes and obviously anything with a high sugar content. However, one problem that was almost insurmountable was the continual lack of energy. He was unable to walk very far or to carry things – this obviously prevented him from doing even the most routine of household tasks, and he found shopping a real challenge.

In 1997 his nephew, who is a pharmacist, suggested he start to drink aloe vera in order to boost both his immune system and his energy levels, and also to help control his glucose levels. In the last six years Sanjay has found that drinking aloe vera has had a profound effect on his health, as he confirms.

> When I was first introduced to the aloe vera gel drink, I was very open minded about using the extract from a plant that was well known in Indian medicine for its healing properties. However, even I did not expect to experience so many benefits. My digestive system seems to work better than ever and I have much more energy, which means I can be more active and not worry about getting too tired (something a lot of diabetics suffer from). I am also not as prone to colds and other infections as I used to be. Interestingly, when I told my doctor how I control my diabetes and I mentioned aloe vera, she simply did not believe me. Now I never mention it – I just go for my annual check-up and don't bother speaking to her!

Claudia: eczema

Claudia, who is in her fifties, had been plagued by eczema for over twenty years, and like so many other problems it seemed to get worse when she was under stress. It was particularly bad around her waist area and this meant that wearing anything other than very loose fitting clothes was almost impossible. She was constantly asking her doctor for a solution to what was becoming a very uncomfortable, debilitating and highly stressful problem. The medicated creams she was prescribed worked occasionally, but she was very aware that long term use of steroid creams could be harmful. Luckily she read an article in a magazine about aloe vera and eczema, as she recounts.

> When I saw that article, it seemed that all my prayers had been answered. I was reading about people with similar problems to mine, who had found no long term success with the medications that had been prescribed. Subsequently, they had been introduced to a range of aloe vera products and the results seemed almost too good to be true. My husband and I both talked with the people mentioned in the article and I ordered a couple of products, one an aloe vera gelly for the skin, and the other a very rich healing cream – a combination of aloe vera and bee propolis. I was determined to use the products as soon as possible and applied them both after my bath that night. Within hours I could feel an improvement. The angry red rash that was often around my waist was much less obvious and there was no itching or pain. I told my husband, who examined me, and he couldn't believe how much it had improved – and that was after only one application! I was conscious that it could be a 'flash in the pan' and maybe it couldn't be repeated (much like some of the other 'cures' that I had taken or been given).
>
> I was determined really to give the products a proper chance to work, and I have to say that I am so glad I did, because all these years later my eczema is still under more control than I ever thought possible before 'discovering' aloe vera. I still have a lot of stress in my life but I have found that through a combination of drinking aloe vera and applying the topical skin care products, I am not so prone to the problem, and if I ever do have a flare-up, it is not as serious or as painful as it used to be before and I soon get over it.

Alex: eczema

Alex is only nine months old but he is covered in eczema. His face, arms, legs and torso seem to be one big red sore as his mother, Jana, explains.

> We are hoping that like many other infants, Alex will grow out of his eczema. Unfortunately in the meantime he can be very distressed, and the main problem is that when the eczema gets itchy, he starts to scratch. We have been told this can sometimes lead to a serious infection. A couple of months ago, a friend from work told us about an aloe vera cream that she had been using for years to help heal and manage eczema whenever it

'reared its ugly head' with her children. She told me it was almost like a natural antibiotic cream and had no side effects. We bought some within a few days, and applied it on the eczema after we had done a series of patch tests on Alex (as recommended by the person who supplied the aloe vera products). The results were astounding. Not only had the eczema been dramatically reduced, but Alex was sleeping better because there was less itching. What had been like angry red wheals on his body had almost disappeared after only a few weeks of applying the aloe vera products. To say I am hooked on aloe vera would be something of an understatement. All mothers with small children should take note and make sure they have some of these products available.

Leigh: HIV

Leigh is a young man who was diagnosed HIV positive in the early 1990s. At first he seemed to fall prey to colds and flu and generally felt low in spirit. He was prescribed antibiotics on several occasions. These made him quite sick, and he felt uneasy taking so many. Then came a change for the better as he relates.

I discovered aloe vera through a friend who invited me along to a talk. At the time I hadn't any money so I didn't buy anything. Very soon after that I fell sick again with a chest and sinus infection. Because of my condition, I also have bad problems with my gums, skin irritations and fungal infections, and, worst of all, I would wake up with a sickly stomach that made me start my day feeling worried and of course sick! One thing that stuck in my mind from the presentation was that by drinking aloe vera it started the healing process from the inside out, so I decided to give this aloe vera stuff a go. I started first with aloe toothgel, which immediately seemed to neutralise the acidity in my mouth and removed a lot of the yellow fur from my tongue. My gums improved quickly and have been fine ever since. Soon after starting the aloe vera drinking gel, I began to notice that if I took if first thing in the morning, twenty minutes or so after waking up, my morning sickness became treatable. I also found that it helped me empty my bowels in a more comfortable and complete way. I'm now able to control my bowel movements, so I can at least feel assured and have no fear of accidents through diarrhoea. Unfortunately in the past I had had some mishaps that, as you can imagine, made me feel awful.

The aloe vera gelly tube has a multiplicity of uses. Before aloe vera I had problems with thrush. Applying the gelly to my penis has stopped the red blotches from forming. I also use it between my toes, it soothes a sore bottom from too much wiping, haemorrhoids, sore nipples, and it also sealed a small cut on my finger, totally stopping any bleeding (this could have become a scary experience).

I could go on and on about incidents where I've been amazed at aloe vera's uses. Essentially, it has brought me much needed relief and a healthy mind. My energy level is much higher, enabling me to swim and be much more active, thereby improving my lifestyle. Aloe vera allows small irritations and problems to remain small. I have not had any courses of antibiotics since I started on it, and, very importantly, my T cell count is up by 100 (which can be medically explained). The choice to go with aloe vera is the one thing that has changed my life for the better. It has been quite difficult actually to put these ailments on paper, as it really made me sit and think about my situation. This is something that I very rarely do, but I decided that if anyone out there gets half the relief that I have had from aloe vera, then it's worth it.

Sarah: IBS

Sarah is a thirty-five-year-old international franchise development consultant, who has suffered with IBS for over fourteen years. Eight years ago she was introduced to aloe vera after years of suffering. She despaired of ever finding anything that could help ease her discomfort and thus improve her quality of life. Here she recounts her story of what living with IBS has been like.

I now believe that I originally developed IBS when I was doing night shift work and I was also under a lot of personal stress. For over ten years I, like so many other sufferers whom I have met and talked with, tried literally everything the doctors could prescribe. The treatments included bulking agents, a drug to help with bowel spasms, peppermint capsules and a homeopathic diet that became so boring and unpalatable I couldn't remain on it for longer than two months. Unfortunately none of these treatments worked for me and as I became more desperate, my condition seemed to worsen. I continued to suffer from severe constipation and diarrhoea, bloating, bowel spasms and severe abdominal pains. My condition was becoming progressively worse and it was having a seriously detrimental effect on both my work and personal life. It was an absolute godsend when I was introduced to what I subsequently christened my 'magic elixir' – because of what it did for me and the effect it had on me and my life. It was almost magical.

I was told that the aloe vera gel drink – a potent unflavoured drinking juice – was not sold for its taste and that I would need to take it consistently every day for between three and six months before I could expect to see any significant changes. I was taking one or two tablespoons consistently twice a day, morning and night and, within a few weeks, I started to see a slight calming effect. They were absolutely right though, it didn't taste very nice (an understatement!), and it was about eight weeks before I really started seeing a significant difference. I was less tired, the bloating and spasms became less frequent and the pain and discomfort seemed to ease. Previously I had lost about ten kilos and was well under my proper body weight, due mainly to the chronic diarrhoea I had suffered with. I managed to regain and stabilise my weight after being on the 'aloe regime' for about three months. It certainly helped stabilise the problem and seemed to boost both my immune system and energy levels. I still take aloe vera gel on a regular basis and although I work in a very high pressure industry, where deadlines, international travel and stress are everyday occurrences, I am still able to manage my IBS very effectively. Before I 'discovered' aloe vera, I was plagued with IBS on a daily basis.

Now, I may have a flare-up only once or twice a year, and that tends to be because I have over indulged myself on spicy foods or red wine (my favourites!). If that ever happens, all I have to do now is increase my intake of aloe vera immediately afterwards for a few days until the condition normalises. The most important effect aloe vera has had on my life is that I now enjoy a totally normal, if sometimes a little hectic, lifestyle where IBS is spelt with a little 'i-b-s' – I control it, it no longer controls me!

Linda: IBS

Linda had been an IBS sufferer for nine years when she was introduced to a new brand of aloe vera drinking gel. Within weeks she felt better and, to give some idea of the beneficial effects, she explains here what living with IBS had been like. Her symptoms are typical of those experienced by many IBS sufferers, as she describes.

The causes and effects of IBS vary from individual to individual. I personally react badly to alcohol, spicy food, rich sauces and citrus fruits, made worse if I feel under stress. The effect of these on me is severe distension of the gut, causing a lot of internal pressure and, in some situations, extreme pain.

> From this I would suffer either bad constipation or diarrhoea, each causing as much discomfort as the other. I tried various so-called remedies, including prescriptions from the doctor for a drug to help with bowel spasms, peppermint oil capsules and a bulking gel, none of which ever seemed to have any positive effect. I spent more money going to a homeopathic doctor, whose prescribed diet definitely seemed to help. However, after nearly two months of being unable to touch alcohol, spicy foods and other enjoyable food and drink, I couldn't stand it any more! I really believe that because of the very nature of IBS, if the medication or treatment regime is inconvenient or restricts your eating or other pleasures, it is unlikely you will stay with if for long. What I have experienced with this aloe vera gel drinking juice is that despite the fact that it doesn't taste too great, it is very convenient and, most importantly, I can now enjoy the food and drink that used to upset me so badly. I take about two full tablespoons morning and night (i.e. four tablespoons per day) and I have experienced a huge difference in the way I feel. I have been taking aloe vera for nearly four years and in that time I have felt better and fitter than at any time in the last nine years. I can quite confidently say that aloe vera has enabled me to enjoy a more or less pain-free life.

Jane: IBS

Jane, who lives in Cambridge, read about the benefits of aloe vera for IBS in her local newspaper, and found that it cleared up the problem in only a few months. However, she also found that aloe vera helped her in other ways.

> Being over seventy years old I had a few complaints, and asthma was something I had contracted in 1986 and was being treated for with steroids. To my surprise, I realised I was using my inhaler less frequently. The aloe vera gel drinking juice was also keeping the inflammation down, which helped me through chest infections. The ultimate happening was a hip replacement in 1996, combined with sensitive skin resulting from steroid treatment. My legs became very dry, scaly and sore, and once again I turned to aloe vera products – in this case, aloe liquid soap and aloe moisturising lotion, which I found invaluable.

Diana: IBS

In 1995 Diana was suffering a very stressful period in her life and at the same time developed very severe stomach cramps and headaches. Thinking the worst, she consulted her GP who suspected IBS but suggested she visit a consultant who in turn ran a series of tests on her stomach. There appeared to be no medical reason for the extreme discomfort and he therefore diagnosed IBS and prescribed a course of tablets. Diana explains what happened next.

> By a stroke of luck, the following day I read an article in the newspaper on the benefits of aloe vera, featuring someone who, like me, suffered very severely from IBS. As the address given was very near to my own office, I made an appointment and went directly there by taxi and obtained the aloe vera gel that same day. Within a few days of taking aloe vera I felt better and have never looked back, though very occasionally certain foods may trigger an attack. Not only has it helped my IBS but my general health and well-being have also greatly improved. I have recommended aloe vera to many of my friends and relations, not only for IBS but for various other reasons, and they all confirm they would not do without it now. Surprisingly enough, my husband has also had symptoms similar to IBS for the last couple of months and is at present going through various tests for elimination. I started him on aloe vera immediately and he is greatly improved, but of course, to be on the safe side he is continuing with his tests. I have also used aloe vera gelly and aloe vera heat lotion, which in turn were great for stings, sunburn and muscular pains.

Mary: IBS

Mary has had chronic IBS for ten years, and during that time has suffered from severe constipation, diarrhoea, stomach cramps, bloating and general discomfort. When she had her first two children, before she was introduced to the aloe vera gel drink, these symptoms became worse. Anybody who has been pregnant will know that trying to go to the lavatory can be very uncomfortable, but, as Mary explains, with IBS it's even worse.

> I used to get spasms quite unexpectedly, and if this happens when you're out you have to find a loo very quickly. I used to get panic attacks at the prospect of not being able to find a toilet, so it tends to restrict what you do and where you go. About a year before my third child was born, I read an article in a national newspaper that suggested aloe vera could help with digestive disorders. I haven't looked back since.

> KEY TIP
> I have taken aloe vera gel (it's a powerful drinking juice) every day and my third pregnancy was so much easier. All the bloating and spasms disappeared within a couple of months of starting the aloe vera and I was able to go to the loo without any discomfort. Talk about a major breakthrough, the relief was just brilliant!

All through my third pregnancy and since being on aloe vera I had much more energy and consequently never felt as tired as I did in my previous pregnancies. Additionally, if I ever get a tummy bug when I'm abroad on holiday (and this is much less frequently than I used to), I seem to recover much more quickly now than I ever did before. I now have three young children and a fairly hectic business and social life that can be very demanding, both physically and mentally. Taking aloe vera has changed my life for the better – I am so much improved that even my husband, who has watched the transformation, has now started to take this plant 'elixir'. I have recommended it to all my friends as a health tonic, and if they do have any sort of digestive disorder I have suggested they use aloe vera. I am Jewish and the aloe vera gel drink that I take has the kosher mark. For all you pregnant ladies out there, whatever religion you are, I recommended you try it, but just make sure it's the pure 100 per cent stabilised aloe vera drinking gel.

Ann: IBS

Ann is an IBS sufferer and had been drinking aloe vera regularly until her brother's unexpected death made her forget all about it. Her story is as follows.

We shared the same house and for many weeks I was in total shock and not eating. However, I gradually started to pick up the pieces and returned to eating better, but no doubt due to all the stress my IBS returned with a vengeance. Strange as it may seem I forgot all about the aloe vera gel until I started using the fridge again and suddenly spotted it after about a week. I promptly started back on it and the results were fantastic. My IBS eased off and I was able to eat more normally again. Another benefit that has occurred is the improvement in the condition of my skin. I had started to get small painful boils outside and inside my nose – something I had never had before. These, thankfully, have completely gone, leaving my skin soft and clear. I really do feel so very much better in such a short space of time and I am now not as depressed as I have been.

Lucy: IBS

Lucy's story is one of continual illness over a period spanning a quarter of a century! However she has finally got to grips with her problems and her life has since changed beyond all recognition, as she recounts.

I had suffered with a number of seemingly unconnected ailments for over twenty-five years and I just felt that nothing would help, that I was destined to be 'ill' forever. The problems included PMS, thrush and IBS. My joints were painful and swollen and I also suffered from severe bloating and stomach spasms. I was constantly overweight, and sometimes with the bloating I looked six months pregnant. I wheezed a lot and I never seemed to enjoy a good night's sleep, because of the continual pains in my joints. As a result, I felt constantly tired – it was like a vicious circle. I had also been on prescription drugs for many years. I took aspirin and cortisone for the pain, hormones for PMS and anti-fungal medications for thrush. To add to the problems, I also developed ulcers. I became so disillusioned with being constantly ill and the fact that conventional medications were obviously not working that I finally decided to take control of my own condition. I forced myself to become a student again and I learnt about complementary and alternative therapies. I began to practise yoga and found that it helped relax my body and mind! I learnt more about diet and decided to improve that part of my life radically.

I cut out red meat, tea, coffee, sugar and most processed foods, and began eating more wholefoods, and I started taking vitamin supplements. It was a bit like 'cold turkey'. There I was – a 'chocaholic' – banning myself from my favourite vice!

Although there was some improvement, it was not until I saw a therapist after a particularly nasty bout of IBS and candida that my health improvement accelerated into the fast lane. She specialised in food allergies and colonic irrigation and explained in great detail that my constant illnesses were due to the fact that I had so many accumulated toxins in my body and was effectively too weak to fight them. She also informed me that I was allergic to wheat and yeast, both of which I had eaten for years, and both of which were actually making me ill. She recommended a detox diet and advised me to start drinking aloe vera and taking vitamins. Within less than a year, my condition improved dramatically. I had lost over twenty-eight pounds, I was no longer troubled by migraines and PMS, and I was finally able to sleep properly at night. Several years later I am almost unrecognisable from that 'ill' person I once knew. I know it's never easy to change your diet, especially as radically as I did, but I would say to everyone out there who reads this and recognises or has experienced the same problems, it really is worth making the changes. I wish I had taken control of my life earlier and I wish I had started drinking aloe vera twenty-five years ago! Why – because I am finally enjoying my life again. I really feel that I wasted all those years just taking more and more medications and accepting my condition.

KEY TIP
Drinking aloe vera has made a huge difference to me but it's as much to do with your own attitude and single-minded determination to improve your own condition and not always accepting the opinions of one particular doctor or therapist. You must take control of your own situation.

Anita: lupus

In 1977, following the birth of her late son, Anita became unwell and was diagnosed with some form of arthritic condition, but it took another eight years before she was properly diagnosed as suffering from lupus, a condition that can sometimes prove fatal. She recounts her story.

It took eight years of consulting specialists before I eventually knew the real cause of my illness. I became a patient of one of the world's leading lupus specialists and was prescribed steroids (steroid substitutes made me feel even worse) and painkillers, which I had to take every day. Six years ago I was almost suicidal. I had put on over thirty-five pounds in weight and I could hardly walk because of the pain. I often collapsed in the street and was spending at least twenty per cent of my time in bed and shuffling to and from the en suite bathroom on my behind because I could not walk. Life was becoming more and more unbearable. About six years ago, a good friend of mine who knew how ill I was suggested that I try drinking something called aloe vera. I had never heard of aloe vera in the context of a drink, let alone something that may help me with the condition I had.

Anyway, she finally persuaded me to give it a go and I began taking this rather strange tasting health drink. Nothing startling happened for the first few weeks but I had been told not to expect any major changes for several months. After about ten weeks, something significant did happen. I realised that I had stopped dropping things and within a few more weeks I was able to walk up the stairs without leaning too heavily on the banister rail. These were major advances for me after so many years of continual and steady deterioration in my condition.

Although I had not been taking the product consistently or as originally instructed, when I saw the changes I decided that I had to take this product much more seriously. After only fourteen weeks I realised that I had not had a day's illness for over a month. It was incredible – aloe vera was really helping me get my life back. I then also started to take other nutritional supplements from the same company, and I weaned myself off painkillers, and also managed to reduce my steroid medication from forty-five milligrams per day to only five. I still have lupus but my hair is no longer falling out, my nails are long and strong, I have lost over two thirds of the weight I put on and I take only five milligrams of steroids and two paracetamol per day – and my aloe vera, of course! There is absolutely no question that aloe vera has been responsible for helping me keep my condition under control and has allowed me to lead much more of a normal life over the last few years. Lupus no longer rules me, I rule it!

Ginny: chronic sarcoidosis

Chronic what? you may ask. Well, at one point this condition, which is not exactly a 'household name' illness, nearly destroyed Ginny's life, as she explains.

Over seven years ago, I was diagnosed as having chronic sarcoidosis. I was doubly shocked – not just because I had been diagnosed with a serious problem – but also because it was something I had never even heard of. Chronic sarcoidosis is a multi-system disorder that the medical profession can offer no firm explanation as to how or from where it's contracted. The doctors did tell me that about fifty per cent of cases are diagnosed as benign, and are monitored until the disorder burns itself out after about two years. Another twenty-five per cent will suffer side effects and are given steroids to reduce inflammation and assist recovery. In the final twenty-five per cent of cases, the illness can run for years with damaging and sometimes fatal consequences. It can affect any part of the body, especially the eyes, lungs, skin, lymph nodes, liver and joints. With me it was my lungs and joints that were worst affected, and because my lungs were not working effectively, I was left continually exhausted after the slightest exertion.

The medical treatment focused primarily on the use of increasingly higher doses of steroids, which helped with the inflammation but had severe side effects. My weight increased dramatically and my face and neck swelled up. Eighteen months into the illness, the problems with my lungs seemed to be under control (because of the steroids) but the constant fatigue was becoming worse and I was beginning to develop symptoms similar to those of rheumatoid arthritis, which began to affect all my body joints. Because of the pain, discomfort and constant fatigue, I was unable to cope with normal everyday activities and I had to give up work as a result. My condition seemed to be deteriorating despite the use of steroids.

I also suffered quite serious and unpleasant side effects from the other drugs that were prescribed in an attempt to control the sarcoid. Furthermore, the stress of illness always has an affect on family life, and ours was no exception. My worsening condition called for desperate measures, and fortunately for me (someone, somewhere must have been looking out for me!) a friend introduced me to aloe vera soon after. Within only a week of taking this potent aloe vera drinking gel on a daily basis I began to notice a discernible difference in my joints – the pain was no longer so intense.

Within two weeks, the pain had been reduced still further. I seemed to have more energy and the constant fatigue I had endured for so long was on the decline. After only a month on the 'daily aloe regime' (four to six fluid ounces per day), the pain in my joints was reduced to a dull ache, the fatigue was less noticeable and I also had more energy. The real plus for me was that I was able to cut back on my steroid intake for the first time in three years, and hospital tests showed that the sarcoid was under control. I lost weight and that horrible puffiness that had plagued me for years disappeared – I started to look and feel like my old self again, which pleased both my daughter and my husband.

I am still taking aloe vera every day (I would never give that up!), and thankfully I am now able to lead a totally normal life, which is something I had been unable to do for years. Both my family and I owe the 'humble' aloe vera plant a huge debt of gratitude. It has completely changed my life (and that of my family) for the better, and has given me the chance to grab my life back from this horrible illness. I am now healthier than I have been for years and although I still have the illness, I no longer 'suffer' from it! I am now in control of my condition.

John: sinus infection

Having had his nose broken several times during the course of his rugby career, John had become quite prone to sinus and ear problems. Ten years ago, while in the Middle East on holiday, he contracted a severe chest and ear infection that spread to his sinuses, and over the next three years he was on various medications, including numerous courses of antibiotics and nasal sprays. Nothing seemed to work. He had a computerised axial tomographic or CAT scan and it was then that the doctors suggested he should have an operation to have his sinuses drained. Two unsuccessful and painful operations later and he still had the sinus infection. By this time he was becoming desperate, as he confirms.

> It was nearly three years since I had contracted the original infection and I continued to suffer from severe pain, headaches and general discomfort in the sinus area. My sinuses became blocked very easily and were almost impossible to clear. What's more, it was very debilitating and I could not really see an end to the problem. Soon after this a friend introduced me to aloe vera and said there was a particular product you could use for ear, nose and throat problems. As you can imagine I was extremely reticent about spraying some plant juice up my nose! Well, all I can say is that nearly eight years later I am very glad I did. The pain and discomfort went within days and I have not had any real problems since. I have drunk aloe vera gel every day since and I need only to use aloe activator very occasionally – probably only once or twice a year. I have not had a cold, flu, a sore throat or any ear or sinus problems for over seven years and, guess what – I have not had any antibiotics in that time either.

Jack: skin disorder

While Sheila and her husband were living in Cyprus, from 1987 to 1990, their son, Jack, then aged four, developed a skin problem on his face – extremely dry flaky skin on both cheekbones, just below his eyes. To begin with they tried various mild moisturising creams, but the problem became worse, spreading to the sides of his ears and up into his scalp. When they returned to the UK on home leave, Sheila took him to a GP who looked at the problem and prescribed a steroid cream for his face and another liquid for his scalp. The cream, when applied, turned the dry white flaky skin to bright red, shiny, sore-looking skin, making the problem seem even worse.

Sheila continues the story.

> We persisted with the cream, hoping that in time it would begin to take effect. The liquid was so strong that it was hurting his head, so we stopped using that altogether. The cream didn't help at all, so we took him back to the doctor who then prescribed another treatment – this time a very mild aqueous skin cream, which didn't work either. This was the first of many visits and umpteen different treatments, over a period of five years, during which time the skin problem continued to worsen. We tried all sorts of creams and numerous different products were prescribed, none of which seemed to have any positive effect. During this time he was being teased continually at school because of the dry scaly skin on his face and the dry skin on his scalp, which looked like very bad dandruff. Prior to this problem he had always liked a very short crew-cut hairstyle, but now he wanted his hair kept longer to hide the problem. The children at school began calling him 'dandruff face' and saying that he didn't wash his hair enough. As you can imagine, he was hurt by their taunts and was well and truly fed up with the whole business.
>
> In 1995, we were introduced to a new range of aloe vera products by my sister-in-law, and she recommended that we try an aloe vera cream with bee propolis on Jack's face. It was a relief to find something that was natural and chemical-free. It certainly couldn't do any harm, unlike some of the prescribed treatments that Jack had been given that contained steroids. We put the cream on his face three times a day, when possible, and were astonished at the outcome. Within a week or so there wasn't any trace of dry skin on his face. We couldn't believe that the problem had cleared up so quickly, especially after five years of to-ing and fro-ing to various doctors and trying all sorts of different creams in an attempt to sort it out. Before trying the aloe propolis cream we had been referred to a skin specialist, so we decided to use the cream on his face only, leaving his scalp as it was for the specialist to see, and hopefully diagnose the cause of the problem. We were so impressed by the success of the aloe and bee propolis cream that we took a tube with us, to show the skin specialist what we had used to cure the facial problem. The specialist looked at my son's scalp and suggested he might have nits, much to my indignation, as I knew for a fact that this wasn't the case. She took skin samples and said she would contact us the

following morning. When she phoned – no nits in evidence (we could have told her that!) – she didn't know what the problem was. Another scalp treatment was prescribed, a shampoo that we decided not to bother with as we had no intention of starting the same old rigmarole all over again. We decided to use more of the products from my sister-in-law, namely an aloe jojoba shampoo and also an aloe jojoba conditioner on his scalp, rather than the shampoo prescribed to us by the specialist.

After only a few treatments, we saw an incredible improvement and decided to continue to use the two products. His scalp condition is now totally healed and has remained so ever since, as has the problem on his face.

Maisy: injury

Maisy's holiday abroad was nearly ruined by a silly accident, as she confirms.

On the first day, someone trod on my foot and I lost most of the nail from my big toe. As you can imagine, this was very painful, my toe swelled and I was worried my holiday would be ruined, as I couldn't wear any of my shoes.

Immediately I covered the area with aloe vera gelly and a pad and bandage and didn't touch it for twenty-four hours. The next evening it was well on the way to healing and within a couple of days and several more applications of aloe vera gelly, it was no longer sore to touch – my holiday was saved.

Harold: duodenal ulcer

After several years of unsuccessful medical treatment for the duodenal ulcer he was suffering from, Harold was told that drinking aloe vera may help improve his condition. Initially, he was extremely sceptical, as he relates.

The medication had not helped and I was still suffering extreme discomfort from my ulcer. I had read about this aloe vera juice and quite frankly although I was highly sceptical about the claims and stories about its healing benefits, at that stage I would have tried anything. I started drinking the aloe vera juice and what surprised me was the first apparent benefit – the arthritis in my elbow had virtually disappeared! The pain from the ulcer gradually subsided and there seemed to be a continual improvement in my condition. Within about twelve to fourteen weeks the pain had totally disappeared and I also had more energy. The hernia operation I had subsequently caused little discomfort and the surgical wound healed very quickly – both of which I also put down to this amazing plant. I have gone from being highly sceptical to being a great advocate of the healing properties and benefits of aloe vera. Personally, I just feel better and it has undoubtedly improved my overall health and general well-being.

Ivy: leg ulcers

Ivy was a ninety-two-year-old woman who lived in a private nursing home. She developed leg ulcers on both legs that were quite large and became very painful. Over the five months she suffered with these sores, conventional medical treatment involved the use of proprietary medical gels and dressings. These treatments were given twice each day at a monthly cost of around £240 or £1,200 for the duration of the problem. However, there was no improvement in this time, the ulcers were deteriorating and the practice GP wanted to refer Ivy to the local hospital for treatment. The nursing home manager and senior nursing staff suggested that as a last resort before referral that they try a natural remedy – aloe vera gelly. It was the same proprietary brand that had been used so successfully in a recent clinical trial conducted by Dr Peter Atherton (as referred to earlier in this book).

They discussed this with Ivy's relatives and the family immediately agreed, as did the GP. The ulcers were duly cleaned with sterile water and then the aloe vera gelly was applied and a bandage placed over the ulcerated areas, and then left for three days. The process was repeated again three days later. When the bandages were removed for the second time, the ulcers had both completely healed and the crust over them had dropped off, leaving smooth unblemished skin. The cost of this totally successful aloe vera treatment was about £22 – the price of two tubes of the particular proprietary brand of aloe vera gelly. Ivy's relatives were all amazed at how quickly the aloe vera treatment had worked, as was the GP.

Although a very short case history, it does show the potency of aloe vera's healing properties and the speed at which it can work compared with some conventional treatments.

Wayne: psoriasis

As a sufferer of psoriasis, Wayne had used the normal over-the-counter medications. He had done this since he was fifteen, when he first contracted the ailment on his elbows and knees. These remedies had very little effect and when he was twenty-three, while working abroad, the condition deteriorated and the psoriasis spread to his hands, arms and knees. His hands kept splitting and bleeding, which meant he couldn't work. He consulted his GP several times and was given more creams, which again did not seem to alleviate the problem.

The condition deteriorated further with more cracking of the skin and bleeding, combined with swelling of the hands. He was still unable to work and his worsening condition made his hands so unsightly he wouldn't go out. July 2002 was a turning point in his life. He met someone at a rural show who was selling a proprietary brand of aloe vera products including drinks and skin care products. He decided to try them – feeling that he had nothing to lose – nothing else had ever worked!

He immediately started using an aloe vera drinking gel, an aloe soap and a topical cream with aloe vera and bee propolis, and within only five weeks his hands, knees and elbows had been transformed (see Colour Plates 9–14). The swelling had gone, the cracking had healed and the bleeding had stopped.

Since then Wayne has been able to return to work full time and he is able to go out without people staring at his hands. Aloe vera has helped his psoriasis and changed his life – he says he would recommend the aloe vera products he has used to anyone. He is now clear of the problem but is aware that flare-ups can occur again. This time he will be prepared!

For further details of this story please refer to Appendix 1.17.

Eva: Acne rosacea

Eva had suffered from a facial dry skin complaint since she was a little girl, and when she was nine she was diagnosed with eczema. The hydrocortisone treatment she was prescribed had no effect on her condition but another cream, Betnovate, did help provide some relief from her 'facial fire'.

Within ten years medical opinion had changed and Betnovate was no longer recommended for facial applications. Eva's skin specialist switched her to a basic 'over the counter' skin cleanser. This was satisfactory for several years but by her mid-twenties the facial condition had flared up again and this time it was almost uncontrollable. The specialist decided to reintroduce Betnovate, as nothing else had helped, but it was to be applied sparingly.

In 1993, Eva's condition was diagnosed as rosacea. A biopsy of facial tissue revealed that she had an allergic reaction to gemel – a preservative found in many beauty and daily care bathroom products. She had to avoid all products containing this substance, now known as imidazolidinyl urea, and she also stopped using soap or shower gel on her face. This new regime, which included the occasional use of Betnovate, helped manage Eva's condition and keep the rosacea under control. She needed to use Betnovate only three or four times each year for a few days until the flare-up in her rosacea subsided.

In October 2002 Eva was taken off Betnovate and put on an aqueous cream for washing and moisturising her face. It didn't work. The pictures (Colour Plates 15 & 16), show a typical sufferer. She has suffered more severe skin flaking and even bleeding on occasions. During such flare-ups she can also experience the most uncomfortable 'sunburn sensation'.

In early December 2002 Eva was introduced to a particular proprietary brand of aloe vera and she soon 'discovered' the healing properties of this amazing plant. She used a topical aloe vera gelly and experienced almost instant relief from the burning sensation she had had for years. Within a couple of days of first applying the product twice a day, morning and evening, her face was almost completely normal. In January of 2003, Eva also started taking a peach-flavoured aloe vera gel drinking juice (sixty millilitres per day) to help the healing process from the inside out and to help reduce the frequency of its recurrence. To date, her condition has continued to improve with a substantial reduction in frequency of recurrent 'flare-ups'.

Susan: iron burn

While doing the ironing at home one day, Susan was distracted by a noise in the house and swung around to see what it was with the iron still in her hand. The hot iron hit her left inner forearm and left a severe burn with the triangular outline of the iron clearly visible.

When I first saw the burn a week later it looked 'angry' with some infection and scabbing in the centre, still with a clear outline of the iron – almost like a 'cattle brand' burnt into her skin. She told me that she had not seen a doctor and I immediately suggested that she wash the area and then apply a combination of a topical aloe vera gelly and an aloe cream with bee propolis (a natural antibiotic). Within an hour she told me that she felt the tightness in the area easing.

I gave her a tube of the gelly to take away with her to apply as often as she felt necessary. By the next week the tightness had disappeared, there was no inflammation, the outer part of the burn was becoming less obvious and the whole area was clearly healing well, with some minor scabs still evident in the centre.

Three weeks later, there is still some evidence of the burn mark but little sign of any permanent scarring. She thought it was miraculous that in only a matter of a few weeks there is almost no sign of what was a very nasty and painful burn. She feels that everyone should keep a tube of aloe vera gelly in their fridge in case of such accidents, whether caused by an iron, hot pans, grills, etc. – the kitchen can be a hazardous place!

Case histories from Dr Audun Myskja

The following case histories are those from patients of Dr Audun Myskja or people who have been referred to him in his capacity as a private GP and therapist. They represent a small fraction of the total number of people whom he sees every year at his private clinic in Oslo, Norway.

Linda: neurological disorders: hereditary spastic paraplegia (hereditary spastic paraparesis or HSP)

Linda is a big bouncy girl in her mid-thirties. She strikes people who meet her as a down-to-earth personality with a lust for life and great humour. Meeting her for the first time, it is hard to take in the fact that she has suffered since childhood from a hereditary, progressive disease of the neuromuscular system, called hereditary paraparesis. There are many different diseases of the neuromuscular system. Hereditary spastic paraplegia (hereditary spastic paraparesis, or HSP) is a name used to represent a group of inherited degenerative spinal cord disorders characterised by a slow, gradual, progressive weakness and spasticity (stiffness) of the legs. Symptoms may be first noticed in early childhood, or at any age through adulthood. Initial symptoms may include difficulty with balance, weakness and stiffness in the legs, muscle spasms, and dragging the toes when walking. In some forms of the disorder, bladder symptoms (such as incontinence) may appear, or the weakness and stiffness may spread to other parts of the body.

The rate of progression and the severity of symptoms are quite variable even among members of the same family. Gradual deterioration may occur in some families, with symptoms of the disorder beginning earlier and more severely in successive generations. HSP rarely results in complete loss of lower limb mobility, though mobility devices such as canes, walkers or wheelchairs may be necessary. In some patients, the symptoms continue to increase throughout their life. For others, symptoms may begin in early childhood, worsen for a few years and then level off after adolescence. HSP progresses slowly over the years after onset, leading to a lack of nerve impulses and muscular activity in the extremities. Gradually it becomes harder to walk, the patient suffers reduced circulation to the tissue and muscles and the extremities become weaker. One serious side effect of this condition is that even small bruises or sores can grow to large ulcers, due to a lack of circulation and nutrients.

A few years ago, Linda developed a small sore on her left leg that gradually worsened, spreading to the whole leg, which developed into a large gangrene. The leg had to be amputated and a prosthesis fitted. Three years later, after tripping and falling, she cut her right leg. What had initially seemed to be a fairly harmless wound worsened. No matter what she tried, including pastes, bandages and wound-reducing substances applied at the hospital surgery, the wound continued to deteriorate. The situation was becoming depressingly like the one she had experienced three years previously. When she next went to the hospital for her weekly treatment and check-up, the news was bad. She was told that her leg could not be saved and that it would have to be amputated in two or three months. She was told there was no option but that there was now an improved prosthesis that would allow her to maintain mobility and a reasonable quality of life.

She was sent home with local ointments to continue the treatment, and she was to go back to the hospital in a month's time to review the situation. Linda had accepted the loss of one foot but being without both feet was too much to bear.

She started to look for alternatives and tried different home remedies and treatments to help improve her circulation. But there was no improvement in her condition and the ulcer kept spreading and growing. A friend told her about the wound-healing properties of aloe vera and she felt she had nothing to lose by trying it out. She tried an aloe vera spray applied liberally on the ulcerous tissue, followed by a topical aloe vera cream combined with bee propolis, a natural antibiotic substance from the beehive that also has powerful wound-healing properties. She also drank aloe vera to boost both her nutrient intake and her immune system. She told me some months later that she didn't believe it at first but after only a week she could clearly see fresh tissue growing in the bottom of the wound. The pus around the wound edges was gradually vanishing and fresh granulation tissue was forming daily. She felt elated that at last there might be a cure for her problem. After two weeks she contacted the doctors at the hospital and told them that they might wish to review their decision, just once more. She got an appointment a week later and she described the meeting with the hospital staff. It was hard to put in words what happened the moment they took off the bandage and saw the leg. But there is no mistaking the surprised looks and raised eyebrows when they clearly saw the wound was healing, with fresh tissue spreading like wildfire!

She did not dare tell them what she was taking, but they were saying: 'This is indeed surprising, to say the least. It looks like you'll keep your foot after all. We're very happy for you, but can't explain what has happened.'

Almost three years later, Linda's one healthy foot is indeed still healthy and has only small traces of her former leg ulcer. Linda now leads a full life and never forgets either her daily dose of aloe vera or to massage her leg with aloe vera cream first thing in the morning. It really does beg the question – what if she had known about the healing powers of aloe vera before? Would she have had the first amputation?

Erik: juvenile rheumatoid arthritis (JRA) and Bekhterev's disease

Erik is Korean and was adopted by Norwegian parents as a baby. He is an only child with a strong personality and a great love of the Korean martial art Tae Kwon Do.

When his behaviour in kindergarten became unruly, moving about and refusing to sit still, it was thought to be due to hyperactivity and his rather individualistic personality. However, later on during his early school years, he developed stomach pains that were initially thought to be psychogenic. Only when he developed irregular bouts of diarrhoea, investigations were made and coeliac disease was found after a coloscopy, by a tissue sample taken from the large intestine. Coeliac disease is a condition caused by an inability to digest gluten and often results in bowel symptoms, weight loss or failure to gain weight, and a lack of certain vitamins and minerals with consequential problems such as anaemia and osteoporosis. Diarrhoea and bulky, smelly motions that float often occur in coeliac disease. This results in fewer nutrients being absorbed from the bowel and thus weight loss or failure to grow and put on weight in children. Sufferers sometimes have a swollen or bloated belly. As Erik approached puberty, he was becoming increasingly tired. He felt stiff in the morning and had difficulty in getting to school on time. New investigations showed nothing at first, but after some time specialists at the rheumatic hospital found that he had a mixture of juvenile rheumatoid arthritis (JRA or Still's disease) and Bekhterev's disease. JRA is a disease that causes swelling and pain in the joints. Arthritis can also prevent people from moving their joints properly. JRA normally affects children under the age of sixteen. These children tend to have arthritis in one or more joints and swelling and pain that lasts for six weeks or more.

Although it has a similar name, JRA is not the same disease as rheumatoid arthritis, a disease that affects adults.

JRA has different symptoms and doesn't damage bones as quickly as the rheumatoid arthritis that affects older people. Bekhterev's disease is a chronic and progressive autoimmune disease characterised by arthritis, inflammation and eventual immobility of a number of joints. The disease usually involves the spine and surrounding spinal structures. Its principal location is in the spine and sacroiliac joints. In the spine, the small synovial joints and the margins of the intervertebral discs are both affected. These structures become bridged by bone and the spine is accordingly rigid. Ankylosing spondylitis is a disease of men but there is disagreement among authors as to the male-to-female sex ratio, varying from three-to-one to eight-to-one. Onset usually occurs between the ages of fifteen and thirty-five. Symptoms of the disease are generally milder among females.

In the course of the following year, Erik's condition progressively worsened. His sedimentation rate was increasing and his haemoglobin counts were falling. X-rays showed inflammation in several joints. When he and his parents went to one of his regular control appointments at the haematological department in the central hospital in Oslo, the specialists decided to put him on high doses of cortisone and metotrexate, a strong chemotherapy drug often used in cancer treatment. His parents were afraid that this would damage his health and hamper his growth. I figured that there was time to try other methods before deciding on the treatment with strong drugs and asked them to try a topical aloe vera product locally on his joints, together with doses of about forty millilitres of an aloe vera gel drinking juice, morning and evening.

We discussed dietary measures and tried to find a balance between his wish to live normally, like other boys of his age, and taking into account the combined dietary needs of his coeliac disease and of his JRA and Bekhterev's disease. In addition he started to do special exercises at home to help develop muscle tone and increase joint flexibility. I also showed him and his parents acupressure points that he could use on himself to relieve tension, stiffness and pain. During this time I also liaised with both the principal at his school and his teachers to discuss with them his condition and how the symptoms of his condition could affect his behaviour. He was almost always late for school, often skipped school altogether and had little motivation or capacity for study. Together, we developed a plan to improve the co-operation between home and school, and prevent any continuing misunderstandings.

The first signs of improvement came after only three or four weeks. He was a little less tired in the morning and had less stiffness in his joints. He was able to move freely and sit still for longer periods at a time. As the autumn passed, he had fewer days of absence from school and managed to get there on time more often. His condition improved steadily through the winter and he gradually felt stronger.

At a meeting with his parents and his schoolteachers in March, the school authorities were clear that everything was on the right track.

Erik's school records showed that his absenteeism had decreased and the school principal confirmed that Erik was much more co-operative and seemed much more stable, emotionally. When Erik went to his next control appointment with the specialists at the rheumatic hospital, they found no traces of rheumatic activity and his sedimentation rate was normalised, the haemoglobin counts were up and x-rays showed no signs of inflammation in peripheral joints. I hesitate to recount this as one of the most spectacular cases that I have seen but I have all the hospital records to back up his improvement. Two years on, Erik is an athletic young man who basically functions normally, with only a few relapses into some morning stiffness and low back pain. Perhaps his martial arts training has a greater effect on his health when he takes aloe vera. Drinking aloe vera has been shown to strip tissue of uronic acid and other waste material. I cannot explain what happened but I believe that aloe vera may have been one contribution to the breaking of the vicious cycles in his physiology and thought patterns, which started a self-healing process. Erik does not care about the explanations. He simply wants to live his life and not 'have to think about my health all the time, like an old lady', as he puts it. However, he would not consider a day without taking aloe vera.

Hilda: osteoarthritis (OA)

Hilda is a widow in her late seventies and belongs to the generation of Norwegians who rebuilt the country after World War II. Her children have always said she has always put others before herself. She has always been very active, with gardening and running her house. She has tended to avoid doctors and hospitals, sticking to her regime of hard work, a healthy lifestyle and home remedies. When she started to get a pain in her right hip, she wouldn't admit it at first. She went to see her doctor only when the pain became so severe that it interfered with her sleep and she found gardening and vacuuming very difficult. An x-ray showed moderate osteoporosis and osteoarthritis (OA) in her right hip. OA is the commonest form of joint disease. It is generally considered to be due to 'wear and tear' of the joints leading to damage of the joint surfaces, which causes pain when the person moves that joint. There are many factors influencing its development, including a family history of OA and previous damage to the joint through injury or surgery. OA is very common in older age groups but can also affect younger people.

Symptoms in OA tend to get worse with increased activity, so that the end of the day is the worst time (in contrast to inflammatory arthritis). There may be hard, bony swelling of the joints and a gritty feeling (or even noise) when the joint is moved (this is called crepitus). Treatment is aimed mainly at symptom relief and tends to be based on simple painkillers and anti-inflammatory drugs. Physiotherapy is also valuable in helping to strengthen muscle groups that stabilise and protect the affected joint. When weight-bearing joints such as hips, knees and ankles are involved it is important for overweight patients to lose weight, as this puts extra strain on these joints. Osteoporosis is a disease in which bones become fragile and more likely to break. If not prevented or if left untreated, osteoporosis can progress painlessly until a bone breaks.

These broken bones, also known as fractures, occur typically in the hip, spine, and wrist. Any bone can be affected, but of special concern are fractures of the hip and spine. A hip fracture almost always requires hospitalisation and major surgery.

It can impair a person's ability to walk unassisted and may cause prolonged or permanent disability or even death. Spinal or vertebral fractures also have serious consequences, including loss of height, severe back pain and deformity. Hilda started on non-steroid anti-inflammatory drugs, but she stopped taking them after two weeks, because of stomach pain. The doctor stated that the OA was not advanced enough to make hip replacement necessary at this point. She asked a few friends if they knew of anything else that could help with her pain and disability.

A lady she knew had got relief from joint pains by both drinking and applying aloe vera, and recommended it to her. Hilda decided to try this new approach. She drank fifty millilitres of aloe vera juice twice per day, sprayed her hip with an aloe vera spray and applied an aloe vera gelly on her joints. Gradually the pain subsided and after three weeks she was able to resume normal activities in the house and also started gardening again. X-rays showed that her OA had not changed. Whether aloe vera has contributed to the halt in the progression of her disease we don't know. However, Hilda feels certain that aloe vera has contributed to her relative freedom from pain and the improvement in her quality of life.

Stein: radiation damage

Stein was a hard-working entrepreneur, who had built up a chain of quality bakeries with several dozen employees. As a baker, he often worked the whole year round from early morning till midnight, year in, year out. When he started getting headaches, he thought at first it was due to long-term stress and decided to reduce his workload. He started taking weekends off and even sold a couple of his stores. He felt a little less tired but the headaches continued and became worse. He had splitting headaches for hours at a time and even strong painkillers only partially alleviated his pain. He contacted his family doctor, who knew him as the type of person who never sought help, even for serious conditions. His doctor arranged for an immediate appointment for a CAT scan. The results of the CAT scan, a few days later, showed a brain tumour in the left frontal lobe of the brain that had already grown to the size of a plum. It had developed to a point where surgery was not possible and there was no chemotherapy available that could help him.

Stein decided to start radiation therapy and he was given the maximum dose of radiation to the head for over a month. The radiation reduced the tumour a bit and his headaches subsided a little. His situation, however, did not improve. He had persistent itching and pain because of the severe radiation damage to his skin. When I saw him for the first time, his skin was red and blistery over all of the left side of his head and face. His eyelids were so swollen that the oedema even made it hard for him to see. He tried to stop scratching the swollen skin that constantly itched while we were talking and asked me if I knew of anything that could be of help. I had read the reports on the use of aloe vera for radiation damage to the skin. I started him on an intensive regime of both drinking aloe vera and applying liberal amounts of a topical aloe vera gel to the affected tissue. We arranged another appointment for fourteen days later. When Stein walked through my surgery door two weeks later, I hardly recognised him. I have never so sorely missed my lack of photo documentation. His skin was smooth and clear like a baby. He smiled and greeted me with a hug. He was so excited when he recounted what had happened. He said that his skin started to heal after only three days and that he could feel the burning sensation gradually reducing. The itching had stopped after a week and he felt like a new man. This is similar to the experience of the patient in the Collins and Collins work in 1935. After this incident, Stein remained one of my closest patients and he had no more problems for many months. However, after nine months the headaches started again and a new CAT scan showed that the tumour had started growing again. He started a new course of radiation therapy and this time he continued with aloe vera during the treatment. He had no skin problems during the second course of treatment and enjoyed another twelve months of good health.

Unfortunately, a year later, the brain tumour gradually took the upper hand and he died peacefully after a few weeks of gradually losing consciousness. Throughout the time we knew each other, he never tired of reminding me of the miraculous effect that aloe vera had had on his skin. He also felt that aloe vera had helped boost his energy levels far into the late stages of his disease.

Janet: chronic fatigue syndrome

Janet's commitment to her job as a language teacher and her willingness to help people was always recognised and appreciated by friends and pupils alike. She went through a period where she had many pupils with learning and behaviour difficulties in school, many of them from difficult backgrounds. Janet went out of her way to help them, often crossing the boundary between professional and private life. At the same time she was under a lot of stress, burdened by both financial difficulties and personal problems. She was continually tired and weak and she contracted a virus infection, diagnosed as glandular fever (infectious mononucleosis) or Epstein-Barr virus infection.

Glandular fever (infectious mononucleosis) is a virus infection characterised by a sore throat, fever, enlarged and tender glands and sometimes inflammation of the liver (hepatitis). It frequently causes a prolonged period of tiredness and can be severely debilitating. Glandular fever often starts with a few days of mild symptoms, including headache and tiredness. The major symptoms then develop and may last seven to twenty-one days. They can vary in how badly they affect you but usually include a fever, sore throat and tiredness, along with aches and pains all over the body. This phase of the illness may last a few days to a few weeks and is accompanied by tender enlargement of the glands (the lymph glands or lymph nodes), which are around the body to help defend against infection. Janet did have recurring fevers, swollen glands and felt unable to move for several weeks. When she recovered, a general feeling of illness and lethargy remained. Even getting up to go to the toilet or fetching a glass of water became almost insurmountable tasks – as if she had to run a full marathon. After some weeks of slow recovery, she felt she couldn't let down the people who were dependent on her, so she decided, fuelled by a sense of obligation, to go back to work. After the first few days at work she felt something was seriously wrong. At the end of each day, she felt totally drained and had no energy even to cook.

After a month, she had to take sick leave and gradually recovered, mainly through resting or sleeping eighteen to twenty hours a day. Although she was showing little sign of improvement, she soon became bored and decided after two weeks of rest that she might as well go back to work.

She had received dozens of calls and postcards from colleagues and pupils at school, often with heart-warming messages. The messages showed how appreciated her work at school was and how sorely she was missed. However, when she went back to work her lethargy remained. She started to feel depressed and hopeless about her general health situation. Her GP had said there was nothing to be done about her health situation except to wait and hope for the best. She made a desperate call to our health clinic and asked us for help. When she came to me she looked thin, pale and worn out.

I felt she needed to boost her vitality and gave her exercises that involved vitalising movements (the five Tibetan exercises), body movement, breathing exercises and self-healing meditations. She got a training programme and was put on the strengthening diet with regular meals, including salads, vegetables, meat, fish and rice, liberally spiced up with garlic, ginger, horseradish and stimulating condiments.

We also introduced her to aloe vera drinking juice. She was instructed to take forty to fifty millilitres twice every day. I also taught her kidney massage and acupressure points to combat low vitality. When she came back to see me after three weeks, she described the feeling of being like a flat tyre that had been mended and gradually pumped up again. Gradually she recovered her old self and was able to resume her normal life.

I saw her again a few days before I wrote this case history. Now, a year after our first appointment, she has a new zest and vigour about her. It is hard to say if drinking aloe vera alone would have given the same improvement in her health. In cases like these I find it necessary to look at the whole life situation and lifestyle and build up health and general vitality with the combination of diet, exercise, herbs and plant remedies and mind-body techniques, tested by centuries of experience. However I believe that aloe vera played a significant role in her improvement.

The British veterinarian Peter Green conducted an investigation into horses with chronic fatigue syndrome or lethargy syndrome. It is presumed that this condition arises after virus infections, but blood samples seldom reveal a certain cause for the horses' lassitude. In contrast to humans, these horses show leucopenia, or low count of white blood cells, revealing that the tired horses have a reduced level of resistance to infections and attacks on the immune system. No matter the cause, which may be viral, bacterial or unknown, the owners report that the horses seem lifeless and dull, and fail in races, show jumping or other activities. The sixteen horses included in this trial had had leucopenia, lethargy and depression for more than three weeks, but no other signs of disease. Many of these horses had tried multivitamins or bacterial wall extracts (e.g. equimmune), without significant effect, but none of the horses included were given concurrent treatments while on the aloe vera therapy. The horses were given oral aloe vera gel, 240 millilitres daily, for three to five weeks. Consistently in all horses but one, the white blood cell count rose and all horses but two returned to eventing or similar activities. This shows that horses given aloe vera had an improvement significantly stronger than horses with the same or a comparable clinical condition that tried other treatments or no treatment.

Dr Green ascribes this clinical effect of aloe mainly to the acemannan component, a potent immuno-stimulant that has been known to enhance macrophage phagocytosis and release of interleukin-1-alpha, tumour necrosis factor and prostaglandins (PGE2). Acemannan further activates T cell production of cytokines and makes immune cells more efficient in their functional activity.

Is this an adequate description of what went on in Janet's body during her recovery? Taking all factors into account, horses or humans, I think it is safe to say that aloe vera *might* have made a significant contribution to Janet's recovery.

Hilda: Crohn's disease

Hilda is in her mid-thirties and is a natural carer. She has worked in health services with old, mentally handicapped and disabled residents since her early twenties. Latterly, she has been studying natural and alternative therapies, in order to expand her knowledge and ability to help people. Despite the fact that Hilda has worked hard to help other people, she herself has suffered from poor health for some time. Even in her late teens she started feeling that something was wrong with her health. She often felt weak and had to rest after school. As a baby, she had suffered from colic for the first year of her life. Now, in her thirties, she again started getting stomach cramps several times a week. She was put on different types of diets, none of which seemed to help her much.

Gradually the cramps became worse and she started to suffer from moderate to severe stomach pains, often lasting hours at a time. Initially, the pains were occurring at irregular intervals and were ascribed to stress. But when she started getting diarrhoea and had to go to the toilet several times a day, only to pass watery liquids, her mother felt that something was wrong. Hilda went to see the family doctor who immediately realised the seriousness of the situation and arranged a hospital appointment. The resultant examination showed a distended abdomen and blood samples showed that she was anaemic, probably due to the loss of blood. At first, an x-ray of the colon did not show any definite pathologies but as investigations continued over the following months, Hilda's condition deteriorated. After a coloscopy showed that there were spots of severe inflammation in large parts of the colon, the small intestines were investigated and it was found that she had Crohn's disease. This is presumed to be an autoimmune disease, closely related to ulcerative colitis and maybe caused by the immune system reacting to bacteria in the colon. Shortly after Hilda's diagnosis was confirmed, she was prescribed steroids. Initially, her condition improved on this regime but after a couple of years she gradually started to deteriorate again. She became unwell and started suffering from painful stools mingled with blood, loss of weight and appetite and a general feeling of weakness. This time, an increased dose of steroids did not improve her situation.

When her mother contacted me, her general health had deteriorated. She had recently been admitted to the hospital, without much improvement in her condition. Even after treatment with painkillers, she had so much pain that her mother feared for Hilda's sanity and health. She had an appointment at the surgical department of the general hospital that treated her. This consultation was due in August, and the gastroenterologist's conclusion after coloscopy was that the activity of her disease had increased to a point where it was necessary to have an operation. A large part of the intestines would be excised and she would have to live with a colostomy. She got an appointment at our clinic to see if anything could be done about this decision.

Hilda panicked at the very thought of a colostomy and spent several sleepless nights picturing herself with a plastic bag hanging from her stomach, cringing at the thought.

I put her on a diet consisting mainly of vegetables, rice and fish and taught her meditation and visualisation concerned with her condition, and aimed at the alleviation of her symptoms. I also taught her how to use acupressure points especially for the intestines. Furthermore I put her on an aloe vera drinking juice (forty to fifty millilitres, twice daily). We arranged another appointment for four weeks later. When I saw her again I noticed she had much rosier cheeks. When I first met her she looked sickly and was unusually pale. She told me that she felt much fitter and had a suspicion that her condition might be slowly improving. When she went back to the hospital in November to prepare for the operation, the surgeons were surprised to find that the coloscopy showed a drastic reduction in the activity of her disease. The operation was postponed and a control at the surgery a month later showed that Hilda's clinical condition had been stabilised. She has continued faithfully with aloe vera and her other self-healing techniques. As I'm writing this passage, more than three years after first meeting Hilda, she has still not had to have surgery. She has had her ups and downs, suffering periods with some pain in the abdominal area, but thankfully these have been few and far between. She is now making a new life for herself as a natural therapist, combined with part-time work in the health services.

Hilda will never reduce her aloe vera intake because she knows that she becomes weaker and the stomach pains quickly return. She simply doesn't want to 'experiment with her health'.

Sonia: constipation

Sonia was in her late fifties when she contacted me. I was lecturing in a town on the west coast of Norway and she insisted on speaking to me after the lecture. She told me she wished to see me, in order to find out if I could be of help with her chronic pain syndrome. She had suffered from back pain since puberty. Her problems increased when she had a slipped disc and she had hoped to get rid of her pains when she had an operation. Instead, the pain worsened after the operation and two other operations in the same low back region two and five years later did not improve the situation. She had developed scar tissue, which created its own pain syndrome on top of what she already suffered. Exercise had a limited effect. Pushing herself increased her pain and she seemed to be in a vicious circle of pain and dysfunction.

Gradually she became increasingly immobile, had troubles walking even short distances, and became a chronically disabled patient. When I met her, she had been in a wheelchair for several years. She had, in a way, adjusted to the chronic pain but the side effect of her immobility, which was causing her more of a problem than the pain itself, was constipation. The fact that she suffered from constipation was not surprising, since she ate little and had little body movement. In addition, she took medicines for her pain containing codeine. We know that one of the possible side effects people have when using these drugs may be constipation. The constipation was causing persistent bloating and a feeling of being unwell. The only way for her to reduce the constipation was to increase her intake of laxatives. At the time of our first consultation, she was using thirty laxative tablets every day and even on this regime she was still suffering from constipation.

I introduced her to aloe vera drinking juice and we started carefully on very small daily doses, so as not to cause disturbances in her failing digestive system. We gradually increased the daily dosage to thirty millilitres, then to sixty, then to ninety per day.

At the same time I taught her abdominal massage to reduce pressure in the abdominal cavity, and acupressure points for constipation. We had another consultation the next day, to determine that she had understood the instructions and was able to follow up what we had agreed on. She lived in another town, so we couldn't easily arrange a further appointment. A month later, she called me as we had agreed and she told me that the aloe vera juice had helped her constipation like no other remedy she had ever tried through the years she'd been suffering. Week by week she had reduced her dosage of laxatives. At the time she called, she was down to only three tablets daily. After this small 'miracle' her condition stabilised, though it was still hard for her to be completely without laxatives.

Two years later, she is still on the aloe vera regime and she is almost totally free of constipation. She tells everyone she meets about her aloe vera success story. When I met her, she had a sceptical attitude towards all natural remedies. Now, due to the overall improvement in her health and well-being, she is one of the most devoted aloe vera ambassadors I know.

Carl: hereditary diseases (Osler's disease or Telangiectasia hereditaria)

When Carl grew up, his boyhood was marked by his mother's strange and unpredictable symptoms. She often suffered from nose bleeds and splitting headaches. He did not dare to ask her for help, even in his early years, as she always seemed to be tired and plagued by splitting headaches. No one knew the reason and she died of a sudden brain haemorrhage when she was in her forties. Carl grew up as a healthy boy and had a successful business career, starting in his early twenties. He didn't connect his problems with his mother's fate when he first started getting headaches and nose bleeds. After he had been admitted to a hospital twice with nose bleeds that were almost impossible to stop, he was diagnosed with Osler's disease, also known as Telangiectasia hereditaria. Growing up, he had never understood the cause of his mother's failing health but now it seemed all too obvious. She had had the same disease, in the same way as her mother before her, who had also died at an early age, with similar complaints. The doctors told him that his life expectancy would be similar to his mother's and grandmother's and that he should make the most of his life, given the short remaining life span he could expect.

Carl was then in his early forties. He tried to accept his fate and live life to the full in his remaining years, choosing to minimise his business activities, in order to live a quiet life with the people he loved. He sold the impressive family home in the city suburbs and converted their lakeside cabin in a rural forest to a permanent residence, finding more peace and happiness out of the rat race.

We met on a ferry while on holiday with our families. From the first meeting, Carl struck me as a wise and gregarious person, with a 'larger than life' air about him. He told me about his life and it was obvious he had lived it to the full and seen more of the world than most other people I had met. He had apparently once smuggled Mohammed Ali away from waiting crowds and police escorts on first saying hello to him, in order to take him to a private party – a snapshot of a life spent all over the world, in the company of kings and paupers. It seemed his life had been both hard work and one big long party.

We immediately 'hit it off' and he was soon telling me about his health problems. People in the region knew of my reputation as a doctor with knowledge of both ordinary and natural forms of treatment, and he asked me for advice and help. This knowledge was put to the test the day after when we played volleyball. A ball hit Carl in his face and blood started spurting from his nose like oil from a drilling rig. He was sent to the hospital immediately but it was almost impossible to stop the bleeding. The doctors at the local hospital feared for his life. Thankfully, after three days, the situation was stabilised and he was discharged. We started talking about a health programme to increase his odds for survival. He always went for regular check-ups with his doctors at the central hospital but there was no curative treatment to offer. He took steroids for symptom relief and had regular blood transfusions at the hospital. Over the previous two years before we met, he had been regularly admitted to the hospital with acute haemorrhages that were both more frequent and more severe. I taught him lymph drainage for his deficient circulation and acupressure points that could be effective in preventing bleeding. I also searched through my pharmacy of natural remedies and found that only aloe vera had proved to have specific actions on the mechanism of blood clotting and worked as an adaptogen. This meant that it could also help the veins and tissues adapt to the clinical situation and that aloe vera could also work to halt ongoing bleeding, at least partly.

I was unsure of the effect of applying aloe vera directly on the vulnerable veins in the nose and upper airways, so he started drinking aloe vera and massaging aloe vera on the acupressure areas in the face connected with the nose and regulation of bleeding. Aloe vera can penetrate skin and tissue and strengthen the process of building up of normal tissue and vessels. At this point Carl had no belief in natural and alternative treatment but he agreed to try it, mainly due to our mutual rapport and the fact that there was little else to try and little to lose. When he called me a month later, he said that his chronic tiredness had been reduced and he had more energy. This was probably connected to the fact that his haemoglobin level had been increasing steadily. It had been down to the level of little over half of the normal value. The month after returning from our holidays, he was again admitted with bleeding but this time it was easier to stop, and he was discharged the next day. He had been treated with steroids and he was gradually able to reduce the dosage of the cortisone drug prednisolon.

The haematology specialist at Carl's hospital was increasingly baffled. Olser's is a genetic disease, and investigating Carl's brain vessels by CAT scans the haematology specialists at his hospital found so many malformations of vessels that they couldn't understand how he could go so long and do so well on the drastically reduced doses of steroids he had started on. As I am writing this, five years have passed since I first met Carl. Now in his mid-fifties, he has outlived his prognosis and has enjoyed a full year without hospital admissions. He is now recommending aloe vera to everyone he knows and he has started using aloe vera topically in his nose and mouth, in addition to drinking the juice. Carl has also continued doing daily lymph massage on his legs and feet, aided by the penetrating herbs in the aloe vera spray. He and his wife have a passion for racehorses and have been breeding them and betting on them for years. Carl's financial success has also been improving over the last couple of years. His racehorses have been doing unusually well at the races, bringing him numerous winners.

No one knows for sure if this is the result of the large doses of aloe vera juice he feeds them every day. He calls it his aloe vera secret, and he is reluctant to share it with his competitors on the racetracks!

Joan: Diabetes mellitus

Joan is an active person who loves being with friends and keeping fit, who now single-handedly runs the Norwegian department of a large philosophical organisation. Originally she came from a healthy family and was the image of health, vitality and energy when she grew up. However, in her mid-twenties, when she worked as a teacher in a school ridden by violence, she was assaulted several times. Understandably, these episodes shocked and paralysed her with fear. She believes that they were the reason for the sudden and unexpected onset of diabetes and high blood pressure three months later. She took several years to recover from her fear and dare to go out shopping without her husband again. Although she has gradually recovered her health, she still has to use insulin injections twice daily and take tablets to keep her high blood pressure down. I met her when I was teaching at a naturopathic school. She was introduced to me by a friend as a case study. Joan told the group of students that her diabetes was steadily worsening and that she had to take increasing doses of insulin to combat her rising blood sugar. When I started examining her it was obvious that she had excessive tension in tissues and muscles all over the body, especially in her legs and thighs. The subcutaneous tissue felt hard to the touch, almost like cement.

I taught her relaxation exercises and referred her to massage and aromatherapy with experienced licensed therapists. I had found reports on aloe vera being able to stabilise blood sugar and reduce the activity of diabetic disease, due to its effect on the glycogen content in the liver. I had also seen scientific reports stating that aloe vera may be able to reduce deposits in blood vessels and lead to slight reduction of blood pressure. So I thought that there was good reason for her to drink aloe vera juice and suggested 100 millilitres daily. At the same time she was to massage the large muscles, aided by the penetrative aloe vera and tissue-relaxing herbs, found as a combination in the aloe vera topical spray. Joan has now followed this regime for nearly a year. At each meeting, she has reported that her situation was steadily improving. She seemed less tense and the skin, tissue and muscles were softer to the touch. Strangely she didn't turn up for our last appointment, and when she phoned a few days later to apologise for her temporary amnesia, she told me that she had just forgotten about it because she felt so much better. She has been able to reduce her blood pressure medication from two different drugs to one at the same dose as before. Her long-term blood sugar level is down and she has also reduced her daily dosage of insulin by eight to ten units per day.

In Joan's case, as is true for many other cases, I think that her improvement may be a combination of many factors, especially when it comes to the reduction of her blood pressure. There was no family history of hypertension. Thus I believe that her hypertensive disease had developed as a consequence of her state of shock, stress, fear and inability to relax. The combination of massage, aromatherapy, relaxation, breathing exercises, meditation and self-massage that she chose, seemed to work well for her and we cannot be certain whether aloe vera contributed to the improvement of Joan's hypertension. On the other hand, the stabilisation of her diabetes may be due, at least in large part, to her continuing intake of aloe vera juice.

There are several scientific reports, from investigations on rats, mice and humans, opening up the possibility of a substantial effect of aloe vera on the activity of diabetes – though aloe vera can of course not cure diabetes. I have recently spoken with Joan and it's now a year since she started taking aloe vera. She just wanted to tell me she's feeling good and that her condition has been stable lately. She is continuing with her relaxation exercises and her daily aloe vera intake. Joan now calls aloe vera her 'life insurance'.

Dora: diverticulitis

Dora, who is now in her mid-fifties, had generally been a fairly strong, active and healthy person who was seldom ill. In her late thirties she started to feel unwell and her overall health deteriorated. She had medical treatment for a minor heart condition and was troubled by pains in her joints and muscles. However, her main problems seem to be digestive. She had suffered from constipation since her teens and she started developing severe stomach pains, accompanied by fever.

After a couple of years of a patient 'wait and see' attitude, an x-ray of the colon was taken. It showed that she had developed diverticles throughout the colon. This means that the pressure on constipated material had led to small sacks of colonic mucosa forming as sacs, almost in the form of raindrops, throughout her colon. Her constipation continued being a problem and this led to depositing of waste material in the diverticles, predisposing, and often leading, to infection. This type of infection is called diverticulitis. When she contacted me, she had been on different antibiotics for some time. After a full history and examination, we discussed her current lifestyle. It was obvious that because of the pain she had to live an increasingly sedentary life and any undue movement only increased her pain. The lack of exercise and reduced appetite was also contributing to her worsening health. For a person who had always enjoyed an active, outdoor lifestyle and had a good appetite, the new 'regime' had a terrible effect on her situation. She was eating less and was unable to take any exercise, and her constipation became worse.

Like most Norwegians, she was fond of cakes, bread and potatoes, and always regarded government nutritional advice as being sound! This policy was based on maximising the amount of carbohydrates in people's diets, with a focus on such staples as bread and potatoes. Blood samples and skin tests showed that she had a mild allergy to wheat proteins and also that she might be absorbing carbohydrates in bread and cakes. We reviewed her diet and made gradual changes so that it included green leafy and root vegetables, brown rice, fish and some lean meats, combined with cleansing and stimulating spices like garlic and ginger. I also introduced her to aloe vera drinking juice, gradually increasing the dosage to thirty and then to fifty millilitres, twice daily.

She was used to being available to others constantly, and so had to learn how to give herself the space to employ the mechanism for creating health in body and mind: the combined use of the principles of *activation* and *relaxation*. I have given her a combined programme of physical exercises and progressive relaxation, as her muscle pains had created a vicious cycle of gradual progression of tension in the abdomen. On this new regime her constipation gradually improved and she has now regained normal bowel movements.

In the last year Dora has had only one episode of diverticulitis, but this relapse passed much faster than her earlier episodes. Dora's case illustrates the same point as that of many others. One cannot necessarily rely solely on aloe vera. It should be taken every day as an integral part of a new and healthier regime. Other lifestyle factors must be taken into consideration, such as diet, exercise, emotional conditions and mental and spiritual disciplines. In this way, the different therapeutic regimes can combine to produce the synergy of self-healing.

George and Donna: Epstein-Barr virus (mononucleosis)

Over the years, I have had several patients with mononucleosis. In the late eighties I saw my first two cases. At this time I knew little about the consequences of mononucleosis and similar serious viral infections, having learned that they are mainly benign virus infections that run their course with no after effects. However, in 1988, I had to change my viewpoint when I ran into two similar cases within a month. Both had been under severe stress. George was an executive in a large firm who worked long hours, late nights and weekends to keep up with the increasing demands of his job and the looming threat of redundancy. Donna had given up her family, friends and her job to be with the 'man she loved', against the advice of her nearest and dearest.

When she discovered that her family and friends had basically been right, she fell apart. She had no job, no money and no friends, and she moved to a small apartment on her own. Both George and Donna contracted serious mononucleosis when they were under stress. Trying to boost their recovery, they pressured themselves to hard physical exertion straight after the peak of their mononucleosis, while the disease was still active. Both collapsed shortly afterwards and were bedridden for weeks. Physically, they were both unable to function normally for years, and Donna had to live on a minimal disability pension. After this double experience I have been very careful with my mononucleosis patients. Medical reports confirmed my stumbling experiences with these patients. They must have:

- ample and frequent sleep
- regular meals
- mild exercises like short walks, followed by periods of rest

I have found that one needs to ensure a gradual rehabilitation after an Epstein-Barr virus infection, rather than try to put the patient straight back into a previous daily routine. This leads to good long-term results and is not generally a long-term health issue. I have had several patients with comparable attacks and courses of the Epstein-Barr infection, and have been able to compare patients who took aloe vera drinking juice with patients who didn't. Consistently, the return of normal function, vitality and energy levels is faster and more complete within the first half year after the disease in the patients who took aloe vera, compared to those who did not.

The course of the disease has seemed to be longer in the group not taking aloe vera. In medical terms this may be plausible. There are several substances in aloe vera that have been identified as having antiviral properties, such as acemannan and the anthraquinones. Therefore, I recommend anyone who is going through an Epstein-Barr virus infection to take aloe vera drinking juice as a supplement, to curtail the course of the disease and speed up recuperation.

Elena: ear infections

The most common of these are the middle ear infection (otitis media), and are often treated with antibiotics. External ear infections are less well known to most people. In this ailment, the external auditive canal is affected, often with an eczematous infection, sometimes affecting both skin and tissue, the outer ear and ear drum.

These infections are treated with local antibiotics and steroid eardrops, sometimes also with oral antibiotics. It is hard to understand why these infections are so hard to treat and so often return. Some researchers hold the view that the condition is actually an immunological disease rather than an infectious one. Elena came to me to ask for help after a series of different local and oral antibiotics that alleviated her symptoms for only a few days, before the itching and pain returned. Most of her symptoms were on the left side. I asked her to try onion poultice, a traditional folk remedy that has helped in some of these cases. This helped for a week, then the symptoms returned. I then decided to try aloe vera drops locally. The week after she started applying these drops to her left ear (in a concentrate of aloe especially helpful for eye, nose and ears), she called me to tell me her symptoms had gone. The symptoms returned again a few weeks later and this time we combined the aloe vera drops with aconitum eardrops, and this succeeded in halting her relapse.

Elena has finally found a remedy that helps whenever the infection recurs, and this is now happening less frequently. Sometimes if she has a particularly severe infection, she will combine the aloe vera drops with antibiotics – if the aloe and aconitum alone do not seem to give her relief. However, like many patients, she cares little about what helps and how it helps, the important thing is that it *does* help.

Martin: eye inflammations

Normally, eye infections are best treated with local antibiotic drops, and products such as Chloramphenicole are usually quite effective. Similarly, we have eye drops that work well for most cases of eye inflammations that are caused by allergies. However, I have had cases where none of the regular medication works, particularly in small children. Martin was such a case. He seemed to have inherited allergies from his mother, and during the autumn and winter months he would always have a runny nose and eyes. Allergy tablets and local anti-allergic drops only reduced his symptoms slightly, and he was always tired because of his interrupted sleep. His nose was always blocked, he had to breathe through his mouth, and he tended to swallow a lot of mucus. At a hospital appointment, arranged by the family, it was suggested that he start a course of steroids to help alleviate the problem. His parents were naturally worried about this development and asked me for help. I said that I basically agreed with the decision to start cortisone treatment but that we had some time to try a more natural alternative. Martin was only six years old, and I believed it would be better if we could avoid the steroid treatment for as long as possible. Because of his sensitivity, I tried Bach flower remedies to give him protection, and I taught the parents acupressure massage in the face and on the body. He also started taking marine oils, and I started him on a course of aloe vera drinking juice and aloe vera drops locally.

Gradually, his symptoms subsided, and it seems he has started to outgrow some of his airway problems. His sleep has improved, and now two years down the line he has still avoided the steroids! Whether his improvement would have come without aloe vera is hard to determine. The fact is that he used two different aloe vera products – one internally and one topically – and they seemed to help manage the problem. His is one of several cases where aloe vera seems to have contributed significantly to the improvement of symptoms in the upper airways of people who suffer with allergies.

Brenda: fibromyalgia

Brenda is now in her early forties. She has three children and works as a secretary. Since her late twenties she has suffered pains in most parts of her body, starting in the neck and shoulders, spreading to her arms, lower back and thighs. Her quality of sleep has been reduced and often she can sleep for ten hours and wake up feeling more tired than when she went to bed. Brenda has also had problems with stomach pains and irregular stools. She has tried several drugs, with little effect. This has tended to be the general experience for many patients with similar symptoms. Drug treatment that works and has no side effects is hard to find. The same goes for physiotherapy. Many patients report a worsening of their pain after massages, especially if they are massaged hard and deep in the tissue. Psychomotor physiotherapy, focused on breathing techniques and body feeling, has generally been more positively evaluated.

Relaxation exercises and movement to music have been found to improve the condition in a group of fibromyalgia patients investigated by a Norwegian research team in the late nineties. Based on her history and this knowledge, I gave Brenda a regime of exercises, using body movements like those of tai ji, and combined these with visualisation and inner fantasy journeys to music, and with the use of movement to music. She had to learn to take more time for herself and learn to distinguish when she started tensing her muscles. I also gave her an aloe vera spray to try on one side of the body. In this way, she would be able to distinguish whether it could be of help to her, as her pains were symmetrically localised on both sides of her body. After fourteen days of this improvised trial, she came back and said she felt better on the side on which she had applied the aloe vera spray. This interested her because normally massages, no matter what type, made her feel worse, not better.

She agreed to start a regime of external application with the aloe vera spray on the tender points known to be diagnostic in fibromyalgia patients. I also asked her to take aloe vera drinking juice at a rate of eighty millilitres a day. Brenda felt the difference the aloe vera made, especially when she stopped taking it! Her symptoms were exacerbated within a couple of days. Aloe vera was an integral part of a regime that helped get her body working normally and recover her energy levels. Since the first time she tried spraying aloe vera on only one side of her body, she has carried out this experiment many times. She pointed out to me that she could feel the difference, even when she changed sides again after a few days. Brenda is now back in business and is convinced that aloe vera is the single most important factor contributing to her improvement.

Mo: gingivitis

Mo attributes his current health problems to the time he spent when he was younger and travelling the world, often eating a poor diet and sometimes experimenting with different drugs. Mo is now an artist and has settled down, and is married with three children.

His lifestyle has improved his health dramatically, but one problem he still suffers from is gingivitis. This is a painful inflammation of the gums and tooth pockets, and every morning and evening, while brushing his teeth, his gums bled. Day and night, the pains continued, and he had even had to have implants because of the damage to the gums. Often he was unable to sleep because of the pain, and nothing he tried in the way of remedies seemed to help.

I had recommended the use of aloe vera on similar conditions with considerable success. I decided to put him on a regime using an aloe vera toothgel, massaging his gums with a topical aloe vera gelly and gargling with a concentrated aloe vera liquid. In addition, he was to take aloe vera drinking juice. His wife had been taking aloe vera drinking juice for general fatigue problems and had felt increased energy and a reduction of lower back pain. This was after taking sixty millilitres per day for three months. Mo came back after a month and told me his gums had not felt or looked so good since he was a teenager, and that he would continue to use all the aloe vera products. He is committed to a strict oral hygiene regime that includes regular meals of healthy foods, self-massage of the gums and jaw, and, as he puts it, 'my indispensable aloe vera'.

Ali: haemorrhoids

Ali runs a business selling clothes and football memorabilia. He has a shop and a café and works long and irregular hours. For years he has had problems with pains in his abdomen, suffering from constipation, bloating and sometimes nausea in the upper gut area, and he also developed haemorrhoids both externally and internally. Haemorrhoids are very common. They are said to be more common in countries where the diet has become based on foods that are more processed and lower in fibre. The main contributory causes tend to be when the pressure in the abdomen is increased, for example straining when going to the toilet. This causes the blood vessels to swell and become engorged. It seems that the people most at risk of developing haemorrhoids are those who have more causes for raised abdominal pressure, such as:

- those chronically straining with constipation
- during or after pregnancy. The baby may actually press on the main blood vessel that returns blood to the heart (the vena cava)
- overweight people
- people with heavy lifting jobs

Useful aspects of prevention are:

- avoid becoming overweight, and lose weight if you are
- eat a high fibre diet
- exercise regularly

Ali had followed many of these rules but he was still suffering from severe recurring piles. Defecation was so painful for him that he could sometimes sit for an hour or more, trying to get out the small and hard lumps that gather in and above the rectum. He often had trouble sleeping at night because of the pain in the anal region, where normal local medical remedies had no effect. He had one successful operation, only to have the haemorrhoids return within two years.

His wife has been drinking aloe vera juice for several years and suggested that he start taking the juice to help regulate his bowel movements. Traditionally, we know that in folk medicine drinking aloes acted as a laxative and purgative. The modern day aloe vera drinking juices tend not to have the same degree of laxative effect, but can help regulate bowel movements in a gentler, cleansing way. It was no surprise that within a few months Ali's constipation had improved and his bowel movements became more regular and much less painful.

He also used a topical aloe vera aloe gelly directly on his haemorrhoids, and this helped to reduce the pain almost immediately (aloe vera contains several natural analgesics or painkillers). He also knows that if the haemorrhoids come back, he may require further surgery. He is able to keep his condition stable by using aloe vera both internally and topically. He has regulated his diet and lifestyle, ensuring that he eats regularly and that his food contains more ample fibre. He exercises daily, and his wife, who is a therapist, gives him localised massage to keep tissue circulation stable and healthy. I believe that this new regime will keep him free from any new outbreaks of painful haemorrhoids in the coming years.

Lisa: hepatitis

Lisa came to me with a condition she had suffered from for several years – chronic hepatitis, type C, of uncertain origin. She asked me if I could help her to supplement her medical treatment with natural remedies. I had some previous experience with similar cases and put her on daily doses of yarrow as herbal tea and poultice, artichoke extract as herbal tea, sow thistles in tablet form, and aloe vera drinking juice, fifty millilitres twice daily. After a month of this regime she was less tired and her liver values had improved from previous blood samples.

Particularly in the cases of hepatitis that may have a viral and contagious origin, an increasing number of sufferers from these diseases are now taking aloe vera drinking juice to boost their immune systems and improve well-being – in the hope that it will help combat the disease. Judging from the cases I have seen and read about, it is sometimes necessary to consume large doses, even up to half a litre per day, to achieve a substantial effect. There is a significant cost involved when consuming such quantities on a daily basis, but the question really is, what price good health? I am finding that more and more people are willing to pay the price in order to regain their health, zest and vitality.

Paul and Laura: Herpes simplex

Paul and Laura are brother and sister, and both were still at kindergarten when I first met them. Their mother had called me because she was increasingly concerned about their general health. She felt that both of them had weak immune systems and she also confirmed that both of them had been unwell for some months. When I first saw them, they both had recurring Herpes simplex around the mouth. Local treatment had been tried, with little or no effect. They had been treated with antibiotic cream when there was secondary bacterial infection, but the blisters kept growing around the mouth. I asked them to try a topical aloe vera gelly, locally. Their condition cleared almost completely within two weeks, and they had no further problems throughout the summer.

Their mother put them on a regime of more fruit and vegetable in their diet, and they also took aloe vera drinking juice (like many small children, they did not like the taste of the ordinary juice, so they used a peach or cranberry-and-apple flavoured juice instead), and flower remedies and massage. They were also encouraged to spend more time playing outside and less time watching TV or immersed in video games. This regime seemed to work and they had no recurrence of the Herpes simplex, and suffered only a couple of minor short-term colds.

Aloe vera does not always work in these conditions, where virus or candida is rampant, and we have no certain way of knowing which patients will respond. However, I would advise any sufferers of herpes or similar viral infections to try aloe vera. It will not interfere with ordinary treatment and will seldom have any side effects. Some aloe vera manufacturers are so confident of the quality of their products that they even give all customers an unconditional sixty-day full money-back guarantee if the customer is not totally satisfied!

Arne: muscular pain

Arne was a natural athlete. In his youth, he was involved in track and field and cross-country skiing. Even after his career as a top athlete ended in his thirties, he was still very active. He had a physically vigorous outdoor job and often ran or went skiing in his spare time, because he liked to push his body to the limit. He started his own business that unfortunately failed and he had to go back to his previous occupation. This business failure and the break-up of a long-standing relationship was a traumatic time for him. He was alone, his business had gone and he was at low ebb. Much of his motivation had vanished too, and although he still continued exercising – his only real pleasure now – he felt totally listless. He was used to having a 'lactic acid feeling' of stiffness, tenderness and tiredness in the muscles throughout his body after training sessions, when by the next day he had totally recovered. Like so many people who enjoy vigorous exercise, Arne felt it to have a cleansing effect on his body. Now, to his dismay, the pain and stiffness didn't subside the day after a hard training and workout session. Instead, he developed chronic muscular pain and stiffness in his joints. Whether he rested or exercised, it didn't seem to make any difference. He became increasingly worried about his health and consulted a sports physician he had known for several years.

Nothing untoward was found from the x-rays or blood samples, and he didn't want to take regular medications for his pains: he felt they might weaken his immune system and cause other problems. He contacted me after friends told him that I was a doctor and was also involved with natural and complementary remedies that could perhaps help his condition. I had seen a video featuring the American chiropractic physician, Gregg Henderson, stating that one important benefit of drinking aloe vera juice was that it helped to strip tissue of uronic acid and other waste deposits and rebuild normal connective tissue. I advised Arne to use an aloe vera spray and an aloe vera gelly topically (on his skin) three times daily, and to drink aloe vera gel at the dosage of forty to fifty millilitres twice daily. I also suggested that he reduce his exercise regime and did not over exert himself. I felt that one of his personality traits was a tendency to put pressure on himself, and I stressed the need for a change of regime to include relaxation and self-massage. I also suggested that he give himself a break and start to take a more positive attitude towards himself.

This new regime had an almost immediate effect on him. His pains subsided within two months and he was soon able to resume his previous training regime. He was however conscious of the need to maintain a balance in his life. Arne is convinced that drinking aloe vera is the main reason for his improvement. As a doctor I have to take a more scientific view and consider all aspects of his life. I was aware that his personal life had become more stable and he was less stressed than before, so this could also have had an effect.

It is impossible to say if this change is as important a reason for his improvement as taking aloe vera, but I was sure of one thing, and that was his condition improved much faster than I had expected. I believe that the aloe vera regime, both internal and topical, played a significant role in the healing process. The most important thing is that Arne has recovered his previous fitness levels and is also mentally fit.

John: thrush and cancer

John was an accountant, married with a family. He had been a patient of mine for several years, suffering from asthma. One autumn, when he suddenly lost weight, I became increasingly worried. I sent him to hospital after the onset of increasing dyspnoea (shortness of breath). A chest x-ray revealed lung cancer and a bronchoscopy showed he was suffering from a particularly aggressive and fast-acting type that treatment with chemotherapy or radiation could do little to halt. He had been a non-smoker and was baffled that he should be suffering from such a disease. After only a few weeks, it became clear that the cancer was extremely severe and his life expectancy was short, so he spent more and more time with his family and closest friends. I visited him several times at home, and although he suffered little pain, he did have some serious breathing difficulties, and was compelled to breathe mainly through his mouth. One of the consequences of this condition was that he was more prone to infection and he contracted thrush in the oral cavity.

Thrush is the widely used term for a common fungal infection caused by the yeast candida albicans, and it usually takes the form of minor vaginal or mouth infections. Sometimes it can also affect the body more widely, and on occasions it can be quite serious. Oral thrush may cause soreness and redness in the mouth and throat, and is characterised by a white discharge on the surface. Babies, especially those being bottle fed, may suffer from it, as well as adults, especially with cancer and other debilitating diseases. After John was prescribed anti-fungal medication – four times daily – his condition improved slightly but he still had soreness in his mouth, and also had some difficulties swallowing. I decided to introduce a concentrated form of aloe vera liquid for local application and gargling. He also agreed to start drinking aloe vera juice at a dosage of thirty to forty millilitres, twice daily. Within a few days of this new aloe vera regime, the soreness in his mouth had disappeared and he was again able to swallow normally.

His appetite seemed to be restored and he was again able to enjoy the little food and drink he could manage. A few months later he died peacefully, but his family told me that even in the short time he was taking aloe vera it helped him and enabled him to eat and drink more normally. This was important to him in his last few months. One positive impact of John's case was that it showed how the combination of regular anti-fungal medication and aloe vera really helped him in those last few months, making his remaining time more comfortable.

I personally will always choose or recommend a complementary approach rather than an alternative one. We need positive contributions from both the regular health care system and complementary therapies, such as aloe vera, to achieve an optimum effect for the benefit of the patient. My hopes are that there should not be any opposition or an either-or situation. Rather, patients and their families should be able to choose what they consider to be the most effective options from the best of both regular and complementary treatment. In this way simple and harmless solutions may be found that lead to alleviation of symptoms and a heightening of the health potential. In most cases, like John's, we cannot obtain miracle cures but we can, and should, aim for that little edge of improvement, that slight alleviation that may mean the world to the patients and those close to them.

Albert: psoriasis

Albert is a strong and seemingly healthy man, who has a demanding and physical outdoor job. However, like so many others in his family, he has suffered throughout his life from psoriasis. Psoriasis is a common condition affecting the skin. It causes red, scaly patches and can also affect the joints, nails and eyes. Psoriasis can be localised to just a small patch or a single dimple on one of your finger- or toe-nails, but sometimes it can affect the majority of your skin surface and your joints and your eyes. It is estimated that up to two per cent of people (one in fifty) have psoriasis to some degree.

Albert had tried all sorts of treatments, including several cortisone ointments, ultraviolet radiation and many other types of baths, creams and ointments through the years, with little effect. From his mid-forties, his seriously debilitating psoriasis, combined with his progressively worsening lower back condition, led to him being retired as disabled. At such an early age and for such a powerful man, this was a devastating blow.

His psoriasis seemed worse when he was at home with little to occupy or distract him. The red, scaly plaques itched constantly and he was unable to sleep because he could not stop scratching. Gradually, the plaques spread to other parts of his body – almost like a contagious disease. A close friend who worked with one of the largest aloe vera manufacturers told him that some highly positive clinical research had been done on the use of aloe vera on psoriasis. Albert immediately felt that he had nothing to lose by trying this 'new' idea. Nothing else had worked so he decided to start using the aloe vera immediately. He used aloe vera gelly on his skin and drank aloe vera juice every day. Like several other psoriasis sufferers I know who have started taking aloe vera juice, his condition became worse during the first few weeks. Yet although he was lying awake, itching and scratching more than ever, he saw that the eruptions in the skin were different from his usual psoriasis outbreaks – the skin was redder and fresher around the plaques. He decided that he had suffered from psoriasis all his life and that this new treatment seemed to be doing something, so he was going to stick with it.

Over the next year he continued taking aloe vera and had recurring outbreaks of severe itching from his psoriasis plaques, but gradually the symptoms and side effects subsided. Today, Albert considers himself to be much healthier than he can ever remember. He still has psoriasis but it is not as debilitating as it once was, and it does not interfere with his quality of life as it used to. He was so impressed with the benefits of aloe vera that he became a distributor for an aloe vera manufacturer.

Part of the reason for his success as a distributor is his own story. He revels in showing his clear skin, obvious vitality and his new-found quality of life. He is one of the very few patients that I have come across who has been able to free himself of the shackles of the disability pension system, and has regained his self-esteem through his new work. Other fellow sufferers and people whom he has met have joined him in his new venture.

In the last few years, I have come across several people on disability pensions who have been suffering from various chronic conditions for years, who have improved both their health and wealth with aloe vera. They have effectively got a new lease of life by taking aloe vera and have established a new career marketing its products. They have left their disability pensions behind and believe that taking aloe vera has contributed significantly to their enhanced health and well-being. One important point about Albert's case is that he persisted with aloe vera, even after he had a temporary worsening of his symptoms. He actually went for weeks without seeing any improvement. This has given me the courage to persist with a couple of other cases where I would normally have given up and reverted to treatment with steroids. It seems that psoriasis is such a far-reaching autoimmune condition that it may take patience and perseverance to get results. However, you must always be careful not to self-diagnose and always consult your doctor.

Sigurd: seborrhoic eczema

Every day, as part of the usual renewal process, the scalp sheds skin cells. Usually there are so few we tend not to notice them. It is a different story when a fungal infection is involved. Depending on the intensity of the infection, the symptoms can range from simple scalp scaling to seborrhoic eczema. In such circumstances, dandruff is more than just a cosmetic problem. Normally, the sebaceous glands keep the horny skin layer supple and, by maintaining a certain skin pH value, protect healthy skin from bacterial and fungal infections. The functioning of this protective coat can be disturbed by changes in the production or make-up of sebum as well as an over- or under-functioning of the sebaceous glands. Bacteria and fungi find an ideal culture medium on a scalp that has become vulnerable. The yeast fungus (pityriasis), normally part of the natural skin flora, is seen as the main cause. However, when it is out of control, it causes itching and inflammation. As a self-protective measure, the scalp reacts with an increased build-up of horny tissue in the epidermis. Often this process is incomplete and the cells are shed in entire cell formations – dandruff. If the problem is only mild, one tends to talk of simple scalp scaling. In contrast, reddening, itching and scaling are the classic symptoms of the seborrhoic eczema that spreads in those parts of the body containing sebum. The eczema may be wet and may appear on the face, neck and upper body. Normally, using suitable drugs, both the itchiness and the fungal infection can be stopped.

In Sigurd's case, he had suffered from an itchy scalp for years and it was diagnosed as seborrhoic eczema. He used regular, prescription, anti-fungal ointments and shampoos, sometimes combined with steroid creams and other liniments. All these forms of treatment reduced the itching and inflammation in the scalp but relief was always temporary. Over the years, Sigurd had tried many natural remedies, but like the medications, none of them had any lasting benefit.

A friend recommended that he try aloe vera, and he decided to drink aloe vera juice and also use an aloe vera and jojoba oil shampoo. Over the next two months, his condition gradually improved and his scalp was much healthier than it had been for years. Sigurd believes that the improvement is entirely due to using aloe vera and is the reason why he now suffers from only the occasional minor outbreak of dandruff and itching. Whenever he has stopped his 'aloe vera regime', his condition worsens within a couple of weeks.

While this condition is not 'life-threatening', it can cause discomfort and embarrassment, so I was glad to see such a quick and seemingly permanent solution to his problem.

Paula: skin rejuvenation

I had known Paula – a successful businesswoman – for many years, and was well aware of her love of the sun. Like so many Scandinavians who have to endure long, harsh winters, she was a great sun worshipper and spent as much time as she could in the south of Spain. She loved sunbathing and always felt better when she was tanned. Most people look healthier when they are slightly tanned and she was no exception. She always tried to 'top up' her tan with weekly visits to a tanning studio, but unfortunately did not use moisturising creams and oils to prevent her skin drying out. In her early forties, the signs of skin ageing rapidly became more visible. Wrinkling, dryness and brown sunspots were increasingly evident and were undoubtedly due to the continued exposure both to the sun and the tanning studio.

She tried regular moisturising creams but didn't see any changes over the next few months. Although she felt healthy, she was developing a complex about the condition of her skin and tended to socialise less than before. When we met, I persuaded her to reduce her sunbathing regime and suggested she start facial massage and the use of acupressure points. I also referred her to a skin specialist who used aloe vera based skin preparations.

She started using this new cosmetic regime twice daily, and within only two months her skin had changed for the better. She continued her skin rejuvenation programme and six months later confirmed that the sunspots were barely visible. This is a similar experience to that of Ivan Danhoff, one of the world's leading authorities on aloe vera. Aloe vera is increasingly used as an ingredient in skin and beauty care products, as well as in many other daily applications. When using an aloe vera based preparation on the skin, and especially on the face, it is essential to use a product with a high percentage of stabilised aloe vera. It really is an issue of quality and efficacy, and our advice, as we have said in other parts of this book, is to use only those products that meet the standards laid down by the IASC.

Ari: injuries, sprains and strains

I had researched the effects of aloe vera and, over the years, I had tried out many different preparations. My personal interest in this remarkable plant was triggered by an injury I suffered when I was playing soccer on a hard pitch. After a strong tackle, I landed on my left knee and suffered a severe contusion of the knee. I was unable to straighten it out and had to be carried back home.

Luckily nothing was broken, but I was in a lot of pain and the injury around my knee joints and deeper tissue was so severe that I thought it would take about three weeks to heal. A friend who came to see me brought an aloe vera and herbal spray with analgesic, anti-inflammatory and skin-penetrating properties. I obviously had nothing to lose so I started spraying it on immediately. The first thing that I noticed was that the pain subsided almost instantly on applying the spray. I tried spraying regular water on the same site and noticed, in contrast, that this had no effect on the pain. I repeated this experiment several times. The morning after, I continued spraying, and to my continued amazement the normal granulation tissue seemed to be growing. I had never known such a large wound to heal so fast.

Because I had suffered a similar injury several years before, I knew that my normal rate of wound healing was average, i.e. about two to three weeks. Yet in only three days I was able to walk and within a week there was no trace of the injury. Following my personal experience, I systematically gathered case histories and research evidence that seemed to indicate that aloe vera indeed was not just 'any tropical plant': in many conditions it could be as effective as regular drugs. Personal experience such as this is hard to refute, and I have had no trouble with my knee since. Sprains and strains are a description of what happens to the muscles and other non-bony structures connected to our bones when they are put under excessive pressure or strain. The result is swelling, pain, bruising and loss or impairment of function of the affected area. The first thing you notice is pain that is often severe. This is usually at the time of the injury, for example 'going over on your ankle' or 'twisting your knee'. Sometimes the damage can be caused by repetitive and less major strains, and the pain becomes apparent the following day or possibly even later. Swelling is often obvious and usually very tender.

The area affected may be inflamed and rather warmer than usual. Bruising usually appears, often away from the area most affected, as blood that's released from the damaged soft tissues (muscles, ligaments and tendons) seeps out along the muscles and other structures before getting to the skin. Shortly after my own recovery, Ari came to see me. He was something of an adventurer, so when he was asked to go mountain climbing by a friend he leapt at the chance. Inexperience can sometimes be dangerous, as he soon found out. While traversing a cliff face, his right foot slipped and he landed on the side of his foot. No bones were broken but he sustained a sprained ankle, with huge swelling. He had to walk on crutches, and the anti-inflammatory drugs he took were not that effective. He contacted me after two weeks, because there did not seem to be any improvement in his condition. After my own experience and as something of a newly converted 'zealot' as to the benefits of aloe vera, I decided to try out the aloe vera spray on his ankle. I suggested that he use the spray several times every day and that he might also talk to a reflexologist. Over the next two weeks, he gradually improved, and six months later his ankle had totally recovered.

The experience with Ari consolidated my belief that aloe vera has a significant 'healing' contribution to make in the handling of sports injuries and other types of sprains and strains.

Alan: mouse arm/tendonitis

Alan was in his early thirties and worked in the IT industry. He came to see me for a 'sick note' because he'd developed a severe pain in his right elbow that was causing him severe discomfort, crepitation and stiffness.

It was obviously a case of lateral epicondylitis or tennis elbow – in this particular case it was more fitting to call his condition 'mouse arm'. Tennis elbow or lateral epicondylitis is a condition where the outer part of the elbow becomes painful and tender, usually as a result of a specific strain, overuse or a direct blow. In some cases the condition may develop without any specific cause. Tennis elbow is similar to 'golfer's elbow', another similar condition, but one that affects the other side of the elbow. Any movements of the elbow or movements that involve lifting, with the hand on top, tend to hurt. Although called tennis elbow, lateral epicondylitis is much more commonly seen in people who are overusing their arm doing other things. It could equally well be called 'plasterer's elbow', 'mechanic's elbow', 'painter's elbow' or even 'computer worker's elbow'.

The most common cause is overuse of the muscles that are attached to the bone at this part of the elbow, that is the muscles that pull the hand backwards (the wrist extensors). All the extensor muscles of the hand attach to the elbow at the outer part (the lateral epicondyle). If they are strained or overused they become inflamed and this means they can become swollen, painful and tender to touch. Sometimes the inflammation is caused by a direct injury or blow. Sometimes, especially when the cause is a direct injury or strain, the muscles can actually be partially torn. Rarely does the inflammation occur without any definite cause, and this may be due to arthritis, rheumatism or gout. Sometimes the problem is partly or completely due to a neck problem that is causing pain in the elbow via the nerves from the neck.

I first referred Alan to an orthopaedic surgeon. There was some benefit from taking non-steroid anti-inflammatory drugs (NSAIDS) and local steroid injections – these tended to give pain relief for only a couple of weeks. However, when the symptoms returned, this time with increased severity, the doctors were reluctant to administer any further injections. Alan wanted to try natural remedies and I taught him stretching exercises for the neck (sometimes one of the causative factors in this condition), exercises to reduce tension in his muscles and tissue, and the use of acupressure points. I also showed him how to apply aloe vera spray and massage it in locally to reduce the tension and inflammation around the tendon. Alan followed this regime for two weeks and was soon able to return to work. An important part of his ongoing recovery was learning to work intermittently and take breaks with ergonomic exercises for five minutes every hour. Our bodies have changed little since the days of our ancestors the cavemen, and our anatomy is not designed to sit at a computer with one-sided movements all day, with few breaks. I think it is important to state that no amount of aloe vera would keep him free of pain if he continued to sit and work with the computer mouse for hours at a time without interruption. In the majority of cases, aloe vera must be combined with a holistic view of a patients' activities, work and lifestyle.

Paul: peptic ulcers

One of the paradoxical situations with aloe vera is that one of the most widely documented properties of it is its ability to heal stomach mucosa and particularly inflammatory alterations of the mucosa, as in gastritis and peptic and duodenal ulcers.

At the same time, normal regular medical treatment of this condition with H2-blocking agents [special drugs used to treat peptic ulcers] has in most cases made both treatment with aloe vera and surgery obsolete. The new drugs are efficient and have few side effects. As with anything in life, there is always an exception to the rule.

I found this to be case with Paul, who had worked with alternative medicine for years and was highly sceptical about taking any regular medication. When he started suffering from stinging pains in the upper abdomen and began passing black stools, he realised he would have to see a doctor. He was referred to a gastroenterologist who diagnosed a peptic ulcer located near the duodenum. Ulcers are small, open craters or sores that develop in the lining of the stomach or the duodenum, the first section of the small intestine. The term peptic ulcer is generally used to describe both types of ulcers. The bacterium, helicobacter pylori (or H pylori for short) is often deemed responsible for the outbreak of ulcers. Current medical opinion suggests that anyone with ulcer symptoms should, at some point, be checked for the presence of H pylori. The importance of this finding is that, in many cases of H pylori positive ulcers, antibiotics can actually heal the ulcer. Some ulcers are caused by different factors such as certain medications and illnesses. Peptic ulcers occur only in those areas of the digestive system that come in contact with digestive juices secreted by the stomach. These juices include stomach acid – basically hydrochloric acid – and an enzyme called pepsin that breaks down proteins. While many people with duodenal ulcers have an overabundance of digestive juices spilling down from the stomach, most of those with gastric (stomach) ulcers have normal or even below normal amounts of stomach acid.

Medical researchers, therefore, believe that poor resistance levels of the protective mucous membrane that lines both the stomach and the duodenum may contribute to the development of a peptic ulcer. Duodenal ulcers tend to produce pain in a small area between the breast bone and the navel. The pain may vary from a hunger pain to a continuous gnawing or burning sensation. Sometimes, the pain is felt during sleep and may be strong enough to awaken the ulcer sufferer in the middle of the night. Usually, however, the pain of a duodenal ulcer occurs two or three hours after eating, when the stomach is empty. Other common symptoms include a bloated feeling immediately after eating and weight gain due to the tendency to relieve pain and discomfort by overeating.

Gastric ulcer pain may be felt in the same place as the pain of a duodenal ulcer or even slightly higher up. There may also be sensations of feeling full, indigestion and heartburn. Sometimes pain occurs when the stomach is full, causing a loss of appetite and weight. The pain of both types of ulcer tends to be relieved by medications that neutralise stomach acid or prevent its secretion. Paul did not, however, wish to take regular medication because he was afraid of any possible side effects. He also felt, rightly or wrongly, that his faith in natural remedies would carry him through. I suggested that the side effects of regular medication in his case were negligible and that it would not be easy to cure his problem in any other way. Paul still insisted on going the natural way. I taught him simple meditation and relaxation exercises to help reduce stress, and I also put him on a diet based mainly on brown rice, cooked vegetables and fish. I also put him on aloe vera juice at a dosage of fifty millilitres twice daily. A month later, hospital tests showed that his ulcer was completely healed.

Several other patients of mine with gastritis have chosen both routes. They take normal medications if their problems are severe, and combine this with aloe vera and digestive herbs like yarrow, dandelion and chamomile in periods of lower activity. One advantage with aloe vera is that it can, in principle, be combined with any known medical treatment.

There seems to be a synergy between the different ingredients in aloe vera and there also seems to be a synergy between aloe vera and some drugs, including the H2-blocking drugs that help combat ulcers.

Jenny: viral infections

Over the last few decades, there have been many claims that there is a silent epidemic of slow-acting virus infections in modern Western society. We do know that viruses, in contrast to most bacteria, are opportunistic and can retreat into cells in inactive forms, and can then become active again when the body's defences are weakened.

Kindergarten workers and schoolteachers that I know often talk about the increasing numbers of children who are neither really sick nor really well, and this is particularly the case in the winter months when outside temperatures are well below freezing. Many children spend weeks or months at a time with snotty noses, lack of energy and recurring sub-febrile episodes. It is not easy to investigate the presence of viruses, but I have often taken blood samples from these children. In a large number of cases I have found viruses like adenovirus or influenza viruses. Another type of virus may be active while these children are experiencing their symptoms, but in many of the adults who have experienced sub-febrile episodes, nightly sweats and general lassitude, virus infections can often be hard to identify clinically.

I have tried aloe vera on many of these children and I have been able to compare the course of the clinical situation with children who did not take aloe vera. Judging from the reports from the parents, and from my own experience, there seems to be an indication that aloe vera, with its antiviral properties, can shorten the course of a virus infection. It is one of the few natural substances that can help with recuperation after a long-standing virus infection, and can possibly even shorten the course of the disease. Jenny was the youngest of three children in a family I had known for a long time. She was what I called a 'winter child': pale, weak and snotty during most of the winter months. Strep tests and blood samples proved negative, and the paediatrician who specialised in allergic disorders did not find asthma or any overt allergies when he examined Jenny.

One autumn, her mother asked me if she could try natural remedies to boost her health and resistance to disease. We agreed to try a regime of fish oils, vitamin C, echinacea drops and aloe vera drops, locally combined with aloe vera juice at a dosage of fifteen millilitres twice daily as a supplement. Jenny's overall health soon improved on this regime and, for the first time since she was two years old, she had a winter without antibiotics. Her parents decided to keep her on this regime all year round. I took away the echinacea drops, as recent research shows that this works only for the first one to two weeks of acute disease, and is thus best reserved for acute infectious attacks. Aloe vera has a mild and definite immune bolstering and antiviral effect, and it makes good sense to include it as an integral part of any health regime to ensure an infection-prone child remains healthy.

Katrina: wound healing and scar tissue

Katrina was a beautiful, adventurous little girl with long blonde hair, who always played with her friends. She was fascinated when she saw a few older boys cutting sticks with a knife. When they ran off to play football they left the knife behind and Katrina rushed over, picked it up and started doing what the older boys had done – she cut some sticks. However, the knife slipped and badly cut her index finger, causing a deep wound. I was on call in the area and treated it.

Over the years, I have seen many similar wounds, but on this occasion, when I stitched it, I decided to try aloe vera locally prior to putting on the surgical dressing. I had heard of aloe vera's wound-healing properties and believed it may help speed the healing process.

When she came back to have the threads from the sutures removed, I was impressed to see the relative lack of scar tissue. After the removal of the sutures, a few days later, there was barely a trace left of the deep wound. Some of my patients have in later years even reported that scar tissue can be reduced through massage with aloe vera gelly, even months after the original incision.

Molly: warts

Warts are small growths of the skin, caused by a virus, that can spread over large areas of the body and become a cosmetic embarrassment. They have a rather rough surface and can often be unsightly. They do not usually hurt, though they may itch. Warts may affect any part of the body but are most commonly seen on the hands.

Warts on the feet are known as verrucae. Here the pressure from body weight causes them to be flatter and grow into the skin more and they can be extremely painful.

Sometimes people have many warts or verrucas, while some others have only one or two. It may be that they can be picked up from direct contact or in swimming pools or changing rooms, but warts and verrucas do not spread rapidly through a family. Many doctors believe that people are more susceptible at certain ages.

I remember in my early teens, when I was called 'the wart king'. My fingers were gradually overgrown and covered with warts. When all tested and tried cures failed, they were surgically removed, leaving large amounts of scar tissue, visible to this very day. I had little success with warts later in my general medical practice with the usual local ointments from the pharmacy. Neither did I have much success with old wives' remedies, like binding a woollen thread around the ankle or walking twelve times around the graveyard at midnight – surprisingly!

I had read many reports on aloe vera's anti-viral action and decided to try a topical aloe vera preparation on Molly, a girl in early puberty who had a large outbreak of warts on her fingers. She applied aloe vera gelly several times a day and over the next two weeks the warts were reduced. After a month they were barely visible. I didn't always have the same degree of success with all my 'wart patients'. However, I do believe that the combination of aloe's anti-viral action and the natural film formed over the wart by the aloe vera gelly has been more effective on warts than regular anti-viral ointments and jellies.

Sunniva: burns

My first exposure to the healing powers of aloe vera was in the eighties when we bought an aloe vera plant and kept it at home. I had read about its healing effect on sunburn and skin damage but I had never had the occasion to try it out. A young girl we knew came to visit us and we had a meditation together, with candles between us. During the meditation one of her hands slipped down into the candle flame. She was in such a deeply relaxed state that initially she did not feel the candle burning her skin. She screamed only when she realised what was happening. I saw that she had second degree burns over a large part of the palm of her hand.

I remembered the aloe vera plant, ran upstairs to tear off a leaf, and then applied it several times. She told me she felt instant relief, so I gave her a couple of leaves to take home. She came back the next day for me to look at her hand and, to my surprise, the wound was already beginning to heal. The pain had also subsided and no local antibiotic treatment was required, as there was no infection. After a week, the burn was totally healed. Since then I have seen her several times over the years and I was always curious to look at her hand and see whether there was any scar tissue on her palm. There wasn't and this incident proved to be my first successful experiment with aloe vera as a therapeutic intervention.

In summary

There are many other people who are taking aloe vera to help manage conditions and illnesses such as ME, MS, diabetes, AIDS and even some cancers, as well as many others. We would stress that while some people may have found aloe vera has 'cured' their particular problem, nobody should ever think of aloe vera as a 'cure-all' or 'panacea' for all ills.

The scientific evidence outlined in Chapter 8 demonstrates that aloe vera has potent healing benefits – both internally and externally – across a broad spectrum of illnesses, diseases, disorders and ailments. For improved overall health and general well-being and to help boost their immune systems, we would suggest that everyone, including children, start drinking the best quality aloe vera gels and juices on a daily basis.

If there is ever a problem with the 'acquired' taste, remember – the best aloe vera is not sold for its taste, it's sold for its benefits. Just mask the flavour with a low-acid, fresh fruit juice. For a healthier skin, use only the highest quality aloe vera skin and facial preparations. Remember too that aloe vera toothgels (without fluoride) and aloe vera deodorants (without aluminium salts) can also contribute to healthier tissue in those areas.

KEY TIP

Aloe vera is one of those amazing gifts of nature that can help you start to take more control of your own lives and health. However, aloe vera is not a 'doctor' in a bottle. It is important that you should still consult your doctors and not attempt to self-diagnose, unless you are qualified to do so.

6

Nutrition: you are what you eat and absorb

Well fed and badly nourished – a conundrum of the twentieth and twenty-first centuries, or a reality?

FEW PEOPLE would probably disagree that there is enough annual food production worldwide, but that inadequate and inequitable distribution means that some have too much and many have too little. We, in the developed world, are slowly beginning to realise that more does not necessarily mean better. In essence many people in the developed world are overfed and badly nourished! You may well ask – why? how?

In the last fifty years, food conglomerates in the so-called developed economies seem to have found ever more efficient ways of stripping our food of valuable nutrients and presenting it to us in an ever more processed (more fats, more salt, more sugar!) and packaged format (and at the same time asking the consumer to pay more for it!). This at the same time ensures that it stays in our bodies for longer than is either necessary or healthy, clogging up our digestive systems, fermenting and decomposing. These actions often produce harmful toxins and can lead to numerous ailments, diseases and other medical disorders, and even death through cancers and other serious illnesses.

Recently, at the first major conference on child obesity in the UK, delegates were warned that childhood obesity had reached epidemic proportions. A survey (National Diet and Nutrition Survey, 2002) had found that children are now eating twenty-five times as many sweets and drinking thirty times as many soft drinks as they did in the post-war 1950s. Some obese children already have clusters of symptoms, including high blood pressure, and raised levels of blood fats that may clog arteries and cause changes in insulin levels. A study from the Royal Hospital for Sick Children in Bristol (2001) found signs of type two diabetes in children as young as thirteen (type two diabetes is almost exclusively triggered by being overweight and having a diet high in sugars and fats). High blood pressure in childhood could also lead to an increased risk of strokes.

Obesity levels are increasing in pre-school children. In diet surveys, eight per cent of eighteen-month-old children ate no vegetables, and sixteen per cent ate no fruit. By the time they were three and a half years old, seventeen per cent ate no vegetables or fruit. At eighteen months, only twelve per cent of children were eating the full recommended daily amount of fruit and vegetables, and by the time they were three and a half, this had decreased to eight per cent. Diet education was a critical factor in the survey. It was found that eleven per cent of seven-year-olds whose mothers had a low educational level were obese, compared with only just over four per cent in cases where mothers were educated to degree level. Children with poorly educated mothers were also less likely to eat fish, wholemeal bread, yoghurt, cheese, fruit, fruit juices and cereals, and more likely to eat chocolate, white bread, chips and drink soft drinks. They also had a lower intake of fibre and vitamin C in their diets. Breast fed children are also less likely to be obese in later life, and once again there was a correlation between the higher prevalence of breast feeding in educated women than in their less well educated counterparts. Another major reason was linked to the dietary history of women – if poor, this was likely to be passed down to the next generation.

Scientists from Glasgow University presented evidence that sixty per cent of seriously overweight youngsters, between five and ten years old, were already displaying signs of early heart disease. The Glasgow study also found a direct link between obesity and the increased risk of cancer. In non-smoking women, every extra 14 pounds in weight (6.4 kilograms) doubles their chance of dying from cancer. In men the risk is increased by fifty per cent. The study also found that one in five adults in the UK is obese, as are four per cent of all children.

Another study by Child Health in London (UK) and the London Metropolitan University, revealed that children's waistlines (stomachs!) have expanded by 2.5 inches (6.25 centimetres) in the last decade – fuelled by a combination of a diet of junk food and an increasingly sedentary lifestyle. The risk to children's well-being is not just their overall health. Individuals who carry weight on their fronts, rather than elsewhere, apparently have an increased risk of heart disease. The British Heart Foundation has confirmed that it is increasingly concerned about the higher incidence of childhood obesity. The problem is often trying to persuade young people, especially children, that what they eat, drink and do today can have a significant bearing on their health in later life. Coronary heart disease affects around 2,000,000 people in the UK and is the UK's number one killer – one person dies every three minutes!

Not a particularly comforting or pleasant picture, is it? Yet it is becoming more and more of a reality in many developed countries!

Nowadays, many doctors and nutritionists believe that much of the sickness and many of the so-called 'modern' diseases, like cancer and arterial disease (some experts believe that these two between them are responsible for up to seventy-five per cent of all deaths from illness in the UK), can be linked to poor diet and a sluggish, overworked and ineffectual digestive system. It has been reported that thirty-five per cent of all cancer in the Western world is due to an unhealthy diet – even more than the level attributed to smoking (circa thirty per cent). We all need plenty of roughage or fibre in our diet, and as I explained in my first book this would traditionally have come from fruits, grains, vegetables, pulses and so on. So let's use the example of brown, unpolished rice again. Naturally, each grain has a husk that is rough-coated, and this is where many of the nutrients are stored. When eaten and chewed well the nutrients are extracted by the time the rice has been broken down in order to pass through the colon. There, the colon's muscles move in gentle waves (peristalsis), pushing the rice (as was) along to the bowel. The husk provides the bulk and roughage that trigger the peristaltic movement, so cleaning the sides of the colon and the bowel and ensuring complete elimination, which means that everywhere is left clean and tidy with no bits left behind to cause or allow bacteria to form.

Now take a bowl of white rice, or any one of our many types of overprocessed or nutritionally deficient foods, with their chemical additives and synthetic preservatives. In relation to rice, while being processed the husk and much of the nutrition value is removed – this is what is meant by 'polished' grains of rice. All that is left are a few nutrients (most of the remainder is likely to be lost in the cooking) and a lot of sticky starch. The roughage has been discarded along with most of the nutritional benefits. This refined or processed food is consumed, and then – because of its lack of roughage and its rather sticky or sludgy consistency – it can become trapped in the digestive system and toxins can build up and be absorbed by the body.

There are very few nutrients available to the body from the consumption of such food, so there's little nutritional benefit, and by the time it has been eliminated, the debris it leaves behind can result or be instrumental in the development of serious digestive and related problems.

There are numerous disorders of the digestive system that can lead to poor absorption of nutrients and that can also be linked to diet, or, rather, poor diet, including perhaps even bowel cancer. Obviously, if someone is living on a diet consisting only of highly refined and processed foods like white rice, white flour and pre-cooked meals from the supermarket, as well as not eating sufficient roughage from vegetables, fruit, bran and so on, the above scenario is repeated daily. Over many years, the cumulative effect can be devastating. The body simply gets exhausted from trying to extract a small quantity of nutrients while struggling to eliminate the waste.

Of even more concern is the fact that all the chemicals (and free radicals) from pesticides and fertilisers used on cereals, vegetables and fruit are having a cumulative, continual and highly detrimental effect on our immune systems – but that's another story! It's no wonder that under this constant daily bombardment of chemically refined food our systems become tired and depleted, and it shows in our skins. Eat too much chocolate and 'stodge', add too much stress – which demands a quick boost of extra nutritional energy for the body – and the skin soon becomes greasy or dry, puffy, blotchy or spotty – I could go on!

KEY POINT
The food we put into our bodies has the vitamins, minerals, proteins, carbohydrates and everything usable extracted from it, so that the body can turn them into energy to fuel every system inside our skin.

Put aloe vera into our bodies and we have a potent natural health tonic. Aloe vera juice is an unpolluted, organically grown, fibrous pulpy juice, rich in valuable nutrients with powerful anti-oxidant and detoxifying benefits to boost our immune systems and increase our energy levels, and increase the bio-availability of essential vitamins and other nutrients.

KEY TIP
Look for the effects of aloe vera working from the inside out.

Because of aloe's deeply penetrating action on the skin, working first on the digestive system, then from system to system, it gradually helps the body to flush out the impurities and toxins and to restore balance to both overworked and sluggish areas.

In time the inner health starts to show on the outside – often with clearer skin, more energy, fewer colds and so on.

How much do doctors know about nutrition?

I believe on average in the UK, trainee doctors spend less than three months studying the subject of nutrition (any health professional or doctor who reads this and disagrees, please let me know if this information is wrong), and this is over a five- to seven-year learning period. This is both astounding and disturbing.

There is a growing realisation among healthcare professionals and nutritional therapists alike that a significant percentage of cancers and many other killer diseases (some believe this figure to be as high as seventy per cent) may be linked to diet and nutrition. It is increasingly acknowledged by such authorities as the UK Department of Health, the FDA in the USA, and cancer specialists at both Harvard University in the USA and Oxford University in the UK, that diet accounts for at least thirty per cent of all cancers. Bearing this in mind, one has to ask the questions, what is being done to improve the situation and what can you, the reader, do to improve your own personal situation? This chapter is not intended to be the definitive guide to nutrition. There are many highly qualified people who write papers and books on the subject every day. I simply want to encourage you to start thinking more seriously about what you eat and drink and whether your daily diet and nutrition regime should be altered to improve your lifestyle and overall well-being. You should also check that any additional nutrients and supplements that you take are of the right quality and are in a bio-available form.

I was pleased to read an article recently in the *Daily Mail* (Tuesday 4th February 2003) entitled 'Eat to Beat Cancer'. Information in the article was extracted from a new book of the same title by Dr Rosy Daniel (she is from the

Bristol Cancer Help Centre) and Jane Sen (*Eat To Beat Cancer*, Dr Rosy Daniel and Jane Sen, Thorsons, 2003). In it they talk of the food that we eat in the Western world, the way we produce it and cook it and the link to many illnesses and cancers. They advocate that what we need to do is switch from a high-protein, high-fat diet to a more natural way of eating, based on fresh fruit and vegetables, cereals and pulses. They say that as we have grown more affluent, our diet has become richer in both fats and proteins and is more highly flavoured with salt, sugar and other additives. Our bodies however have not evolved as quickly and cannot keep pace with these 'new' eating habits. We are basically unable to cope with the stresses this 'new diet' places on us, and because of this we are seeing a significant increase in cancer, heart disease, skin disorders, joint and bowel disorders and diseases like diabetes and possibly even those diseases affecting the brain.

I firmly believe that aloe vera can play a significant part in improving your overall nutrition and well-being. However, it is not some 'nutritional panacea' that you can switch on and off like a light to make up for the lack of a regular healthy diet and lifestyle. When I read one of Patrick Holford's books, *The Optimum Nutrition Bible*, I really began to understand the words of Dr Carl Pfeiffer (who is referred to in the book) when he said:

> It is my firmly held belief that with an adequate intake of micro-nutrients – essential substances we need to nourish us – most chronic diseases would not exist.
>
> Good nutritional therapy is the medicine of the future. We have already waited too long for it.

This statement came from a brilliant scientist who, at the age of fifty-one, had a massive heart attack and was given a maximum of ten years to live, provided he had a pacemaker fitted. He chose not to do so and then spent the next thirty years of his life researching and developing optimum nutrition. Now, let's put it to someone who knows about nutrition.

Patrick Holford, UK pioneer of optimum nutrition

I asked Patrick Holford, one of the key pioneers of optimum nutrition in the UK, and the founder of the Institute for Optimum Nutrition in London, to contribute to this chapter. I did so because I believe his views on diet are illuminating. He is well qualified to discuss the importance of nutrition and the role that aloe vera can play in establishing and maintaining a healthy, nutrition based lifestyle. I am convinced that if more of us listened to what he and many complementary therapists are saying, and also acted upon it, we would not only lead a healthier, more active and more enjoyable lifestyle, we would also be better nourished and more able to cope with both the pleasures and rigours of modern day life. Here are his comments:

'Let food be your medicine and medicine your food'

> Every single cell in your body is made from the food you eat. For this reason nutrition is considered the cornerstone of health. The words of Hippocrates over 2,000 years ago are probably more relevant now than they were then and should be enshrined in all advice on health and nutrition.
>
> *Patrick Holford*

> As the science of nutrition advances, we discover more and more naturally occurring substances in food that are both necessary for good health and can enhance our resistance to illness. First there were carbohydrates, proteins and fats; then vitamins and minerals; then enzymes; then essential fats; then antioxidants and now 'phyto-chemicals', a catch-all phrase for chemicals found in plants which have positive effects on our health and resistance to disease.
>
> *Patrick Holford*

Nutraceuticals or pharmaceuticals?

> Paralleling the increasing realisation that what you eat has the greatest effect on your health is the increasing realisation that the causes of most of the diseases we suffer from stem from the fact that we are moving increasingly further away from our natural design. Currently, the conservative estimate is that seventy per cent of the diseases we die from are diet related! Many of today's diseases are being shown to be the accumulated result of toxic agro-chemicals, drugs, food chemicals and eating a highly processed diet. Yet in most cases, the treatments recommended by the medical profession are based on a cocktail of pharmaceutical drugs – substances which are completely alien to the human body – which can often be toxic and can have highly undesirable side-effects. At the thin end of the wedge, modern day living and eating are causing fatigue, decreased resistance to disease and

stress and a whole lot of other 'minor' health problems that make life less than satisfactory.

Patrick Holford

KEY POINT
'Recently I rang up two doctors who had been in general practice for many years.
One told me, "I'm convinced that nutrition will be a major part of medicine in the foreseeable future. I'm getting substantially better results with improved diet and supplements than I used to with drugs."'

KEY POINT
'The other said, "The evidence for nutritional therapy is becoming so strong that if the doctors of today don't become nutritionists, then the nutritionists will become the doctors of tomorrow."'

Instead of using pharmaceutical drugs with undesirable side-effects, the medicine of tomorrow is turning to nutraceuticals, nature's pharmacy of nutrients found in living foods, to correct the body's chemistry and restore well-being. A plant such as aloe vera contains such a cocktail of proven health-promoting substances that to isolate each ingredient and then treat it like a drug to cure a specific illness is not only impractical, it is nonsensical. Aloe vera contains over 200 different constituents, including vitamins, minerals, enzymes, antioxidants, polysaccharides, important phyto-chemicals and other ingredients (these have been described earlier in this book). Recently, the effect of one antioxidant, namely vitamin E, was shown (by a large-scale medical study carried out by Cambridge University) to be three times more powerful at reducing the risk of a heart attack than the best available drug.

Just think what the effects would be of a lifetime of eating living foods, fruits, vegetables and nature's most action-packed health promoters like aloe vera. Plants like this provide a whole cocktail of essential vitamins, minerals, amino acids, antioxidants, enzymes and phyto-chemicals that work together synergistically to promote good health. Not surprisingly, the proven beneficial effects of aloe vera are very diverse, making it an excellent all-round tonic.

Patrick Holford

KEY TIP
'You don't have to be ill to benefit from aloe vera! The essence of all these nutritionists' thoughts is that with the right foods we can avoid many of the debilitating modern illnesses – and that aloe vera is a "Super Food" among them.'

Research by Dr Jeffrey Bland has shown that aloe vera juice improves digestion and the absorption of nutrients and enhances elimination of toxic substances. As well as all the nutrients within the juice, there is a special factor that is attracting a lot of attention. This is a complex type of carbohydrate called a polysaccharide. As we have seen earlier in the book, polysaccharides are a major building block for the human body and they also help to boost the immune system.

In animal studies, the polysaccharides in aloe vera have been shown to be powerful anti-cancer agents, stimulating the production of macrophages, which fight off cancer cells.

Patrick Holford

KEY POINT
'A lack of polysaccharides means the gut wall becomes too "leaky", thus letting through large food molecules, often resulting in allergic reactions. So anyone with an "irritable bowel" or an "inflammatory bowel" condition like colitis can benefit from drinking aloe vera.'

The increased 'leakiness' of tissue means an increased risk of infection and allergy, so people who are allergic or are prone to frequent infections can be helped by drinking high quality aloe vera.

Patrick Holford

KEY POINT
'Polysaccharides also seem to be natural anti-inflammatory agents, so they tend to help calm down inflammatory diseases like arthritis, asthma or eczema.'

You are what you can digest and absorb

Many raw foods contain the enzymes needed to break the food down and these enzymes are often destroyed by cooking. Aloe vera is especially rich in digestive enzymes, so unlike cooked food that taxes the body, aloe vera assists the body to break foods down. Since it also helps to promote a healthier digestive tract, it also improves absorption of nutrients.

Patrick Holford

KEY POINT
'Aloe vera is itself a rich source of nutrients including the vital anti-oxidant nutrients, vitamins A, C, E, selenium and zinc, to name a few, which are proven to protect us from heart disease and cancer, to boost the immune system and slow down the ageing process.'

Aloe vera also contains two essential fatty acids that are needed by the brain and nervous system, the skin and almost every organ of the body. Once again, cooked foods contain mainly damaged or 'hydrogenated' fats, while processed foods have, as ingredients, these or saturated fats. These hard fats are the ones that can kill, while the essential fats have the power to heal. I believe tomorrow's medicine will be about using nutrients instead of drugs. It will be about taking a different approach or 'looking through a new pair of glasses' that will reveal the true causes of diseases. In most cases these lie in faulty or poor nutrition, pollution, stress, and lack of exercise – the greatest cause of all, being ignorance and inadequate education about diet and nutrition.

As Thomas Edison, the great inventor, said, 'The doctor of the future will give no medicine but will interest his patients in the care of the human frame, diet and the cause and prevention of disease.'

Patrick Holford

KEY TIP
'As modern science is now proving, nature already has the answers. Living foods, such as aloe vera, uncontaminated by man-made chemicals, contain all the ingredients we need for promoting good health and improved vitality.'

Nutraceuticals and glyconutrients – what are they?

The medicines of the future?

The word 'nutraceuticals' is an unofficial term that comes from a combination of the words 'nutrition' and 'pharmaceutical'. The term describes natural food-based substances (nutrition) that have pharmacological (healing) properties and benefits for the body. Nutraceuticals is a relatively new term (past decade), used by the Food and Nutrition Board of the Institute of Medicine for all natural, standardised, non-toxic, dietary supplements designed to optimise health through improved nutrition.

A 'glyconutrient' is a new and more specialised type of nutraceutical. These nutrients support the process that our individual tissue cells use to recognise and communicate with each other. Glyconutrients are not disease or ailment specific, they are not a magic bullet, but the body has an extraordinary ability to heal itself when supported by the proper nutritional regime. Unlike other nutritional supplements, glyconutrients provide the monosaccharides identified as essential for good health.

The efficacy of glyconutrients has been established by the world's leading scientists and researchers as the key to proper cellular communication and proper cell function. In 1999, the Nobel Prize for medicine was awarded to Dr Gunter Blobel for his work in the exciting new field of science-medicine – glycobiology. Dr Emil Mondoa is the founder of the Glyconutrients Research Foundation and a joint author of the book *Sugars That Heal. The New Healing Science of Glyconutrients* (Emil Mondoa, MD, and Mindy Kitei, Random House). In the book, Mondoa explains the role of the eight essential sugars, known as saccharides, as the basis for multicellular intelligence...the ability of cells to communicate, cohere and work together to keep people healthy and balanced. He believes that even tiny amounts of these sugars...or a lack of them...can have profound effects on health.

Michael Schlachter, MD (board certified internal medicine and pulmonary disease clinical instructor), Integrative Health and Healing Institute, believes that the biggest revolutionary change in the war against disease is represented by glyconutrients. He determines that if people do not want to become patients (and hence statistics), they need to answer in their own hearts and minds the question, is what you are doing for your health optimal, and if not, what else can you do? He feels that if people do nothing more than to begin to question the present day medical dogma, he has done his job!

Rob Ortramm, MD, immunologist and research scientist, believes that glyconutrients are something that will become mandatory for overall health. He has reached this conclusion because during his research and searches on the use of glyconutrients in numerous disease processes, he has been amazed by the number of quality studies that have shown benefit and promise in a myriad of diseases, ranging from arthritis to diabetes.

Dr AT Fernandez, MD, a medical practitioner for over twenty years (currently working in gynaecology and obstetrics), believes that to practise medicine is a continuous learning curve and that future medical practice will one day rely less on drugs and more on providing glyconutritional assistance to the body to help the natural healing process.

This sounds so like the great Thomas Edison all those years ago!

Much of the information in this section has been sourced from: www.GlycoInformation.com.

Aloe vera and the acid-alkaline balance

We know that aloe vera can contribute in regulating the pressure, temperature, fluid content and basic acid balance in tissue. In recent years, research and experience have shown that aloe vera has an effect on the acid-alkaline balance.

See Bland, J, 'Effect of orally-consumed aloe vera juice on human gastro-intestinal function', *Natural Foods Network Newsletter*, August 1985.

This may be evident in the way it contributes to the stripping of waste materials from tissue. Several investigations have shown that aloe vera drinking juice can help increase pH in the stomach. Aloe vera can also have a weak antibiotic effect and influence the growth of helicobacter pylori, the bacteria that cause ulcers, and it has also shown the ability to reduce fungus growth in the stomach. These factors would suggest that aloe vera is one of the few plants that in some instances can replace drug treatment in the healing of ventricular and duodenal ulcers. Fortunately, in most patients this is not an issue as there are now effective drugs with few side effects in the current medical treatment of stomach and duodenal ulcers. However, there will always be some patients who suffer some degree of side effects from medication, and this is where the influence of aloe vera on the acid-alkaline balance could be important. The theory of acid-alkaline balance claims that the body needs both acid- and alkaline-forming food. If the diet contains an excess of acid-forming foods, this will be neutralised by taking calcium from the bones. Calcium acts as a buffer to ensure the acid-alkaline balance.

What are acid-forming foods? They are not necessarily sour tasting foods like citrus fruits, but rather mainly protein-rich foods with a high content of chlorine, sulphur and phosphorus, such as meat, fish and eggs. Whole grain products are mainly acid forming, with notable exceptions being grains like buckwheat and millet. Alkaline foods have a high content of potassium, calcium and magnesium. They are mainly found in vegetables and also in dairy products. Fruits are alkaline forming, but cultivation with pesticides can lead to many fruits becoming acid forming in the body.

Nowadays, there is little risk of consuming too much in the way of alkaline-forming fruits, unless someone is suffering from a disease with significant biochemical disturbances. To put it simply, the most important thing to emphasise is the necessity of ensuring everyone consumes enough vegetables in their diet. This will ensure the correction of the acid-alkaline imbalance that is believed to exist in most people in today's developed world.

Indeed, aloe vera may be the plant that has the ability to have a direct effect on the regulation of the acid-alkaline balance. This may be one of the explanations for the cleansing and well-being effect that many people experience and report when drinking aloe vera – whatever the medical reasons – so let us explore the subject in some more detail.

We know that pH is a measurement of the acidity or alkalinity of a substance. The pH scale runs from nought to fourteen and indicates the level of free protons (H+) in a system. At the low end, nought indicates a strong, complete acid that is saturated with highly reactive free protons. The high end, fourteen, indicates a strong, complete alkali with virtually no free protons and, instead, is saturated with highly reactive hydroxide ions (OH-). The middle, pH 7.0, indicates that the substance is neither acid nor alkaline – it is neutral. The pH scale is logarithmic so each step up the scale is a ten-fold increase.

Definitions:

pH = measure of how acid or how alkaline a substance is.
pH scale = scale of measurement for acidity and alkalinity.

acid	neutral	alkaline
1	7	14

All chemical processes have an ideal pH at which they are most efficient. For example, the body functions best with an internal chemistry being slightly alkaline (pH of 7.0 to 8.0). The pH of the blood is even more specific:

blood pH 7.4 = normal; 7.2 = death.

Our internal body chemistry functions in an alkaline environment. Our blood must maintain a pH of 7.4. If it drops below that to 7.2 we die.

The cells of the body in health are alkaline. In disease the cell pH is below 7.0. The more acid the cells become, the sicker we are and feel. The cells won't die until their pH gets to about 3.5. Our bodies produce acid as a by-product of normal metabolism. This is the result of our bodies burning or using alkaline to remain alive. Because our bodies do not manufacture alkaline, we must supply the alkaline from an outside source to keep us from becoming acid and dying.

Human cells produce acid as they function. For example, body metabolism produces certain acids and heavy exercise produces other acids. Body chemistry and the foods we eat also determine the types of acids produced during metabolism. Removing or neutralising that acid is important because the human body works best, and its chemistry functions most effectively, when it is slightly alkaline. The acid-alkaline balancing mechanisms are key to healthy and efficient body chemistry. For example, blood pH in a healthy body is kept in a narrow alkaline range of 7.35 to 7.45. Lactic, uric and various other complex acidic compounds are by-products of metabolism and they push the blood pH toward the acidic range.

Kidneys and lungs are the organs predominantly responsible for keeping blood pH under control. The kidneys, through their selective filtration functions, cleanse the excess venous acids and discharge the waste through the urinary tract. The kidneys also secrete some ammonia into the blood as a buffer to bring the blood pH to normal levels. Oxygen absorbed through the lungs also contributes to maintaining pH balance. The oxygen combines with carbon in certain proteins to create 'carbonates', i.e. buffering agents that slow acidic build-up and bring blood pH into the normal range. As we age, body functions become less efficient. Kidneys and lungs do not work as well as when we were young. As a result, we may get acid-alkaline imbalance. Food is a means of replenishing the alkaline in the body. The main determining factor of alkaline is the organic minerals. One can equate organic minerals with alkaline for better understanding. Foods are of two types, acid or alkaline. This refers to the ash value of a food, i.e. the type of residue that remains after the food is digested and processed. Is it acid or is it alkaline? If there is an acid residue (inorganic acids), the body must neutralise this acid to keep the blood from getting acid. The acid is neutralised with alkaline. Ideally there is adequate alkaline in the diet to do this. However, if there is not, the body must extract alkaline from its cells to neutralise the acid. This, of course, causes the cells to become acid and thus diseased.

Because our bodies are an alkaline entity, in order to maintain health, the majority of our diet must consist of alkaline ash foods. We can remain in good health by consuming a diet that is seventy to eighty per cent alkaline and twenty to thirty per cent acid. The more alkaline the better. If our bodies become too alkaline as a result of eating a high alkaline diet, we will lose our appetite and automatically want to fast, during which time the normal acid metabolic by-products will return the body's pH back to normal.

The breakdown of foods into acid ash and alkaline ash categories would generally be as follows (note: foods in the Acid Ash column are listed in order of least acid to most acid, and in the Alkaline Ash column foods are listed in order from most alkaline to least alkaline). See overleaf.

How do nutrition and lifestyle affect acid-alkaline balance?

In terms of chemistry, when one talks about acidity or alkalinity, one is talking about hydrogen. An acid is a substance that releases hydrogen into a solution, and an alkali or base is one that removes hydrogen from a solution. The amount of free hydrogen is measured on a scale ranging from one to fourteen, called pH, and this denotes the exact level of acidity or alkalinity. A pH value below seven is considered acid and above seven alkaline.

Inside the human body, the acid-alkaline balance is important because many functions in the body occur only at a certain level of acidity or alkalinity. Many enzymes and chemical reactions in the body work best at a particular pH. A small change in pH can have a profound effect on body function. For example, muscle contractibility declines and hormones like adrenaline and aldosterone increase as the body becomes slightly more acid. In addition, different parts of the body have different levels of acidity and alkalinity. Some of these are shown in Table 1. It should be noted that while

TABLE 1. pH of Various Body Tissues

TISSUE	pH
Skeletal muscle	6.9-7.2
Heart	7.0-7.4
Liver	7.2
Brain	7.1
Blood	7.35-7.45
Saliva	6.0-7.4
Urine	4.5-8.0

TABLE 2. Acid Ash and Alkaline Ash Foods

ACID ASH	ALKALINE ASH
SOME RAW FRUITS AND VEGETABLES (cranberries, blueberries, plums, prunes, squash)	RAW FRUITS
	ALOE VERA
WHOLE GRAINS - COOKED	DRIED FRUITS
OVERCOOKED FRUITS/VEGGIES	FROZEN FRUITS/VEGGIES
DAIRY PRODUCTS (cheese, eggs, milk, etc.)	LIGHTLY STEAMED FRUITS and VEGGIES
SUGAR and REFINED GRAINS	RAW NUTS (almonds, pecans, cashews, etc.)
WHITE MEAT (fish, fowl) Raw, rare, well done	SPROUTED GRAINS
RED MEATS (beef, pork, mutton) Raw, rare, well done	
HERBS, SPICES, CONDIMENTS, SPICY FOODS (garlic, hot peppers, onions, horseradish, etc.)	
FRIED FOOD, COFFEE, TEA, SALT, ALCOHOL	
DRUGS and MEDICATIONS, TOBACCO.	

there can be a wide range of pH values for the saliva and urine, the value for the blood is maintained within narrow bounds.

TABLE 3. Factors Regulating Acid-Alkaline Balance in the Body

In the blood:	**Inside cells:**
Bicarbonate	chemical reactions generating or consuming hydrogen
Amino acids	
Albumin	entry or exit of hydrogen from the cell via pumps or diffusion
Haemoglobin	

Because of the importance of the acid-alkaline balance in the blood and tissues, the body has a number of mechanisms for regulating this balance. These mechanisms are shown in Table 3. Many body functions are involved in the regulation of acid-alkaline balance, including respiration, excretion, digestion and cellular metabolism.

In the bloodstream, there are substances known as buffers that act chemically to resist changes in pH. The most important of these compounds in the blood are bicarbonate, albumin, globulins and haemoglobin. Other regulation of blood pH is carried out mainly by the lungs and the kidneys. The lungs aid in acid-alkaline regulation by removing carbon dioxide from the blood. Carbon dioxide combines with water in the body to form carbonic acid, so that removing carbon dioxide is equivalent to removing acid. Respiratory rates can vary depending on the acidity of the body, speeding up under acid conditions to remove carbon dioxide and reduce acidity, and slowing down under alkaline conditions to retain acids and reduce alkalinity. The kidneys also respond to the pH of the blood. If the blood is too acid, the kidney excretes extra hydrogens into the urine and retains extra sodium. Phosphorus in the form of phosphate is required for this exchange. The body obtains this phosphorus from bone if it is otherwise unavailable. When the bloodstream is extremely acid, the kidney uses a different method and excretes ammonium ions, which contain four hydrogens, into the urine. When the body is too alkaline, the process is reversed, and hydrogen is retained. In the digestive process, the acid-alkaline balance is affected by the secretions of the stomach and the pancreas. These secretions are absorbed into the bloodstream and affect the rest of the body. When food is eaten, the stomach secretes hydrochloric acid. In response to this acid, the pancreas secretes bicarbonate, which neutralises the stomach acid so that pancreatic enzymes can work properly.

Normally, after eating, there are transient changes in blood pH, known as the acid and alkaline tides, that correspond to the stomach and pancreatic secretions. Usually the pH of the blood quickly returns to normal. However, if digestive secretions are out of balance, then the whole body can be affected. Other digestive problems that affect the body's pH are diarrhoea, which results in a loss of bicarbonate, and vomiting, which results in a loss of acid. Just as the pH of the bloodstream is kept under tight control, the acid-alkaline environment inside the cells is also regulated so that it remains within narrow bounds. One way that this regulation occurs is by pumps in the cell membrane that cause hydrogen to enter or exit from the cell. Many of these pumps require phosphorus and magnesium to function so that micronutrient nutrition is a factor affecting the acid-alkaline balance. Another way that cells regulate the pH inside the cell is by changing the chemical reactions that occur, so that more or less hydrogen is produced. When the blood is too acid, symptoms include drowsiness, progressing to stupor and coma. Acute acidosis can result from kidney or lung problems, dehydration, ingestion of certain drugs, diabetes or diarrhoea, and is treated by giving an alkaline solution such as bicarbonate of soda.

A particular form of acidosis is ketosis, which occurs in diets high in fat and lacking in carbohydrates, as well as in conditions of diabetes or starvation, when the body burns fats rather than carbohydrates. However, when normal quantities of fat are consumed in a diet containing carbohydrate, the fats cause no problems in the acid-alkaline balance for the majority of people. When the blood is too alkaline, symptoms include cramps, muscle spasms, irritability and hyperexcitability. Acute alkalosis may be caused by impaired kidney function, hyperventilation, use of diuretic or steroid drugs, vomiting or gastric drainage. Acute alkalosis is treated by giving an acid solution such as ammonium chloride or by breathing expired carbon dioxide from a paper bag .

TABLE 4. Acid, Alkaline and Neutral Ash Foods (8)

Acid Ash Foods	Alkaline Ash Foods	Neutral Ash Foods
bread (grains)	cheese	arrowroot
cake	cream	butter
cereal	most fruit	candy
mayonnaise	jam	coffee
cranberries	milk	cornstarch
plums	almonds	lard
prunes	chestnuts	margarine
meat	coconut	vegetable oil
Brazil nuts	molasses	postum
walnuts	most vegetables	white sugar
peanuts		syrup
legumes		tapioca
corn		tea

Before World War II, there was considerable interest in how the food we eat affects the acid-alkaline balance of the body. While today the subject is not receiving much attention in orthodox circles, many alternative practitioners place considerable importance on the acid-alkaline balance characteristics of various diets. In spite of a degree of ongoing debate, it is generally acknowledged that the food that is eaten is a major source of acid and alkali for the body.

Some confusion in terminology has resulted because of the way that the discussion evolved. In investigating how different foods might affect the acid-alkaline balance, various foods were burned to ash in the laboratory and the pH of the resulting ash was measured. These foods were then classified as acid, alkaline or neutral ash foods as shown in Table 4. In addition, various alternative practitioners have referred to acid and alkaline-forming foods, based on the reaction of foods in the body. These categories are shown in Table 5.

TABLE 5. Acid and Alkaline Forming Foods

Acid Forming Foods	**Alkaline Forming Foods**
All meat, poultry, eggs, and seafood	All fruits except those noted above
All foods made from cereal grains including breads, breakfast cereals, crackers, pasta and rice	All vegetables except beans, peas and lentils
Fat including salad oil, butter, margarine, lard etc.	Dairy products including milk, buttermilk, cheeses and yoghurt
Legumes including beans, peas, lentils and peanuts	
Fruits containing benzoic or oxalic acid, including prunes, plums, cranberries, rhubarb and sour cherries	
Chocolate	
Coffee, tea and most soft drinks	
Sugar, syrup	
All true nuts	

The terms acid or alkaline ash and acid- and alkaline-forming are often used interchangeably, but as can be seen from these tables, the terms are not always synonymous. Using the more scientific definitions, alkaline ash foods are those that contain large quantities of magnesium, calcium, potassium and/or sodium – minerals that form alkaline compounds. Most fruits and vegetables are considered alkaline. Acid ash foods are those that contain chloride, phosphorus, or sulphur – minerals that form acid compounds. These acid ash foods include meat, fish, poultry, legumes and grains, which all contain high levels of phosphorus, and mustard and eggs, which contain sulphur. In addition, fruits such as plums, prunes, cranberries, rhubarb and sour cherries are also acid-forming because they contain either oxalic or benzoic acid, organic acids that are not completely broken down in the body.

Individual digestion and metabolism also plays a role in determining whether a food leaves an acid or alkaline residue. For example, certain foods containing organic acids, such as citrus fruits and tomatoes, which normally leave no acid residues, may be incompletely metabolised in some people and are acid-forming for these individuals. This is quite frequently the case where stomach acid is low or thyroid activity is subnormal. There are other metabolic and lifestyle factors that affect the acidity of the body and the reactions of foods. Infection, smoking and alcohol consumption tend to make the body more acid. Conversely, exercise will tend to make the body more alkaline, but if it is continued beyond a comfortable level it can become acid-forming, as lactic acid levels build up. Furthermore, the dietary content of trace elements also affects the acid-alkaline balance. Adequate magnesium and phosphorus are necessary for cellular pumps. Zinc is necessary both for secretion of acid in the stomach and for excretion or retention of acid by the kidney. In addition, many other nutrients, the B vitamins for example, are necessary to oxidise completely carbohydrates and fats. It has been recommended by Edgar Cayce and others that the diet be comprised of eighty per cent alkaline-forming foods and twenty per cent acid-forming. In more practical terms, the recommendation was four vegetables and two fruits to one starchy food and one protein food. It is not clear whether these proportions apply for all people. By contrast, Dr Weston Price found that the traditional diets of the healthy primitives he studied were higher in acid ash foods than in alkaline ash foods.

The traditional diets were higher in minerals than the more processed modern diets. Dr Price's research confirms the importance of nutrient-dense, unrefined, properly prepared foods. Moreover, genetic differences may play a role in what constitutes an appropriate balance in the diet. For example, it is known that Eskimos handle fats far more efficiently than other populations and do not suffer from ketosis from very high fat consumption as other groups do. The fact that Cayce's recommendations seem at odds with those of Dr Price can be explained by the fact they were aimed at a different population group, living in a different climate with a different level of activity. In people of European descent in the USA, manipulation of the acid or alkaline nature of the diet has been used along with other measures to treat disease conditions, particularly dental caries.

In the 1940s, Dr Harold Hawkins, a professor of dentistry at the University of Southern California, studied the effects of foods on the pH and mineral content of the saliva, urine and bloodstream. Dr Hawkins found that the pH and mineral composition of the saliva and urine were affected by diet but that the pH of the bloodstream was more influenced by digestion and other metabolic and lifestyle factors. As a result of his studies over many years, Dr Hawkins was able to construct a diet that was adequate for most people and to treat those with dental problems and other disease conditions using primarily diets adjusted to balance saliva and urine chemistry. Like Dr Price, Dr Hawkins stressed the importance of animal protein and whole grains along with adequate fat and vegetable intake.

The acid-alkaline balance is an important factor in the health and efficient functioning of the body. Diet is one factor that influences the acid-alkaline balance both through the acid- or alkaline-forming nature of the foods that are eaten and through the nutrient content that affects metabolism. Nutrient rich traditional diets provide the essential factors necessary for excellent metabolism, efficient acid-alkaline regulation and optimal health. Today, a number of alternative practitioners advocate a diet based primarily on fruits and vegetables – one that minimises 'acid-forming' foods such as meat, fish and grains. While the inclusion of fruits and vegetables in the diet is important for many reasons, including the fact that these foods provide alkalinising minerals, for most people it is not necessary to minimise acid ash foods such as meat and whole grains in order to maintain acid-alkaline balance. In fact, a diet in which these acid ash foods are absent can lead to deficiencies that can undermine the body's ability to maintain the proper blood pH. Meat and other animal foods provide protein. Red meats provide zinc and properly prepared whole grains provide phosphorus, all of which are needed for the regulation of the acid-alkaline balance.

Fat-soluble vitamins found in organ meats, shellfish and good quality butter help maintain the health of the lungs and kidneys, the two prime organs involved in the acid-base regulation. Weston Price's research indicates a nutrient-dense diet that supplies both alkaline-ash and acid-ash minerals in liberal amounts is key to the health of the entire organism, including the complex systems that regulate the acid-alkaline balance.

In her new book entitled *500 Of The Most Important Ways To Stay Younger Longer* (Cico Books, 2003), Hazel Courtney talks of the need to maintain a good acid-alkaline balance in the body. She says that cells function best when alkaline, and ideally our bodies should be seventy per cent alkaline and thirty per cent acid.

However, the average person is eighty per cent acid and twenty per cent alkaline, so most people need to eat more alkalising foods such as honey (pure honey), watercress, carrots and celery. Added to that list should of course be aloe vera juice as it raises pH levels in the gut – as was found by Jeffrey Bland in his ground-breaking research (see Bland, J, 'Effect of orally-consumed aloe vera juice on human gastro-intestinal function', *Natural Foods Network Newsletter*, August 1985).

Aloe vera, because it is one of the most alkalising, natural substances we know of, can be an integral and important part of a healthy diet/lifestyle programme to ensure an effective acid-alkaline balance. This is especially due to its effect on tissue, regulating pressure and circulation and thus ensuring a proper balance of body fluids.

The impact of the modern diet

There is no question that the impact of so-called 'fast foods' and 'convenience' foods in the more developed and affluent countries of the world has exacted a heavy price on the health of the hundreds of millions of people who live there. The fact that we have food in abundance but spend a larger proportion of our disposable income on 'convenience' foods and foods containing too many fats, sugar and salt, fizzy drinks and other items like cigarettes (that damage our health), has resulted in an unfortunate and highly concerning state of affairs. We in the developed world, in spite of our riches (and really because of them) are now better fed than ever before and worse nourished. Since the end of World War II, the provision of cheap and highly plentiful food has been one of the key political agendas of most governments. How it was produced and what was used to produce this food was of secondary importance. Only now are we reaping the grim results of such a policy. This approach may have been necessary and even beneficial at the time, but unfortunately it has not evolved since to cope with the widely publicised damage that has been done to the health of both people and animals, and the environment.

In general, the food we eat and the water we drink now contains literally thousands more chemicals than it did fifty years ago. Our bodies and our digestive systems in particular are being bombarded with an array of synthetic chemicals (including pharmaceuticals) and toxins, and we are fighting a continual detoxification battle to rid ourselves of those that are detrimental to our health. We are continually exposed to health scares such as bovine spongiform encephalitis (BSE) and Creutzfeld Jakob disease (CJD), and a recent epidemic of foot and mouth (a disease not seen in the UK for over thirty years) caused widespread damage and suffering to humans and animals alike across the UK, and in some parts of western Europe. Outbreaks of dangerous e-coli, salmonella and other serious infections seem to becoming more common. We are told that the fish in our rivers are changing sex because of the hormones in the water. We are probably even eating genetically modified (GM) foods without being aware of it or being told about it!

Literally, every day, when we open a newspaper, watch the television or listen to the radio, there is another scare of some type related to the food we eat, the water we drink or to the environment. We eat meat that is fed with and contaminated by antibiotics and growth hormones. Our vegetables and fruits have the residues of so many pesticides and other chemicals present on the skin (and sometimes in the core) that the only safe way to eat them is to ensure that the skins and the cores are totally removed.

We eat too much of the wrong grains; too much refined sugar and other foods; too many fats and salt, and last but not least, too much cow's milk and dairy products. The latter is an excellent example of how misinformation has dominated the nutritional thinking of successive governments, no doubt heavily influenced by vested interest pressure groups. I have always been amazed by the fact that humans are the only animal species that consumes another animal's milk on a regular and ongoing basis, and we, in the UK in particular, are very high consumers of dairy products.

The UK is responsible for over one third of the total consumption of dairy products in the European Union, though we have less than one fifth of the total population. We, in Britain, are continually told that milk is essential for our intake of calcium, and without it we cannot have healthy teeth and bones. Not so. Calcium and magnesium are found in nuts, seeds and vegetables (cabbage, broccoli, carrots, cauliflower, etc.), and other essential minerals like manganese, chromium, magnesium and the important anti-oxidant mineral, selenium, are present in higher quantities in various fruits and vegetables than they are in milk. Milk is a food that is specifically produced by animals for their young, and cow's milk (it's good for calves!) is the source of an increasing number of cases of both allergies and food intolerances among both adults and children in the more affluent and developed countries of the world.

KEY TIP

There are many health professionals who strongly recommend that cow's milk should not be fed to children who are less than one year old. There are also numerous people who find that when they reduce or eliminate dairy products from their own or their children's diets, the eczema is eased, the sinus problem is alleviated, the asthma improved and that person's general health improves, in some cases dramatically. These improvements also tend to happen quickly.

Many complementary therapists are also now recommending the use of coral calcium.

Recently, a book written by Professor Jane Plant, who is an eminent British geo-chemist, put forward the argument concerning the possible link between milk and dairy products and breast cancer in women (and prostate cancer in men). She suggested that the hormones and chemicals that are present in milk and dairy products are the causal link. She had first developed breast cancer in 1987, and when, in 1993, she was diagnosed with cancer – for the fifth time – it had now spread to her lymph system and she had a secondary tumour on her neck. She was given only a few months to live and decided immediately to take control of her disease. Her book, *Your Life in Your Hands* (see Appendix 2), details what she has done over the last decade to regain her health. She describes how, by radically altering her diet and totally eliminating milk, dairy products and all processed foodstuffs that contained them (and she found that many did), together with red meat and most other animal products, and by adopting a more 'Chinese style' diet, based on soya (tofu), vegetables and many other anti-oxidant foodstuffs, the tumour that had been threatening her life (and had not been reduced by chemotherapy) shrank and then totally disappeared – within only a few weeks!

The research and work that she and her husband had both done in China was instrumental in making what for her was a lifesaving 'discovery'. They had checked the statistics (using age-standardised incidence rates per 100,000 people) and discovered that in rural China only 11 women out of every 100,000 contract breast cancer, and for prostate cancer it is 0.5 men out of every 100,000. In the UK the incidence of this type of cancer is apparently seventy times greater! (Source: *Your Life In Your Hands*.) In the Western world, the risk of a woman developing breast cancer during her lifetime varies from around one in eight in the USA (up from one in twenty since 1960!), to one in twelve in the UK and one in twenty in southern Europe (where milk and dairy products form a much smaller proportion of the diet in these regions).

With regard to mortality rates, the figures are that in China only 1 in 10,000 women die from breast cancer every year, but in Britain alone, deaths from breast cancer are currently about 13,000 per annum (deaths from prostate cancer – for which there is interestingly much less publicity – are about 10,000 per annum!). She also found out that Japanese women living in Hiroshima and Nagasaki (both cities were devastated by atomic bombs in World War II and radiation sickness was prevalent in the population thereafter for many years) had rates much the same as women in urban areas in China!

After pondering these facts for some time, they both came to the conclusion that the common denominator was that Chinese people (and Japanese people) do not drink milk or eat significant amounts of dairy products. This only happens when they move to a more urbanised culture and are then exposed to and influenced by more so-called Western eating habits. As a result of her own personal experiences and her research, Professor Plant now believes that the link between milk and dairy products and breast cancer is as compelling as the link between smoking and lung cancer. She apparently also discovered that as far back as 1989, yoghurt had been implicated in cases of ovarian cancer in the USA, after detailed studies conducted by Dr Daniel Cramer of Harvard University. Professor Jane Plant's book – *Your Life in Your Hands* – is a detailed account of her illness, the painstaking research that she and her husband conducted to find a 'cancer busting diet and lifestyle' and the way in which she has quite literally saved her own life! I have read her book and would recommend that anyone who is concerned about breast cancer or prostate cancer should both read this book and share it with anyone they know who is suffering from either disease. Let them make up their own minds about Professor Plant's opinions and conclusions. They should also consider adopting a healthier 'cancer busting' diet immediately, if they are not already following a healthy, anti-oxidant-rich regime.

She has developed what she calls the 'Plant Programme'. It is not simply a diet, it is more a way of life. It consists of seven food factors and five lifestyle factors, designed to prevent and overcome breast and prostate cancer and protect against osteoporosis and other ailments that we are told (no doubt by vested interest groups or those influenced by them) are always linked to a dairy-free diet! Without wishing to be over-dramatic, such changes may help people improve or even save their own lives! However, as Dr Audun Myskja has commented earlier, there are undoubtedly times when conventional medication and treatment may be required or may be the only option. The choice of treatment should be that of the patient once they have an objective view of the options available to them.

Undoubtedly, it has suited successive administrations in the UK (and probably in many other developed countries) to promote milk, being one of the cheapest food sources available to the mass of the population. It is also a significant source of employment and, for the companies involved in the dairy industry, it is a huge revenue earner. Little or no consideration is ever given to any possible or resultant health problems, and any relevant research seems to be studiously ignored, as is the promotion of healthier alternatives. However, following the publication of Professor Plant's book, hopefully more health professionals will not only study her findings but will also give some urgent consideration to the need to develop some diet alternatives for future generations, which do not necessarily focus so exclusively on dairy products.

Milk: a health myth or an important food?

The choice is yours!

There are many people who believe that the influence of the dairy industry worldwide in promoting its products (both wet and dry) causes more health problems than it contributes to good health and nutrition.

There are those who believe that dairy products (whether pasteurised or unpasteurised) can have serious health risks to certain parts of the population in both the developed and the developing world.

There are those such as Professor John Hermon Taylor in the UK, one of the world's pre-eminent researchers into the causes of Crohn's disease, who is at the forefront in the development of a vaccine to prevent the disease.

There are those such as Tim Page who runs the Chronic Crohn's Campaign in the UK (see Chapter 5, and Appendix 1.9), who firmly believes that one of the main causes of Crohn's disease can be laid firmly at the door of dairy products.

Other campaigners such as Robert Cohen (see www.notmilk.com) are vehement in their campaign against the dairy industry and the products it promotes as being good for your health.

Readers should look at both sides of the coin and make up their own minds.

They should also remember that aloe vera can play a significant role in the overall process of developing and maintaining good health and well-being, as well as in the healing process to fight against illness and disease.

Wheat and gluten

There is also something of a myth about wheat being good for you (normally in the form of bread), but increasingly, over the last few decades, more and more people have developed allergies to grains, and in particular to wheat with a high gluten content. More and more independent health professionals are convinced that the increased number of chemicals (pesticides, herbicides, hormones, antibiotics, preservatives, etc.) in our food chain, the nutrient deficient, over-processed foods and drinks that are making up a higher proportion of our diets, and the damaging 'oxidants' or 'free radicals' and other toxins, are combining to make a lethal 'cocktail' – a scenario that the human body is struggling both to deal with and counteract.

Perhaps this is why we have seen such a huge increase in the number of people suffering with eczema, asthma, arthritis and many other diseases and disorders – where the immune system simply can no longer cope, and is why cancer of all types seems to be so prevalent now. Nowadays, virtually everyone seems to have been 'touched' by this 'epidemic' – either directly or indirectly. The increasing links between diet and diseases are not simply coincidences that can be dismissed out of hand by governments, public sector health professionals, large food conglomerates and industry focus groups. They are real issues that must be addressed if we are to reduce the scourge of diseases such as cancer, diabetes, heart disease, etc.

In his book *Food is Medicine* (Duncan Baird Publishers), Pierre Jean Cousin refers to diet 'playing a fundamental role in the health of the heart and blood vessels'. A good diet can help to keep the cardiovascular system (heart and lungs) working efficiently during a person's lifetime, whereas a bad diet is likely to be a major risk factor for heart attacks and strokes, high blood pressure and thickening of the arteries. The Western diet, which as we have said before tends to be high in sugars, salt and saturated fats, promotes the deposit of these fats in the arteries, thus increasing the risk of blood clots and heart attacks. Improving diet can substantially reduce the risk of future health problems and can even halt or reverse arterial damage and even restore arteries to good health. Many scientists, nutritionists and even doctors now agree that diets that have increased levels of high-fibre foods and oily fish, potassium-rich vegetables and herbs such as ginger and garlic (and one could argue aloe vera too, which is rich in minerals, vitamins and soothes, cleanses and protects the digestive system), green vegetables and fresh fruit will help lower blood pressure and maintain better health. Other foods such as blue fruits (blueberries, etc.), yellow, orange and red vegetables that are rich in health-promoting anti-oxidants, can also help promote better health.

The role of supermarkets, fast food companies and the media – good or bad?

One area that should concern all parents, health professionals and governments is the increasing influence that supermarkets, fast food companies, the media (especially TV) and advertisers have on our eating habits and lifestyles and that of our children and younger, more impressionable people in general. A recent survey conducted in the UK (source: Sustain) examined the relationship between the percentage of advertising spent on various foodstuffs (and drinks) and their relative importance in a healthy diet for children. The findings follow research by the UK government's Department of Health and the Food Standards Agency, which revealed 'the appalling diet of many children' and suggestion that Britain is 'on the brink of an obesity epidemic resulting from poor diet and a general lack of exercise'. The survey showed that as much as ninety-nine percent of the food products advertised during children's TV viewing time were potentially unhealthy – i.e., promoting high value-added, processed products with high salt, high fat or high sugar contents (all ingredients that the government has identified as being detrimental to children's health). Some recent studies in the UK have shown that the salt content of some savoury snacks (such as crisps) has nearly doubled in the last ten years.

The seemingly unstoppable and cynical exploitation of children in the UK and many other developed countries by so called 'junk food firms' and advertisers has resulted in a massive explosion in the market for products that are arguably 'nutritionally deficient' and 'potentially harmful'. It is no coincidence that advertisers spend millions on researching target markets or groups, and many more millions persuading those target groups to purchase their products. Children as a target market are both vulnerable and easily persuaded: advertisers know that children will continually pester their parents (and generally persuade them) to buy the latest junk food (or toy) – the 'nag factor'. I know because I'm a parent with children who has regularly experienced this phenomenon, and *I* have a marketing background!!

When one considers the results of the survey and the breakdown of what the media spends on food and drink promotion, it is easy to contemplate that we are sitting on a health time-bomb in relation to diet-related diseases and illnesses twenty or thirty years down the line. The financial costs to this and other nations will be astronomic compared to what they are now unless there is a complete rethink of the role of media in relation to advertising. In the USA, for example, the US surgeon general estimates that obesity-related healthcare costs taxpayers almost as much as smoking-related illness. Many European countries have strict guidelines regarding children's advertising, and some ban it altogether – so at least they have already identified the potential risks. The results of the survey are quite startling and show the power of TV and why advertisers use it. The survey looked at what percentage of a child's diet each food category should be and what percentage of advertising for children that category takes.

Fatty and sugary foods (seven per cent of diet: seventy per cent of advertising outlay); bread, cereals and potatoes (thirty-three per cent of diet: sixteen per cent of advertising outlay); fruit and vegetables (thirty-three per cent of diet: nought per cent of advertising outlay); milk and dairy products (fifteen per cent of diet: ten per cent of advertising outlay); and meat, fish and alternatives (twelve per cent of diet: four per cent of advertising outlay). (Source: Sustain.) It is obvious from these figures that the more processed the food and the more high-value-added, the more the profit margin to manufacturers and the more the advertising financial outlay and revenues to media companies. That is why so little is spent advertising fresh fruit and vegetables, fresh meat, fish and poultry or grains and seeds.

The survey also compared the percentage of advertising outlay on children's products between TV and other media. Interestingly 95.6 per cent of all snacks advertising was TV; 97.1 per cent of all food/confectionery advertising was TV; 63.2 per cent of all drinks advertising was TV; 95.4 per cent of all toy advertising was TV. (Source: Sustain.)

These are all high-value-added consumer goods where manufacturers want to maximise young consumer targeting and influence, so they use the highest-impact medium – television. Unfortunately it would seem that the foods that are the most nutritionally 'suspect' are also the ones that are the most heavily promoted. The only way to prevent that happening in relation to our children and younger people, in general, is to introduce controls that would help parents and health professionals seize back the 'diet and nutrition initiative'.

Over the last twenty or thirty years the food purchasing and eating habits of people in the developed economies of the world have been systematically 'hijacked' by manufacturers and advertisers with short-term, cynical, vested interests – most of whom are backed by or have large institutional investors. It is these same organisations that also fund the large pharmaceutical and drugs companies that sell us hugely expensive treatments for the illnesses, cancers, etc., often caused by bad diet. It's very much a win-win situation for them and a lose-lose situation for the vast majority of the general public. That is of course unless you decide to make a stand and say enough is enough and declare that 'your life' and that of your children is 'firmly in your hands', and not in those of some faceless, unaccountable vested interest institution or organisation. Maybe more foodstuffs should carry 'health warnings' in much the same way as cigarettes now have to (given that so many deaths can now be attributed to an unhealthy diet!). For example, if all the heavily advertised sugary drinks and other 'nutritionally deficient' food products for children had to include both the potential health risks attached and the percentage content of the sugars and salts, fats, hormones, antibiotics, additives, added water and growth hormones etc., in a large typeface on the front of the label, very few people would buy them. The companies concerned would have little choice but to reformulate them to make them more acceptable, i.e. more nutritious and less detrimental to both children's and adults' health. There are well recorded cases of this happening already in the UK.

What if fast food chains had to declare what the source of their meat products was and the percentage of meat, fat and water content? What if milk and other dairy products had to carry a health warning about possible chemical residues, or that there could be a possible link to breast or prostate cancer? Would so many people think it was the only source of bio-available calcium and other essential minerals and vitamins available?

In his book *The Optimum Nutrition Bible* Patrick Holford compares the diet of the caveman, the peasant, modern man, and the ideal modern diet and its make-up in terms of the balance between fat, protein, carbohydrate and sugar:

modern diet	**ideal diet**	**caveman diet**	**peasant diet**
fat (40%)	fat (15%)	fat (18%)	fat (13%)
carbohydrate (28%)	carbohydrate (70%)	carbohydrate (65%)	carbohydrate (70%)
protein (12%)	protein (15%)	protein (17%)	protein (12%)
sugar (20%)	sugar (0%)	sugar (0%)	sugar (5%)

(Source: *The Optimum Nutrition Bible* by Patrick Holford.)

Let's ask ourselves the question, 'how far have we really developed?' It would seem, from this information, that both the caveman and the peasant had more nutritionally balanced diets than the average person, living in a developed country, has today. Why are we so well fed and badly nourished? The source of these key constituents is also of prime importance. With fats, it is infinitely more healthy to have a diet rich in unsaturated fats such as olive oil (extra virgin), seeds (flaxseed, sunflower, etc.) and oily fish (salmon, sardines, etc.) than in saturated fats from meat and dairy products. The best quality protein sources are soya, lentils, beans, corn, broccoli, peas (non-animal) and fish, eggs (free-range), meat and cheese (using only organic animal sources). Carbohydrates can be obtained in sufficient quantities from vegetable produce such as sweet potatoes, sprouts, peppers, watercress, etc., from fruits such as apples, berries, bananas, citrus, etc., from whole grains such as oats, rye and breads, pasta or pulses. (Source: *The Optimum Nutrition Bible.*) We must all take more responsibility for our health and say NO more often to 'junk foods and drinks' and advertisements that promote them. We should all adopt a healthier diet regime and one that focuses more on a diet that is not only more nutritious but where we also consume fewer and fewer processed foods and drinks.

KEY TIP

Remember, healthy does not have to mean boring and bland! In fact a lot of organic foods are chosen simply because they taste better.

KEY TIP
The role of natural products like aloe vera is more important in a modern diet as our bodies struggle to get rid of the toxins and other undesirable substances that most of us accumulate in our bodies.

Aloe vera, which has been around for thousands of years, is, in our opinion, one of those 'key' or 'essential' natural products that people should take on a daily basis. Aloe vera can:

- soothe and heal the digestive tract
- help break down trapped matter
- help detox the body
- help regulate the digestive system
- cleanse the liver, kidneys and colon
- boost the immune system
- provide a wide range of health-giving and healing nutrients to assist in new cell production

Aloe vera should become an essential and integral part of every family's daily diet and nutrition regime. This may also comprise products such as alfalfa, wheat grass, seeds (such as flax or linseed, pumpkin, sunflower, hemp), oily fish, beans, nuts, lentils and other pulses, fresh organic fruits and vegetables. Healthy foods are and should be available to everyone wherever they live.

The more we care for our diet, the more we care for ourselves and for our overall health and general well-being.

References

Bedani, A, DuBose, T D (1995), 'Cellular and whole-body acid-base regulation' in *Fluid, Electrolyte and Acid Base Disorders* (eds Arieff, AI, DeFronzo, RA), Churchill Livingstone (New York), pp69–103.

Narins, RC, Kupi, W, Faber, M D, Goodkin, D A, Dunfee, T D (1995), 'Pathophysiology, class and therapy of acid-base disorders' in *Fluid, Electrolyte and Acid Base Disorders* (eds Arieff, A I, DeFronzo, R A), Churchill Livingstone (New York), pp104–98.

Berkow, R (ed) (1982), *Merck Manual* (fourteenth edition), Merck, Sharp and Dohme Research Labs, Rahwy (New Jersey), pp945–52.

Beddoe, A F (1984), *Biological Ionization as Applied to Human Nutrition, Principles and Techniques*, Agro-Bio Systems, Fort Bragg (Ca).

Hawkins, H F (1947), *Applied Nutrition*, International College of Applied Nutrition, La Habra (Ca).

Shenker, G R (1997), *The Nutri-Spec Letter*, 8 (7): 1–6.

Rector, F C (1973), 'Acidification of the urine', *Handbook of Physiology*, Section 8: 'Renal Physiology', (eds Orloff, J, Berliner, R W, Fieger, S), American Physiological Society (Washington DC) pp431–54.

Ensminger, A H, Ensminger, M E, Konlande, J E, Robsin, J R K (1994), *Foods and Nutrition Encyclopedia* (second edition), CRC Press (Boca Raton, Florida), pp6–7, 41.

Read, A, Ilstrup, C (1967), *A Diet/Recipe Guide Based on the Edgar Cayce Readings*, ARE Press (Virginia Beach, Va).

Beisel, W R (1990), 'Nutrition and infection' in *Nutritional Biochemistry and Metabolism* (ed Linder, M), Elsevier (New York), pp507–42.

Price, W A (1935), 'Acid-alkaline balance of diets which produce immunity to dental caries among the South Sea Islanders and other primitive races', Dental

Cosmos 1935: 842–46 (Guyton A C, 1980), *Textbook of Medical Physiology* (second edition), W B Saunders.

7

Animal magic – they can use it too!

IN 1996, when I was researching my first book on aloe vera, the definitive information and probably the only credible information on the use of aloe vera for animals was from books that were comparatively old. Although aloe vera had been used for hundreds of years, by farmers, animal breeders, and the like, in countries where aloe vera grows naturally, modern day veterinary practitioners have, to date, been generally unwilling to accept that a plant based extract could be an effective healer. Ironically, the Royal College of Veterinary Surgeons in the UK has on its coat of arms an aloe vera plant! This undoubtedly demonstrates the important role that aloe vera played in the treatment of animals by veterinarians in earlier times.

> KEY TIP
> However, it is really only in the last twenty-five years that health professionals (in both the human and animal sectors) have rediscovered the plant's considerable and well justified reputation as a potent healer and health-giving 'agent', and the fact that it has no toxic side effects.

Historically, in areas where the fresh plants are readily available, farmers would wash out the wound and then wrap freshly sliced aloe vera leaves round the animal's affected leg, as a poultice or dressing, and thereby allow the healing ingredients in the plant (and nature) to take their course and do their work. The aloe vera would help reduce swelling, fight infection, act as a powerful antiseptic and anti-microbial agent, and heal tissue (both flesh and skin), often with little or no evidence of scarring, and would do all of these things simultaneously. It is really only in the last twenty or thirty years in the USA, and only in the last few years in the UK, that any clinical studies have been carried out to verify and expand on this traditional knowledge and practice and the wealth of anecdotal evidence available. Over the years, aloe vera has been used as an effective treatment for numerous internal and external disorders in animals, as well as in the healing of wounds, from quite minor surface abrasions to deep and potentially threatening puncture wounds. Whatever the size of the animal, it can be treated, from small wild animals and birds, to cats, dogs and other domestic pets and larger commercial animals, such as cattle and horses. Interestingly, in the last few years, more and more vets seem to be taking an interest in the potential of aloe vera as a general healer, with the added advantage of not having to worry about any possible toxic side effects.

A few years ago, a friend of ours who owns and runs several hunters bought some aloe vera products from my wife to use on her horses, and was amazed to find out from her vet (he was in practice with one of Britain's leading equine veterinary practices) that they were also using these very same products in the practice. She uses a range of topical products, as well as aloe vera gel drink (the same one that humans take) to help with listlessness and lethargy in some of her horses. We told her it would help give them more energy and boost their immune systems.

The practice concerned is run by Peter Green, who was, we believe, the first veterinary practitioner in the UK to carry out a small but nevertheless statistically significant clinical trial using a particular proprietary brand of aloe vera products, for both topical and internal disorders. Peter Green's paper, entitled 'Aloe vera extracts in equine clinical practice', was first published in the September 1996 edition of *Veterinary Times* (this was after my first book had been written but prior to it being published), and detailed the use of aloe vera to treat 'persistent leucopaenia' and lethargy syndrome found in competition horses. This particular disorder can often be largely unresponsive to conventional treatment and therapy. He also used topical applications of aloe vera to treat various skin diseases, including ringworm. The results were impressive to say the least. Of the fourteen horses treated for lethargy, eleven returned to their previous normal activities with no apparent side effects. The dosage was around 240 millilitres of aloe vera gel drinking juice per day for three to five weeks, and none received any medication, conventional or otherwise, for the duration of the trial.

The results of the topical application of aloe vera were no less impressive with the products being used for the treatment of ringworm, mud fever, plaque urticaria and contaminated wounds. Aloe vera performed as well as any conventional medication, including antibiotics, anti-fungal agents and steroids (anti-inflammatory) and, in some cases, was seen to assist in rapid wound healing without excessive tissue granulation and without additional antibiotic treatment. Peter Green believes that 'there are genuine therapeutic benefits to be gained from the administration of aloe vera extracts.' Further details of Peter Green's paper are detailed in Appendix 3, and reprints are available by mail order from the Aloe Vera Centre (priced at £1.50 plus post and packing: see Appendix 1.1).

I am delighted to say that the animal kingdom and everyone involved with it, including vets, now have what is undoubtedly the definitive guide to the use of aloe vera for itself and in veterinary clinical practice. David Urch, who has over twenty years' experience in clinical veterinary practice, with a particular interest in complementary therapies, has now written a book called *Aloe Vera – Nature's Gift. Aloe Vera in Veterinary Practice* (see Appendix 2).

The book provides animal and veterinary professionals alike, with the most comprehensive guide, practical advice and a unique insight into how best to use aloe vera to help treat and manage a wide range of animal ailments, disorders and diseases – both topical and internal. It also details a number of case histories (with colour photographs) of the relevant treatments for the various conditions highlighted, as well as for some accidents. David details over 200 conditions that affect cats, dogs, children's pets, reptiles like lizards and snakes, fish and birds and also larger animals like sheep, goats, cattle and horses. Based on his personal experience as a veterinary surgeon, he describes (in plain English!) how to use different aloe vera preparations effectively to treat and manage the said conditions. He also outlines step-by-step instructions, with recommended doses, and provides detailed guidance for owners on both animal care and first-aid.

David's book includes many of the common conditions affecting the skin, eyes, ears and the respiratory, digestive, urino-genital, immune and musculo-skeletal systems. Specific mention is made of conditions such as arthritis, burns, chronic post-viral fatigue syndrome, eczema, laminitis, mastitis, mud fever and wounds. Interestingly, in the introduction to his book, David talks about the reticence of his profession (and of the medical profession) to consider the use of aloe vera. This continuing resistance is in spite of the increasing abundance of literature on the subject, the huge amount of anecdotal evidence over the years, and more than 200 clinical trials into the medicinal properties of aloe vera that have been conducted at various research centres throughout the world.

In our opinion, anyone who is interested in exploring new methods to treat animals in a more natural way and in a way that reduces the potential for any toxic side effects, need look no further than this excellent book (and the video and leaflets that accompany it). Whether you are a layperson or an animal health professional, you will find the book interesting, informative and highly instructive. David is also involved in several ongoing trials using both orally administered and topically applied aloe vera in both large animals and domestic pets. His book outlines a new approach to both treatment and healing that is already proving to have substantial benefits for both the animals and their owners. I am sure that anyone reading it will understand the potential that aloe vera has to enhance the healing process for a wide range of internal and topical disorders.

Many other people who keep or are involved with animals are now beginning to realise how effective aloe vera can be as a healer, both internally and externally.

The following research study is just one example of how aloe vera is making an impact in the equine world.

Aloe vera and hoof growth

Ann Hayes, an ex-vet and someone who is herself involved in the aloe vera industry, was kind enough to share this story regarding hoof growth in horses (suffering from cracked hooves) supplemented with aloe vera (see appendix 1.18).

> In 2001, I was approached by a student in her final year at University College, Northampton, studying for a BSc in equine science. She was keen to do as her dissertation the 'Effect of aloe vera on the growth of horns in horses' feet'. David Urch, in his book *Aloe Vera – Nature's Gift. Aloe Vera in Veterinary Practice*, stated that he had 'noticed in practice that the addition of 120–250 millilitres of aloe vera gel drinking juice to the diet of horses increases the growth of the hooves and improved horn quality'. Many people who drink the same type of aloe vera juice on a regular basis often find that their nails grow more quickly and are stronger. Horses' hooves are the anatomical equivalent of our nails, so it was interesting to see if the same effect was seen. Most of the same minerals, vitamins, amino acids and trace elements are present in aloe vera as are in commercially available combination hoof supplements, though in smaller quantities. However, the synergistic action of the constituents of aloe vera meant that a trial to assess its effect on horn growth was warranted. David Urch, consulted about the viability

of the project, gave some very constructive comments and remained in close touch with the study throughout. The UK's leading aloe vera company generously agreed to sponsor the project.

Selecting a suitable group of horses to use in the study was hampered to a major degree by the outbreak of foot and mouth disease. Eventually, a group of suitable ponies was offered by the BHS Rescue Centre at Oxhill, Warwickshire, on a site that could be accessed throughout the foot and mouth epidemic. Ten ponies were selected ranging in age from two to six years and in height from eleven to fourteen hands. They were divided into two groups, balanced by age and height as far as possible. One group was to be fed 120 millilitres of the aloe vera juice daily for sixteen weeks, while the other remained an untreated control group. Both groups grazed together, so they were all on the same nutritional plane. The ponies' feet were trimmed at 63 and 126 days, and at each trimming hoof measurements were taken at various points and a mean hoof volume calculated.

The results showed several interesting features:

1. In just sixty days the difference between the two groups was only minimal. This was as expected, because, like many other natural products, aloe vera takes some time to get to into the system and for its benefits to be manifested.

2. In the second sixty-day period the rate of horn growth in the control group dropped dramatically. This was due to the time of year – late summer – when the pasture grazed by the horses was declining in food value.

3. As expected, the treatment group, during this second sixty-day period, showed a significant increase in the rate of horn growth, a massive forty-two per cent as compared to the control group.

In addition to better horn growth in the treatment group it was observed that the new horn growing at the top of the hoof was smoother and shinier in the treatment group compared to the control group. This suggested that the horn produced in horses supplemented with aloe vera was of better quality than that of the unsupplemented horses, but a much longer study would be necessary to ascertain the exact changes. Furthermore the hooves of the treatment group had fewer sites of damage (cracks in the hoof wall, etc.) than the control group.

The conclusion was that the use of the aloe vera gel drinking juice appears to supply many of the nutrients necessary for the growth of healthy horn, and supplemented animals showed a much higher rate of horn growth: the quality and strength appears to be much greater than that seen in the unsupplemented animals.

Helen: Billy, leg injury

In December 2001, my horse Billy sustained a very serious injury to the outside of his hind leg, and I knew instinctively that it was not going to be straightforward. The wound was about five inches long and extremely deep, the kind of injury where damage to the tendons and ligaments is not unusual. It was however clean and I dressed it with a topical aloe vera gelly product and waited for the vet to arrive. I knew by the look on his face my worst fears were justified. Billy was taken away to the vet college immediately and I was warned he might not come back.

There he was sedated and scanned, whence I was told '...this horse must have nine lives.' Luckily, there was no damage to his tendons or ligaments.

The wound was dressed and I took him home. I was told to expect severe swelling and lameness the next day, to walk him out in hand until it healed, but that the recovery process was likely to take some considerable time. I immediately put him on 240 millilitres of a proprietary brand of aloe vera drinking juice containing glucosamine sulphate, chondroitin, dimethyl sulphone (MSM) and vitamin C. The next morning there was no swelling or lameness and he continued with the 240 millilitres for three weeks, then I reduced it to 120. I also dressed his leg with an aloe vera and bee propolis cream (a natural antibiotic from the beehive), and there was never any sign of infection. In mid-January, my vet came to do some routine work and also took a look at Billy's leg. He was extremely surprised at the rate at which it had healed. The wound had nearly closed up and there was no proud flesh. He knows I use aloe vera and just said to carry on using it as it certainly *was* doing the trick. Billy was back in full work just seven weeks after his accident.

Philippa: Meadow, sarcoids

Philippa is the head nurse at a veterinary practice just north of London. She describes an incident involving her horse, Meadow, a six-year-old mare (see Colour Plates 17–20 and Appendix 1.19):

> Meadow had developed a sarcoid between her front legs and over the first few months of this year (2003) it had been getting larger. I had decided to have it surgically removed after I returned from my holiday to Australia in late March.
>
> A sarcoid is a very common fibrous equine tumour that can develop over weeks or months from small nodules to masses several centimetres in size. They can be malevolent, though metastasis is rare. The accepted treatments are surgery, freezing, injections into the tumour, radiotherapy and toxic topical ointments. Most of the above are pretty invasive, radical and not without an element of risk, and I am thrilled that I have not had to resort to them.
>
> On 7th March, the day before I was due to fly out, I discovered that the sarcoid had burst and it looked a real mess. I really did not want my horse undergoing anaesthesia and surgery while I was away so I instructed a friend to bathe and treat it in my absence. She was only to call the vet if she was really worried.
>
> The treatment regime I recommended was to clean the area with very dilute aloe vera based washing liquid (known as MPD), spray the area with an aloe veterinary spray and then apply a combination of equal amounts of topical aloe vera gelly and an aloe vera cream formulated with bee propolis (the natural antibiotic from the beehive). The application was to be carried out at least once daily.
>
> I arrived back nearly three weeks later on 27th March and, although the sarcoid still looked very large, it was clean and showed no signs of infection, so I continued the regime. Ten days later, when I brought her in from the field, to my amazement the sarcoid had completely disappeared! I was tempted to go to the field to look for it but it was dark and it's a pretty big field (the saying 'looking for a needle in a haystack' came to mind!).

The surrounding tissue was still quite inflamed and reactive. However, this slowly subsided over the next two weeks. At the time of writing this – 28th April 2003 – the only remaining evidence of the sarcoid is just a small scab that should drop off quite soon.

The speed of healing and the way in which the sarcoid simply fell off naturally are undoubtedly the result of the deep penetrative properties of aloe vera and the way in which these high-quality aloe vera products accelerated the healing process. It is evident that the tissue healed beneath and around the sarcoid to such an extent that it simply fell away.

I believe that there will be little or no trace of any scarring in the area or any whitening of the hair – something that can often happen with such problems or injuries in horses.

Kate: Sevenge, leg injury

Sevenge is a sixteen-hand and two-inch seven-year-old French thoroughbred mare, who in November last year had an altercation with a lorry ramp that would have sent most horses to their sickbed for months. It was a typical wet Scottish winter evening, and while going up a slippery ramp into the lorry for the short journey home, she lost her footing, resulting in her off-side rear slipping down the side of the ramp, trapping her leg between it and the door. When she was finally back in the safety of her stable, a vet was called. He said the wound looked fairly superficial and applied a dressing. As you can see from the first photo (Colour Plate 21), which was taken a month after the accident, and after the vet's second visit, it was far from superficial and required stitching and an antibiotic drain. At this point, an amount of proud flesh started to grow, which I was assured would have to be removed at a later date under sedation.

While telling a friend about Sevenge, she suggested I use two products – a particular proprietary brand of topical aloe vera gelly and an aloe veterinary spray. Attending to the back legs of a horse is not always the safest of pastimes and I have to admit that spraying the veterinary formula on an open wound was fairly precarious. We took out the stitches and persevered, and within only two weeks we had gone from a horrible protruding wound to what you can see in Colour Plate 22 – all the proud flesh completely gone. We are now applying the topical aloe vera gelly and keeping it covered in the stable, and as the third colour plate shows (Colour Plate 23), there has been a significant improvement, with the scarring reduced by about fifty per cent.

Sevenge does not take kindly to anything that curtails her equestrian activities. As you can see from the last picture (Colour Plate 24), she is now fully recovered, a big girl who loves to jump and who definitely enjoys the outdoor life. She is as 'tough as old boots', and throughout the whole incident she had only one day off from work, and that was because she was waiting for the vet to turn up.

Mary: Muffin, pony

Muffin is a fifteen-year-old fluffy skewbald Shetland pony, given to an old neighbour of mine as a companion for another old pony. Although Muffin was loved and well fed, the old man had very poor eyesight and was not always able to check for any problems with the horses.

Muffin was kept in a paddock just down the road from me, so I could also check up on him occasionally. Last summer was particularly wet, and one Saturday the old man called round to say Muffin was unwell and could I come and have a closer look at him. At first he looked as though he had a touch of colic or tummy ache, and as he was rather muddy I gave him some aloe vera drinking gel down his throat with a syringe. This is something I would normally do with the onset of colic, as it often just settles the discomfort and gives me time to watch and decide the cause of the problems. As I was standing there, thinking what had caused Muffin to be so distressed, I noticed a group of maggots coming out of his coat around his shoulder. It was a terrible sight and I thought he must have some sort of wound. On closer examination I realised his whole back was a crawling mass of maggots, so I soaked him in an aloe vera veterinary spray. The maggots evacuated non-stop for the rest of the afternoon. I phoned the vet and asked him to leave out some sheep maggot spray in case I needed it, and as it was a weekend I did not want to call him out and incur extra expense for the old man on his pension.

I took Muffin home to my farm and continued to apply the aloe veterinary spray until the area was clear. Obviously Muffin had suffered rain rot or scald under his fluffy coat, and because of his failing eyesight the old man hadn't noticed the damage. The flies then set to work laying eggs on the cracked skin and when it was warm they had hatched out – causing poor Muffin's discomfort. I then knew why he had been rolling around so much getting muddy – he had obviously been trying to get rid of the cause of the discomfort in the only way he could. After soaking his back several times the next day I applied a topical aloe vera gelly to the affected area. His whole back from mane to tail lost all its scarred skin. Within six weeks he was growing new healthy skin and hair and did not have a single scar by the end of the summer! Needless to say I phoned the vet on the Monday morning to say I didn't need the maggot fly spray after all! I have had horses all my life but I had never seen anything like it before. Muffin is now enjoying life again, though sadly his keeper has since passed away.

Retriever: ear infection

My retriever had the beginnings of an ear infection, to which he is rather prone after the swims he takes in a stagnant pond in the woods. I put two drops of aloe activator in each ear and also used it to bathe and clean the outer ears. Within hours I could tell that he was much more comfortable. He had also stopped scratching

After several more treatments within the following twenty-four hours he was completely cured. I now use aloe activator routinely as an ear wash for various animals.

Cat: health tonic

Our nineteen-year-old cat was recently diagnosed with thyroid problems. We had noticed he was less steady on his feet, was drinking a lot, was always hungry, and had very runny stools and problems going to the loo. After two visits to the vet, which included consultations, blood tests and two doses of medication, which didn't seem to make any difference, we decided to incorporate aloe vera drinking juice into his diet on a daily basis. We now give him one dessert spoon of aloe vera gel every day – mixed well into his food. He has a similar mix of wet and dry and fresh food as he has always had, but now he has firmer stools, his coat has improved and he seems slightly more relaxed.

He even brought the remnants of a sizeable bird into the kitchen recently – a gift that we thankfully haven't had for several years – which surprised us as we didn't think he still had the speed or the agility any more. He is also still able to jump onto tables and work surfaces, and is much more lively than he was before the aloe vera. One other thing we have noticed is that his claws seem to be growing much faster – we don't know whether he is scratching less or that they are genuinely growing faster. Maybe aloe vera has the same effect on cats' claws as it does on horses' hooves.

Retriever: chest wound

My dog had been leaping about through the woods on his walk, and when we got home I saw blood dripping from a deep, open wound over his ribcage. It was a gaping cut about an inch long and more than a quarter of an inch across the middle. I washed it thoroughly with aloe vera liquid soap, packed it with aloe vera gelly and stuck a large plaster over it, repeating this four times in the first day. The next day I used aloe activator to clean the wound instead of the soap, and repeated the packing with aloe vera gelly and covered it with plaster. Over the next two days he was kept on the lead for his daily walk, so that the wound could remain clean and dry. On the third day the cushions of flesh were beginning to close together – the 'floor' moving up and the two side cushions meeting. A soft, pliant scab formed, leaving a small drainage hole in the centre that would 'weep' a lot of clear fluid every day or so. It was always odour-free, and although the immediate area surrounding the wound was hot and swollen, the wound itself was pink and clean. It was obvious there was no infection. The dog enjoyed the four-times-a-day ritual and would roll on his back at the first sight of the aloe vera container, with a huge grin on his face. Every day the wound shrank and by the tenth day the scab had hardened and formed a narrow 'frill', rather like the ridge of pastry on a Cornish pasty!

Irish setter: internal disorders

Although I bought aloe vera gel drink for my own use, I also found that it proved very successful for one of our Irish setters. For some years he had problems with an enlarged spleen and hiatus hernia, which caused him to retch, bringing up bile or mucus. In spite of using some proprietary medical syrup the problem had become progressively worse. On the off-chance we gave him some aloe vera gel and since then he has retched only once instead of the customary three or four times a night. Before using the drinking gel, we were beginning to think we would have to put him to sleep, if the condition worsened. Incidentally, aloe vera continues to help me with my tummy problems, too!

Collie: skin allergy

For several years my collie-cross dog had suffered from a pollen allergy in the spring and summer, and the only effective treatment had been steroids. Unfortunately there can be quite serious side effects and these included weight gain and excessive thirst. I now use the aloe veterinary spray on the irritated areas and have managed to cut the steroids down to a quarter of a tablet per day. He has a particularly sore patch on his elbow, which responded well to the aloe vera veterinary spray and it soon healed up.

Golden retriever: skin allergy

My young golden retriever began scratching his chest and within a few days he had created a large raw area that was seeping. I washed the area with a gentle soap and warm water and clipped the hair to improve access to it. There was no evidence of any fleas or insect bites or other damage, so I decided to use some aloe activator to wash the area initially. Then I used aloe veterinary spray to cover it. The advantage with the spray is not having to touch the area physically, which was obviously quite painful. The anti-itching properties of the aloe vera spray seemed to work quite fast because he soon stopped scratching, and within a week or so the sore patch was totally healed and the hair was growing back. Since then, he has had no recurrence of the problem. I have also incorporated the aloe vera gel drink into his diet as a general health tonic, and to help any potential problems with his joints.

Summary

Many more people with animals tell of different aloe vera products that they have used to help treat and heal a wide spectrum of ailments and disorders, from eczema (West Highland terriers seem to be particularly prone to this problem), to arthritis, colitis and other digestive disorders.

Anyone wanting to know more about aloe vera and its use in the treatment of animals can contact the Aloe Vera Centre (see Appendix 1.1).

Below is a listing of some of the common sorts of ailments that aloe vera may help with and some recommendations for the different treatments that can be used.

Aloe vera products and their use in common animal ailments:

- Abrasions: aloe vera topical gelly, aloe vera veterinary spray
- Abscesses: aloe vera activator, aloe vera veterinary spray
- Arthritis: aloe vera gel drinking juice, aloe vera heat lotion on joints
- Bites: aloe vera topical gelly, aloe vera veterinary spray
- Blood in urine: aloe vera gel drinking juice with cranberries
- Bruises: aloe vera heat lotion, aloe vera topical gelly, aloe vera activator
- Burns: aloe vera topical gelly, aloe vera veterinary spray
- Catarrh: aloe vera activator (two or three squirts up nostrils three times daily)
- Conjunctivitis: aloe vera activator
- Convalescence: aloe vera gel drinking juice (100g (4oz) daily)
- Coronet injuries: aloe vera activator, aloe vera veterinary spray, aloe vera topical gelly
- Cough: aloe vera activator, aloe vera topical gelly (down throat several times a day)
- Cuts: aloe vera activator, aloe vera topical gelly, aloe vera gel drinking juice
- Diarrhoea: aloe vera gel drinking juice
- Eye injuries: aloe vera activator
- Grass sickness: aloe vera gel drinking juice
- Inflammation: aloe vera activator or aloe vera veterinary spray followed by aloe vera heat lotion, aloe vera gel drinking juice
- Laminitis: aloe vera gel drinking juice
- Limestone infection: aloe vera activator, aloe vera lotion, aloe vera heat lotion, aloe vera gel drinking juice
- Mud fever: aloe vera veterinary spray, aloe vera activator, aloe vera propolis cream
- Nasal discharge: aloe vera activator (two or three squirts up nostrils three times daily)
- Pain and swelling: aloe vera gel drinking juice, aloe vera activator, aloe vera topical gelly, aloe vera veterinary spray

- Pharyngitis: aloe vera activator
- Puncture wounds: clean with aloe vera activator, pack with aloe vera topical gelly, aloe vera propolis cream, aloe vera veterinary spray
- Rashes: aloe vera topical gelly, aloe vera veterinary spray
- Respiratory problems: aloe vera activator, aloe vera gelly
- Sarcoids/proud flesh: aloe vera topical gelly
- Skin disorders (eczema, ringworm): aloe vera veterinary spray, aloe vera lotion, aloe vera topical gelly, aloe vera propolis cream
- Sore legs: aloe vera heat lotion, aloe vera topical gelly, aloe vera activator
- Sore mouth: aloe vera topical gelly
- Sore throat: aloe vera activator, aloe vera topical gelly
- Sprains and strains: aloe vera activator or aloe vera veterinary spray followed by aloe vera heat lotion, aloe vera gel drinking juice
- Strangles: aloe vera gel drinking juice (approximately 100g (4oz) in feed or water daily). Combine fifty grams (two ounces) aloe vera topical gelly and aloe vera activator and squirt down throat daily
- Sunburn: aloe vera topical gelly, aloe vera veterinary spray, aloe vera sunscreen (SPF30)
- Suspensory ligament: aloe vera activator, aloe vera heat lotion, aloe vera veterinary spray
- Sweet itch: aloe vera topical gelly, aloe vera propolis cream
- Swelling: aloe vera gel drinking juice, aloe vera activator, aloe vera topical gelly, aloe vera veterinary spray
- Swollen joints: aloe vera heat lotion, aloe vera gel drinking juice, aloe vera veterinary spray
- Throat infections: combine fifty grams (two ounces) aloe vera activator and aloe vera topical gelly and squirt down throat twice daily
- Thrush: clean with hydrogen peroxide and pack with aloe vera topical gelly
- Uterine infections: aloe vera activator, aloe vera veterinary spray
- Virus: aloe vera gel drinking juice (100g (4oz) daily)
- Warts: rub in aloe vera topical gelly several times a day
- Wounds: for minor ones apply aloe vera veterinary spray. For severe wounds, clean thoroughly with aloe vera activator and pack with aloe vera topical gelly

KEY TIP

Wash pets' blankets or cushions and horses' rugs, tack and numnahs with aloe vera detergent. This is also good for sponging mats under the feeding bowls of cats and dogs.

8

Aloe vera: research or anecdotal evidence?

The scientific case for the medical use of aloe vera

THIS CHAPTER is not meant to be the definitive guide to all the research data on aloe vera (I have already suggested that someone should compile such a list). It is simply a chronological summary of some of the major research that has been conducted in the last seventy years. It begins with the work done by Collins and Collins in the 1930s that was widely accepted as the first detailed medical study of the uses and benefits of aloe vera. Prior to the 1930s, many important civilisations and many eminent physicians and vets of their day recognised the role and importance of this 'legendary healing plant'. As far back as the first century AD, Dioscorides, the Greek physician and pharmacologist, wrote of the healing powers and general therapeutic properties and benefits of plants including aloe vera. His *De Materia Medica* was the foremost source of botanical reference and pharmacology until the sixteenth century.

Various researchers are now studying the glyco-biological properties, effects and benefits of aloe vera, and other commercial organisations that market glyco-nutrients are incorporating aloe vera into their products (see Glyco-nutrients, Chapter 6).

Aloe vera research through the twentieth century and into the new millennium

1935: Collins and Collins, radiation injuries and Roentgen dermatitis

The first modern medical study on the healing properties and benefits of aloe vera was published in 1935 by CE Collins. Later that year, he and his son (hence the references to Collins and Collins) published a second paper on the use of aloe vera in the treatment of radiation injuries in fifty patients. The father-and-son team highlighted, in both papers, the case of a thirty-one-year-old female patient with severe Roentgen dermatitis. The description of the patient's condition by Collins and Collins was very detailed:

> There was a desquamation over an area of 4 cms by 8 cms. On the left side of the forehead, extending 2cms above the hair line. The medical history showed that in May 1932, she had received what she had been told was a depilatory x-ray treatment. Fourteen months later, she said the skin of her forehead and scalp became rough and scabby and itched continuously (dermatitis exfoliativa). Between July, 1933 and March, 1934, she had consulted three different physicians, all of whom agreed on the diagnosis and who then prescribed boric acid, phenol in olive oil, ichthyol, a five per cent mercury ointment, and zinc oxide, respectively. The condition had become progressively worse until there was extensive desquamation with oozing of serious fluid. The patient stated that the itching and burning sensations were often so severe and constant that she had to wear cotton gloves at night to prevent her scratching the damaged area and causing bleeding. After a review of this history and an examination of the patient's condition, it was felt that a skin graft was indicated and the patient was so advised.
>
> At the time of the examination, the patient was furnished with a quantity of aloe vera (fresh whole leaves) for local application, with the hope that this material might serve as a palliative (i.e. act to allay the itching). Twenty-four hours later she reported that the sensations of itching and burning had entirely subsided. She was instructed to continue the use of the plant material and, when seen from time to time during the next five weeks, the condition was found to be progressively improved. At the end of this time (i.e. on 7th April, 1934), there was complete regeneration of the skin of the forehead and scalp, new hair growth, complete restoration of sensation and an absence

> of scarring. There was at this time a slight blanching of the affected area. When last seen on 23rd July 1934, the area seemed to be completely healed, with no indication whatever of a relapse. On exposure to the summer sunlight, the forehead skin was seen to be pigmenting normally along with other exposed skin surfaces of the body.

Collins confirmed that the results achieved in this case had encouraged them to use aloe vera on a few cases of x-ray dermatitis and concluded the report by saying:

> Since April, 1934, we have treated more than fifty cases of x-ray and radium burns with aloe vera leaves and an ointment known as 'Alvagel', made from the aloe leaf. While all have not been perfect cures, the results as a whole have been most gratifying.

Interestingly, the reaction of many medical authorities at the time to the thirty-one-year-old's incredible healing was almost unbelievable. They felt that, despite the detailed reports of Collins and Collins, her miraculous recovery had nothing to do with aloe vera but was, in fact, due to her fear of the proposed alternative treatment, i.e. skin grafts! Collins and Collins' work really pioneered the medical use of aloe vera and in the 1930s, there followed numerous similar studies, many of which used the same procedures as laid down by this father-and-son team.

1936: Dr C S Wright, x-ray ulceration

In his paper, Wright reported on his use of aloe vera to treat several patients, using the Collins methods. One patient had x-ray damage dating back ten years. Wright concluded:

> My purpose in this case is to present the remarkable improvement obtained in two cases of x-ray ulceration with the hope of stimulating interest in what promises to be a revolutionary method of treatment for early x-ray damage to the skin and ulceration of the skin resulting from x-rays.

1936: Dr A Loveman, Roentgen ray-dermatitis

In his paper, Loveman reported on the cases of two patients, one of whom was suffering from severe Roentgen ray-dermatitis and the other from severe dermatitis.

The first had the problem on the backs of both hands and the other all over both hands. In both cases, other methods of treatment had failed. The immediate application of fresh aloe vera was recommended for both patients. In the case of the first patient, it took nearly three weeks for the pain to subside, but within eight months the whole ulceration had healed. The second patient experienced total pain relief within only thirty-six hours, and within only two months he was completely healed.

1938: Drs A Fine and S Brown, radiology burns

In their medical paper, these two doctors reported on the use of fresh aloe vera leaves in the treatment of radiology burns. They said:

> We have noted in those cases which are receiving prolonged courses of therapy, whereby the skin is becoming irritated and painful, though intact, that application of the leaf is extremely soothing and allays the discomfort considerably. This was noted especially in breast cancer cases, in which the axilla received a large amount of radiation and became quite painful.

1939: Dr F Mandeville, Roentgen dermatitis

In his medical paper, Dr Mandeville reported on the successful use of aloe vera in the treatment of five cases of Roentgen dermatitis and roentgen ulcers and stated:

> All five of the patients have experienced definite relief from pain and discomfort.

1945: V P Filatov, Cutaneous leishmaniasis

In his medical paper, Filatov reported on the successful use of aloe vera in seven cases of Cutaneous leishmaniasis.

1953: C C Lushbaugh and D B Hale, radiodermatitis

In their medical paper, Lushbaugh and Hale said:

> Aloe vera has a remarkably curative effect upon radiodermatitis in the rabbit… .
>
> Treatment was found to hasten both the degenerative and reparative phases of the lesion so that complete healing of an ulcer caused by 28,000 rep of beta radiation was accomplished within two months of treatment, while

> the untreated ulcerations were still not completely healed more than four months after radiation. Aloe vera contains substances that are stimulating both to the delayed development and delayed healing of ulcerative radiodermatitis, and because of the growing importance of this injury, further investigation of the action of aloe vera should be pursued.

1956: S Levenson and K Somova, periodontitis

In their medical paper, Levenson and Somova stated:

> Aloe extract was used for the treatment of periodontitis (a disease which destroys the bonding of the teeth to the bones within the gum) and subgingigival and supergingivival dental calculus.
>
> Over 150 patients, both men and women were treated using an aloe-based injection at the site of each affected tooth. Thirty injections were given over a six-week period.

They concluded that:

> ...normal colour returned to all gum tissue and oedema disappeared. Further, the membrane around the tooth was tightened to help strengthen the support for loose teeth. Besides that, the number of lymphocytes in the blood drops to normal as a result of treatment with aloe vera.

1963: J J Blitz, J W Smith, J R Gerard and D O Dania, peptic ulcers

In their medical paper, Blitz, Smith, Gerard and Dania said that they had used aloe vera gel as the sole medication for the treatment of peptic ulcers in eighteen patients. They concluded:

> Clinically, aloe vera gel emulsion has dissipated all symptoms in the patients considered to have incipient peptic ulcer. Duodenitis, probably representing duodenal ulcer but lacking x-ray demonstration of pathogonomic deformity, treated with aloe vera gel, resulted in uniformly excellent recovery.
>
> In the case of peptic ulcer about which there could be little clinical doubt, and in every instance confirmed by roentgenologic identification of a flick, niche or crater with accompanying hypermotile manifestations, aloe vera gel emulsion provided complete recovery.

1973: Dr M El Zawahry, Dr M R Hegazy and M Helal, leg ulcers, acne, allopecia, sebborhea

In their first medical paper Zawahry, Hegazy and Helal reported on the treatment of three patients who were suffering from chronic leg ulcerations. The first patient, a fifty-year-old man, had chronic varicose leg ulcers that were over fifteen years old, the description of which was:

> The patient had a large ulcer on the medial surface of about 1400 mm square...and a smaller one on the lateral surface of the left leg. The ulcers were deep, foul-smelling and their bases were dirty and fixed. The margins were irregular. On application of extracts from fresh aloe vera leaves, healing began within one week and after ten weeks the lateral ulcer was completely healed. The medial ulcer took slightly longer but was nevertheless healed within eleven weeks.
>
> The second patient, a fifty-one-year-old man, had oedema and pseudo-elephantiasis of the left leg and foot. He had chronic and foul-smelling leg ulcers that were over seven years old, one of which was over 5000 mm square. During the first two weeks of treatment, he experienced throbbing pains (this is probably the so-called 'healing-crisis' that is often referred to when using aloe vera to treat serious conditions such as leg ulcers) in his leg. After that time, the pains subsided and the smaller ulcers healed within six weeks and the larger one showed significant improvements within nine weeks and some slight bleeding as the circulation in the area improved. Although inconclusive, the report seemed to indicate total healing eventually.
>
> The third case was a younger patient, a twenty-two-year-old man, who had suffered burns to his left leg eight years previously and had then developed a leg ulcer on the burn site. The leg ulcer was five years old and had an area of about four hundred and forty square millimetres. It was dirty with purulent effusion and necrotic material at the bottom of the lower part. After five weeks of aloe vera treatment there was good progress of healing of the ulcer and the epithelium moved towards the inside. The area progressively decreased during the treatment.

The three doctors, when discussing their results, noted that there was no recorded, effective treatment for leg ulcers available at that time and thus the healing improvements that they had witnessed represented a significant step forward in the treatment of such conditions. Importantly, they also recognised that there had been a significant improvement in the circulation in and around the ulcerated areas, thus encouraging the healing process. This observation has been supported by many other doctors and researchers when explaining their findings in describing the healing benefits of aloe vera. They also mentioned the importance of polysaccharides, and said:

> We believe that the active principle for promoting healing is the polysaccharides that are present in high concentrations in aloe vera.

In a second medical study the same three doctors examined the effects of aloe vera on patients suffering from acne, alopecia and seborrhea. Three women patients, all in their twenties, who were suffering from 'mixed Acne vulgaris' were treated with aloe vera. Within one month, two of the three were totally healed and acne free and the third showed significant improvement with little sign of any acne remaining. The aloe vera treatment decreased the loss of hair and within one month had totally eliminated the problem. Within three months, two of the patients experienced new hair growth in bald areas and those with seborrhea improved also. Three of the alopecia patients showed new hair growth within a week (similar to that experienced by Catriona, see Chapter 5), and a further ten patients who were also treated with the same aloe vera preparation also showed signs of improvement.

The three doctors concluded:

> No case of contact dermatitis was reported. No active irritation happened to any of the treated patients with seborrhea, acne vulgaris or alopecia. Control cases were few, one for each disease, but no control patient was affected by the vehicle alone.

KEY POINT

'Aloe vera proved to have a powerful stimulating effect on the rate of healing of chronic leg ulcers. We believe improvement in three patients treated can be attributed to improvement in the peripheral circulation that is usually deficient in such patients.'

The drug appears to stimulate hair growth and the drying of seborrheic skin. Improvement was noted after treatment of patients with seborrheic alopecia, acne vulgaris and alopecia areata.

1975: R B Northway, veterinary treatments

In his veterinary paper, Northway outlined his use of aloe vera to treat a variety of animal ailments, including ringworm, allergies, abscesses, otitis externa, lacerations, lip fold dermatitis, cysts and so on (all of these conditions are mentioned in David Urch's book, *Aloe Vera – Nature's Gift. Aloe Vera in Veterinary Practice*. (See Appendix 2.) The 'patients' included four horses, twenty-two cats and forty-two dogs. Northway reported 'good to excellent results' when aloe vera was used to treat various skin disorders. With the exception of eight cases, all showed significant improvements over the four-week duration of his aloe vera trial.

1980s: Dr B Wolfe, Dr E Zimmerman and the Baylor College of Dentistry, Dallas, Texas, dental disorders

In the 1980s, Wolfe, Zimmerman and the Baylor College of Dentistry undertook what to this day is still perhaps the most detailed and exhaustive research study ever undertaken to examine the use and benefits of aloe vera as a treatment for dental disorders.

> KEY POINT
> The study showed that the aloe vera gel used was highly bactericidal against certain organisms, including Candida albicans, Streptococcus viridaus, Staphylococcus aureus and the five most commonly occurring strains of streptococcus mutant found in dental plaque.

Furthermore, Zimmerman discovered that the potent benefits of aloe vera were not evident until the percentage concentration was seventy. In virucidal studies, aloe vera (the aloe vera gel used was ninety per cent) was tested as virucidal against both Herpes simplex and Herpes zoster.

> KEY POINT
> Anti-inflammatory studies revealed that aloe vera was as effective as two commonly prescribed anti-inflammatory drugs of the time, namely 'prednisolon' and 'indomethacin', without any of the toxic side effects.

Toxicity tests on the aloe vera gel revealed that it

> reduced cellular death rates by nearly 70% and it was found to be non-toxic, virucidal, bactericidal, fungicidal, a powerful anti-inflammatory agent, a stimulant of cellular life-extension and to have anaesthetic effects while it heals.

Aloe vera was also found to be an effective treatment for use with dentures to safeguard against soreness. Wolfe concluded in the section on oral pathology in the report:

> Aloe vera is virucidal, fungicidal and bactericidal and can thus be used effectively as a post-operative treatment following oral surgery to help heal sockets, to help treat any oral lesions and herpes ulcerations in the mouth and to use as a massage treatment to help promote healthy gums and dental hygiene.

Finally, he suggested that dental professionals should test the ideas highlighted in the report and also consider what role aloe vera could play within their own dental and oral hygiene practices.

1980s: Dr J Heggers, thermal injuries

Some of the most comprehensive work ever done on the healing properties of aloe vera relating to burn and other thermal injuries (including frostbite) was carried out by Dr Heggers and his colleagues at the Chicago Burn Center in the early 1980s.

KEY POINT
In the medical papers, Heggers and his colleagues state that they believed aloe vera's ability to heal third degree burns and frostbite is related to the presence of certain active ingredients in the plant. These include salicylates, triglycerides and fatty acids such as cholesterol.

They also confirmed the findings of previous reports (Zimmerman, Brasher, Gottschall, Collins et al), that aloe vera contained powerful anti-inflammatory agents that were also non-toxic. Aloe vera was also found to be a potent anti-microbial agent due to the presence of barbaloin.

In his study, Heggers found that aloe vera (at concentrations of seventy to ninety per cent) was as effective as the most commonly used medication (silver sulfadiazine) in controlling infection in burns.

> KEY POINT
> Heggers also confirmed that he believed aloe vera's painkilling properties to be related to the presence of both salicylic acid (an aspirin-like compound) and magnesium (see Chapter 2).

Heggers concluded:

> Aloe vera, therefore has three major properties that are most beneficial in thermal injury. Either due to its aspirin-like effect or the high magnesium content or probably both, acting synergistically it can potentiate an anaesthetic effect. It has a broad-spectrum anti-microbial effect especially against agents responsible for burn wound sepsis. It has anti-prostanoid or, specifically an anti-thromboxane effect. Aloe vera has an abundance of fatty acids that probably supply the necessary nutrients required for normal tissue maturation...These experimental data clearly suggest that a 70%+ concentration extract of aloe vera can be beneficial in a burn wound.

1987: Dr Rosalie Burns, shingles

In her work on the use of aloe vera to help treat shingles, Dr Burns points up the connection between the virus that causes both chickenpox and shingles. It is the same virus that also causes herpes in the mouth and on the genitalia, and she concludes:

> The sap from the leaves of the aloe vera plant is an old folk remedy that relieves pain and speeds healing when spread over the blisters.

1987: Drs H R McDaniel, T R Watson and T Pulse, Dallas Fort Worth Medical Center, AIDS

Since the late 1980s, studies conducted by these three doctors have shown aloe vera to have an important and highly significant role to play in the management of AIDS. Dr McDaniel stated:

> A substance in the aloe vera plant shows preliminary signs of boosting AIDS patients' immune systems and blocking the human immune deficiency virus's spread without toxic side-effects.

The results of McDaniel's pilot study were significant:

> The symptoms of sixteen AIDS patients were significantly reduced when given 1,000 mgs per day of the drug for three months. After three months, six patients with advanced cases of AIDS showed a twenty per cent improvement in symptoms and less seriously ill patients improved on average by seventy-one per cent. Fever and symptoms of night sweats, diarrhoea and opportunistic infections were either eliminated or significantly improved in all patients, with corresponding drops in HIV antibody positive cell cultures and HIV core antigen levels.

In his study Pulse administered up to twenty ounces of stabilised aloe vera juice every day to sixty-nine AIDS patients classified as 'those who would never improve or get better'.

He found that most were able to return to normal work, go back to their normal energy level and their symptoms disappeared almost completely.

Pulse concluded when asked about aloe vera as an AIDS treatment or cure:

> It means that until there is a magic bullet, this is a stop-gap measure and it buys them time at a fraction of the cost of AZT.

It is important to note the aloe vera juice referred to in all these studies is based on 100 per cent stabilised aloe vera.

1987 onwards: Professor R H Davis et al, Pennsylvania College of Podiatric Medicine, Philadelphia, healing mechanisms of aloe vera

Professor Davis and his colleagues have been at the forefront of medical research into identifying the healing mechanisms of aloe vera and what is responsible for its potent anti-inflammatory and healing benefits.

> KEY TIP
> Like many others before them, they have confirmed that the use of aloe vera accelerates the process of wound healing by a factor of fifty per cent or more and that the process is both totally reliable and reproducible.

In one study they compared the respective healing and anti-inflammatory actions of aloe vera and a commonly prescribed anti-inflammatory medication, hydrocortisone.

They found that while aloe vera was demonstrated to have both a positive healing and anti-inflammatory effect, and to have both simultaneously, the hydrocortisone had a positive anti-inflammatory but an anti-healing effect, that is it was seen to inhibit the wound-healing process! In another medical paper Davis et al found that:

> Aloe vera contains numerous strong growth promoting factors ...[and]...certain amino acids, gibberellin and indole-3-acetic acid.

They also confirmed that:

> Aloe vera has an enzyme called 'Bradykininase' which by breaking down 'Bradykinin' reduces inflammation.

This explanation of aloe vera's powerful anti-inflammatory properties is shared by other doctors and researchers, including Dr Peter Atherton in his study 'Aloe vera: magic or medicine?' – which is reviewed later in this section.

Davis et al also share the conclusions of many others that the major active ingredients in aloe vera show an almost unique synergy in their different actions – all of which seem to demonstrate positive healing and general therapeutic benefits. Davis et al found (like Danhof) that aloe vera stimulates fibroblasts. These are the cells that produce collagen – the protein fibres that strengthen new tissue and help heal wounds. The increased rate of tissue repair is achieved without any loss in aloe vera's anti-inflammatory properties. This 'collagen enhancing' activity is probably the main reason why people who use aloe vera on a regular basis seem to have skin that retains its 'youthfulness' and 'suppleness'. Davis et al also believe that a plant growth hormone found in aloe vera – gibberellin – increases wound healing. In one of their medical papers, they say that:

> gibberellin, isolated from aloe vera, increased wound healing more than 100% in mice.

1996: T A Syed, S A Ahmad, A H Holt, S H Ahmad, psoriasis

Syed et al found that following a double-blind clinical trial to evaluate the clinical efficacy and tolerability of topical aloe vera extract (0.5 per cent in a hydrophilic cream) versus a placebo treatment to cure patients with psoriasis vulgaris, the aloe vera results were significantly better. Out of sixty patients (thirty-six males and twenty-four females), split equally into two groups, the following results were achieved. The aloe vera cream had cured 83.3 per cent of patients, compared to the placebo cure rate of only 6.6 per cent. In relation to the clearing of psoriatic plaques it was 82.8 per cent and 7.7 per cent respectively.

The cream had no toxic or other side effects. There were no reported cases of hypersensitivity or dermatitis. The study was followed up on a monthly basis for eight consecutive months and there were no relapses.

KEY TIP
This showed that the aloe vera treatment could be considered to be a safe and effective alternative treatment to cure patients suffering from psoriasis.

1996: Peter Green, aloe vera extracts in equine clinical practice

Persistent leucopaenia and lethargy syndrome is a syndrome found in competition horses, and has proved largely unresponsive to mainstream therapy. Horses affected by this disease have lower than normal total leucocyte counts when compared to similar horses of similar age and condition. They generally have persistent low tolerance to exercise and show signs of lethargy. The condition may relate to a previous or ongoing viral or bacterial respiratory infection, but in many cases there is no history of any previous or causal factor. Without treatment many such horses will simply remain tired and unable to function normally. Normal treatment with antibiotics, vitamins and other conventional therapies have shown no benefit. Green reports:

> We decided to use an orally administered aloe vera gel drinking juice for two main reasons. Firstly we had heard that humans suffering from problems like ME had derived some improvements from drinking aloe vera and secondly that we had read of the increasing amount of research being conducted on the immuno-modulating properties of aloe vera. We treated fourteen cases of persistent leucopaenia and lethargy with the aloe vera gel drinking juice at a rate of 240 mls per day for between three and five weeks. None of the horses in the trial had any signs of other infections or diseases. Some had received previous medications and multi-vitamins but none was given any other medication or treatment for the duration of the trial. Only two out of the fourteen horses in the trial showed no response to the aloe vera treatment. Twelve showed improvements in their leucocyte levels (between 10% and nearly 100%) and an increase in overall energy levels and exercise tolerance. Ten out of the fourteen in the trial returned to

previous tasks, i.e. eventing, point to point, dressage, showjumping, etc. and two were sent to stud! In our experience, these results were significantly better than those obtained using other treatment regimes or rest alone.

Source: *Veterinary Times*, volume 26, number 9, September 1996

For a reprint or copies of this paper, please contact the Aloe Vera Centre (see Appendix 1.1).

1998: Dr P Atherton, leg ulcers

Although this was a small pilot study, it nevertheless demonstrated the significant healing properties of aloe vera in relation to treating chronic leg ulcers (as described by Zawahry in 1973 in this section (leg ulcers)). In this study, Dr Atherton treated seven patients whose ulcers had failed to heal using conventional methods of treatment, including skin grafting, and who had been selected by nursing staff as being able and suitable to be involved.

Each patient was patch tested to determine any allergic reaction to the two aloe vera products to be used and then each was prepared according to the study criteria. Each patient was given an aloe vera drink (in this case a proprietary brand with ninety-eight-per-cent-by-volume content of stabilised aloe vera gel, at the rate of two fluid ounces, twice per day). The ulcers were irrigated with water to remove all debris and then packed with aloe vera jelly (with in excess of eighty per cent stabilised aloe vera gel – the same proprietary brand as the drink) and covered with a waterproof dressing and a pressure bandage. The process was carried out daily wherever possible. Seven ulcers were treated (from four to fifteen years old), six of which were chronic venous leg ulcers, and the last in a patient suffering with systemic lupus erythematosis. Six of the patients were female and one male. The results showed that one patient dropped out because she could not endure the stinging sensation caused when aloe vera jelly was applied (a common sensation that passes within less than half an hour normally). Of the remaining six, one saw no improvement. The other five were pleased with the improvements in their conditions and three were totally healed. The study clearly demonstrated the cleansing effect of aloe vera and its ability to destroy the wound's infecting bacteria. Other benefits experienced by the patients included a pronounced improvement in the 'health' of the patients' hair, skin and nails (these benefits are common 'side effects' of using aloe vera orally and topically on a regular basis).

The study did not analyse whether the healing benefits were more attributable to the aloe vera drink or the topical aloe vera jelly. Other studies are planned to determine and compare the effects of topical aloe vera gelly with a standard dressing.

2001: Professors Baxter and Williams et al, IBS Trial, Morriston Hospital/ University of Wales, Swansea

In 2001, the world's first ever randomised, placebo-controlled, double-blind crossover clinical trial, using a proprietary brand of aloe vera gel drinking juice in the treatment of IBS, was launched. IBS is a common and debilitating problem and a great deal is known about the disease, but effective treatment has remained elusive. Although there has been considerable anecdotal evidence that drinking aloe vera juice can help manage IBS, this is the first time that a rigorous scientific trial has been undertaken anywhere in the world. The trial is under the supervision of the professor of surgery, Professor Baxter and his team, including Professor Williams, and will involve over 200 patients (all of whom have not responded to conventional treatments). The trial is expected to last two to three years.

In the UK alone, IBS is the most common disorder referred to gastroenterologists by GPs, and is estimated to affect around twenty per cent of the people in the developed world at some time during their lives.

2002: Joe A Vinson, Hassan Al Kharrat and Lori Andreoli, Department of Chemistry, University of Scranton, PA, USA, 'Effect of aloe vera preparations on the human bioavailability of vitamins C and E'

One of the most exciting aloe vera studies to be undertaken in recent times is that undertaken to determine the effect on bio-availability of taking two of the most widely consumed nutritional supplements, i.e. vitamins C and E, with two different aloe vera preparations (aloe vera drinking juices), compared with a placebo. The results were significant with the bio-availability rates of the vitamins increasing by up to 350 per cent and above when taken with the aloe vera preparations. More details of this study are available in Chapter 2 and from the IASC (see Appendix 1.4 and 1.5).

In summary

From a scientific point of view, I believe it is now safe to say that:

> There is now sufficient clinical, as well as thousands of years of anecdotal evidence, to show that aloe vera has powerful healing, immuno-modulating, anti-inflammatory and tissue regeneration properties

and

> There is no question that aloe vera can make a significant impact on the prevention, the management and the recovery rate of many ailments, diseases, disorders and so on, but the bottom line is that aloe vera helps the body heal itself.

Indeed, many leading scientists, doctors, therapists, nutritionists and others now believe that aloe vera could have a much more significant role to play in the treatment, management and healing of many conditions, ailments, disorders and illnesses that afflict millions of us throughout the world. The greatest challenge we face is in overcoming the massive medical and political influence and indeed the lobbying powers that the global pharmaceutical giants have. The economic self-interest of pharmaceutical companies is continually and rightly being challenged as more and more of us seek more natural, toxic-free methods of treatment for our particular conditions, and who also realise the value of improving diet and nutrition as a way of helping to combat illnesses and diseases. One exciting new area of research is the work being done to identify the 'glyco-biological effects, properties and benefits' of aloe vera. The potential role of aloe vera in the development of 'glyco-nutritionals' could open yet another new chapter for one of nature's most amazing plants.

I firmly believe that the demand for aloe vera and its 'herbal remedy cousins' will become a tidal wave during the twenty-first century. For example, in 2002 in Germany we saw a massive increase in the sales of aloe vera products. This surge in demand was due to a mainstream natural health TV programme on medicinal plants, and this particular programme focused on aloe vera. More and more medical practitioners are beginning to realise the advantages of using such natural based 'treatments' in certain circumstances compared to the toxic side effects of many (but by no means all) pharmaceutical treatments.

We are seeing the development of almost unprecedented global viruses like SARS that can be transmitted around the world in a matter of only a few days. Such new phenomena may place impossible strains on current health care systems, medical treatment regimes and practices and on the medications that are available today.

Who knows, but the answer could lie in further research into the healing properties of plants like aloe vera (and many others) and natural substances like honey and bee propolis, and others. I believe that we have seen only the tip of the iceberg in relation to the benefits of using such products that, when used on a daily basis, can boost the immune system, enhance the bio-availability of nutrients and give the human body better 'weapons' to fight new infectious diseases and agents.

I am sure that the IASC (and its leading members) will continue to be at the forefront of initiating research into further investigation of the benefits of aloe vera.

In the meantime, I will remain one of the staunchest advocates of the benefits of using aloe vera (and other nutritional supplements) on a daily basis as an integral part of my health and diet regime.

9

How to use, store and maximise the benefits of taking aloe vera

Aloe vera – not a panacea for all ills

IN SPITE of the wide ranging health benefits that can be derived from drinking aloe vera and applying it topically, don't think of aloe vera as a panacea for all ills – in reality there is no such thing. Aloe vera's history and track record as a healer and the significant role that it has played in herbal medicine over the centuries is well documented. However, like most other 'natural remedies', it can often take longer to have any beneficial effect on some chronic symptoms than a chemically based drug, though there are no guarantees that such drugs may work or work any better than a natural remedy like aloe vera.

Aloe vera works harmoniously

The reason for this is that it works harmoniously with the body's own self-regulating systems rather than overcoming them and leaving them depleted. Aloe vera works with the body to increase the absorption of nutrients and the bio-availability of vitamins and minerals and to boost the immune system, with no known detrimental side effects.

Case study of antibiotic drugs

For example, it is now common knowledge that synthetic antibiotics can so successfully override – rather than gently boost – the immune system, that they can kill off both the 'harmful' and the 'beneficial' bacteria in the digestive tract. It can then often take two or three months, or even more, to rectify the imbalances caused and for the beneficial 'flora' to be re-established and continue their role of protecting the body against infections. It is also becoming apparent that the overuse of some antibiotics can lead to fungal infections such as thrush that can be notoriously difficult to eradicate. Doctors have now been warned not to prescribe antibiotics in the same 'cure-all' way that was so prevalent in the 1970s, the 1980s and the 1990s. This is mainly due to the increasing risk of so-called 'superbugs' developing that are totally resistant to all antibiotics – even the most powerful. We are already witnessing something along these lines with the development of the MRSA 'bug' that has apparently developed a resistance to many synthetic drugs.

Interestingly, in recent tests carried out at the University of Wales Institute in Cardiff, Dr Rose Cooper has found that pure, natural honey – even at fairly low concentrations – can inhibit the growth of the MRSA bacteria. There are also many natural antibiotics (such as bee propolis) that boost rather than deplete the body's immune system and act synergistically with other natural products, such as aloe vera, to enhance the body's natural defence mechanisms.

How to get the maximum benefit from aloe vera

The following hints and tips are designed to help you not only as a first-time user of aloe vera, but also to act as a guide to those of you who are actually involved in advising others on the use of aloe vera products.

Give aloe vera time to work

Aloe vera is not some sort of overnight cure. It is important to give it at least three months to six months, so that the body has time to benefit from the more gentle 'synergistic' action of aloe vera.

Seek good advice

Seek good advice from someone who understands both how aloe vera works and who can discuss properties, benefits and potential uses with you.

Consider the dosage

Dosage is very often where people make their first mistake: Always start on a smaller dose and build it up over the first two to four weeks, and do not necessarily start on the optimum dosage straightaway. You may start with as little as one teaspoon at a time, or a dessert spoon or a tablespoon (circa five millilitres, ten millilitres and twenty millilitres, respectively), twice per day when you start – depending on your medical situation or past medical history.

If you have been ill or are still ill, then the smaller dosage is how you should begin and then gradually work up to the optimum daily dosage over the next one or two weeks. I would recommend that you take aloe vera first thing in the morning and then again last thing at night and avoid food and hot drinks for about one hour. The dosage really depends on whether you want to take aloe vera just as a tonic or for a more serious problem such as a skin disorder, a digestive problem or an inflammatory condition such as arthritis. If so, I would suggest that you can either take it little and often through the day (not very practical if you are working!) or in the two large doses suggested earlier. Personally, I drink about two to three small wineglasses per day (a litre bottle lasts about three days in our home!!) as a tonic. It seems to have helped boost my energy levels and my immune system and has kept me free of colds and various other bugs and infections for the last six years. My wife has found that the aloe vera drink with glucosamine sulphate, chondroitin, MSM and vitamin C has helped her knees and neck, which were causing a lot of discomfort. Long may it continue!

Take aloe vera on an empty stomach

Some say aloe vera improves digestion when taken just before or just after a meal. It's really up to the individual to determine how they take aloe vera, how often and how much – our 'job' is simply to guide them. I believe it's best taken on an empty stomach and just before bed.

Beware of the 'detox' effect

While on the subject of digestion, we should also discuss detoxification. This is often a 'thorny' subject and many people simply dismiss it.

However, the process of 'the toxins and other noxious elements' being eliminated from the body is essential and can and often does happen when drinking aloe vera. One of aloe vera's properties is that of a cleanser and purifier (but in a gentle not a purgative way as some rather uninformed observers often claim). Not everyone goes through the so-called 'detox' process or is even aware it is happening, but some people may experience the tell-tale signs, such as unexplained skin rashes, headaches, puffy skin, wind, tiredness, queasiness, aches and pains and so on. If you have a chronic condition like IBS, arthritis, ME, etc., you might find a temporary worsening of your symptoms as part of this detoxifying process. This leads on to the next piece of advice. If you experience any symptoms that arise for seemingly no apparent reason and if you think the cause might be the aloe vera you are taking, please take the following advice:

- don't panic
- contact the person that sold you the product
- take his or her advice
- if you do not feel confident then phone the manufacturer

If there is nobody to ask, you should consider coming off the aloe vera for a couple of days or until the symptoms stop and then start again on a very low dose (possibly just five millilitres per dose), and then gradually build the dosage up again over the following days. You may find that you do not need quite as much as before or that you need to take it at a different time of the day, or that you should be taking a higher dose. Whatever the reason, give your body time to adjust.

Keep your aloe vera drinks in the fridge

Please remember to keep any opened container of aloe vera drinking gel or juice in the fridge. Some brands of aloe vera have very short shelf lives, so please check for details on the container. The major aloe vera brands have drinks and other products that are 'stabilised' to keep the contents fresh for several years. This means that provided the container is kept out of sunlight and stored at room temperature (and I mean UK room temperatures, not those you would experience in hotter climates), if unopened, it does not have to be stored in the fridge.

Travelling with aloe vera

If you want to take aloe vera with you on your travels, do not decant it into another ordinary bottle and stash it in your hand luggage. Take an unopened bottle with you and open it only when you reach your destination. If you do not have a fridge in your room, ask the hotel or whatever if they can store it for you (just tell them it's your medication!!). The other option is to take the proper container (many manufacturers now have special, smaller travel bottles) safely tucked between two ice packs, in a small freezer- or cooler-bag, and then refreeze the ice packs when you get to your destination so as to ensure the aloe vera container is always kept cool but not frozen!

Very often when I am travelling, as soon as I arrive at the hotel, I empty the mini-bar and put my aloe vera drinks in the fridge.

Aloe vera for young children

Young children (from the age of two to three-plus) could be given small amounts of aloe vera gel drinking juice as a health tonic or even for conditions such as asthma (see Chapter 5).

Using aloe vera if you have an allergy/skin problem

If you have an allergy or skin problems, it is good practice to do a 'patch test' first apropos of either the drink or the topical preparation you want to use.

Using aloe vera on wounds/burns

This section would apply only to surface abrasions and minor injuries or burns.

Remember to ensure that a wound is properly cleaned prior to the use of any aloe vera preparation. This is because of aloe vera's ability to penetrate deeply into the skin, and it may carry particles of dirt down with it. Do not use aloe vera on more severe injuries or 'puncture' wounds. You should always seek the advice of a medical professional and any such injuries/wounds/burns should always be examined by a qualified medical practitioner immediately. Aloe vera is non-toxic and is generally considered safe to use alongside conventional methods of medication.

Diarrhoea and detoxification

Diarrhoea, as part of the detoxification process of the body, is only a problem if it lasts longer than a few days. Drink plenty of filtered water every day (see Appendix 1.1, and in respect of water filtration contact the Aloe Vera Centre), and lower the dose of aloe vera for a few days as mentioned above.

Using aloe vera for constipation

Constipation can be improved by drinking more filtered water every day (to help flush through the system, rehydrate the body and soften the stool), and increasing the dose of aloe vera until the bowel is working comfortably again.

Drink water too!

As well as aloe vera, I suggest that everyone (adults and children) should drink plenty of filtered water. Leading health professionals and nutritionists recommend that everyone should drink a minimum of 1.5 to 2.5 litres of good quality filtered water every day.

> KEY TIP
> If you are unfortunate enough to work in an air-conditioned environment all the time, then your water intake should be more because of the drying nature of the working atmosphere. Office workers and airline crews especially should take note.

Safety – first and last

If you are at all unsure of whether you should take aloe vera or any other natural remedy, consult someone who knows about such things. You can contact the Aloe Vera Centre (see Appendix 1.1).

Where to seek advice about natural solutions

As we have said earlier in this book, there are many doctors (and other health professionals) who dismiss out of hand aloe vera and other such 'natural remedies' – they can obviously not give you any objective advice. Talk to a nutritionist or a herbalist or, if your doctor is not 'stuck in the Dark Ages', seek their opinion and then make your decision based on why you want to take aloe vera or what you want to take it for. All reputable companies involved in the manufacture and sale of natural 'remedies' should have doctors and other health professionals on their advisory boards. If you have bought a product from a reputable outlet or a trained person then ask them to check with their medical advisor.

You should remember that if you wish to start taking aloe vera to ensure that you re-read the earlier chapters of this book, especially Chapter 2, Chapter 3, Chapter 4, and Chapter 5.

For more advice you can contact us at the Aloe Vera Centre (see Appendix 1.1).

Can pregnant women take aloe vera?

In the past, pregnant women have always been advised to avoid taking aloe vera internally as a tonic (there have even been numerous highly misleading and factually incorrect press articles on this subject). This was because it was said to cause bowel spasms that could be detrimental to them. There seems to be an element of scaremongering on this issue. I personally know dozens of women who have taken aloe vera throughout their pregnancies and found it extremely beneficial (see Chapter 5).

Those aloe vera products that do not meet the minimum IASC quality criteria (see Appendix 1.4 and 1.5), or have too much aloin content, would not, I agree, be beneficial to pregnant women. They would also not be beneficial to anyone else either! The leading aloe vera brands, especially those products that are based on the pure, stabilised inner gel, with the now accepted therapeutic aloin levels, have been used by pregnant women for years without any apparent or reported side effects.

> KEY TIP
> The case history featuring Mary (see Chapter 5) is a good example of how aloe vera gel drinking juice helped someone with IBS and particularly during her third pregnancy.

Over the last few years, I have met and have got to know countless other women who have been using aloe vera for many years, and who have also taken it throughout their respective pregnancies. If anything, they seem to swear by it because when taken as a tonic it boosts their energy levels, helps with digestive problems like constipation, and can also ease the problem of piles.

Aloe vera is also a rich source of vitamins, minerals, enzymes, amino acids, polysaccharides etc., and it also contains folic acid, which has now been found to be highly beneficial for pregnant women and an essential part of all pregnant women's diets.

> KEY TIP
> Aloe vera also contains folic acid – a substance that has been proven scientifically to reduce the risk of disorders like spina bifida in newly born babies.

Use of aloe vera topically

Aloe vera moisturising lotions and other topical preparations, like aloe vera gelly, aloe lotions etc., are also particularly effective in helping with stretch marks – a problem experienced by most pregnant women.

> KEY TIP
> The quality of the aloe vera you take is, without doubt, the critical factor in whether or not aloe vera will benefit you. Make sure that you always take or use the best.

Using aloe vera with diabetes

In some diabetics, it has been discovered that drinking aloe vera can increase the amount of insulin produced by the body. Anyone who has diabetes who wishes to take aloe vera should be aware of this and should consult their doctor to ensure that their insulin levels are properly and carefully monitored. There are many diabetics now drinking aloe vera gels or juices and finding that their diabetes is more 'under control', that their weight is more stable and that they have much more energy. Again the quality of the aloe vera that is taken is critical as to how much it will benefit you.

Contra-indications – are there any?

To our knowledge, and from the experience of others over the last twenty years or more, there are no contra-indications. Please remember aloe vera is a non-toxic, natural substance and it is also unlikely to react with any conventional medication. However, if you are susceptible to any allergic reactions, it is always better to do a 'patch test' or 'trial' first. Always take advice when using aloe vera internally, especially for the treatment of wounds, sinuses, ears and eyes. Where necessary you can dilute the particular product with boiled, filtered water that has been sufficiently cooled.

10

Aloe vera: last thoughts and what next?

Last thoughts

I HOPE this book has provided you with an even closer, more in-depth and broader insight into the full scope of aloe vera's almost 'magical' healing and health-giving properties, benefits and uses, than any previous publication has been able to do. When I was researching my first book in 1996, I was aware of and had enormous belief in this plant's remarkable history of proven healing. However, my opinion was not shared by many 'conventional' health professionals or by many of those in positions to influence innovations in health care, diet and nutrition. In the past few years that knowledge and belief has been enhanced greatly, and the reason is mainly twofold. Firstly, I have witnessed so many more people benefiting from the use of high quality aloe vera products, either internally or topically or both, to help manage a wide range of illnesses, diseases, ailments and disorders. Secondly, I have now met and spoken to so many specialists, general practitioners, vets and other 'allopathic' health professionals, whose attitudes and opinions have performed what I can only describe as a radical u-turn when they have witnessed for themselves the healing properties and benefits and the many potential uses of aloe vera – both internally and topically.

Suddenly, they all seem to be 'rediscovering' the key role that nutrition and diet plays in improved health and the role that aloe vera (both topically and orally administered) can have in helping to manage and heal many disorders (in both humans and animals). At last, we are seeing something of a breakthrough or a breaking down of the entrenched attitudes that have characterised the majority of the medical profession over the last fifty or more years. Slowly but surely, there is an increasing and wider understanding of the importance of both nutrition and diet and the increased recognition that they are powerful tools in the fight against the growing incidence of immune system disorders and even illnesses and diseases like cancer and diabetes.

When I was researching my first book, the number of companies either involved in the aloe vera industry or producing products with aloe vera, was far fewer than is the case today. It is almost impossible to open a magazine or a paper nowadays without the mention of yet another product containing aloe vera. Many of these new products are what I would term 'recreational' or 'market led' products, i.e. they fit into the modern desire to consume only so-called lifestyle products or have some aloe vera content to entice the consumer, but generally they do not have enough aloe vera content to have any true therapeutic or real healing benefits.

They may have some effect but they are unlikely to have the same level of benefits as the leading brands that have high percentages by volume of stabilised aloe vera gel content, i.e. more active ingredient. While I am delighted with the increased awareness of the benefits of aloe vera, I still recommend that you should drink aloe vera every day if you want to improve your overall health and general well-being. I would also strike a cautionary note. There is always the danger that since the current demand for 'aloe vera' products seems almost insatiable, it will undoubtedly attract poorer quality products onto the market.

Generally, such products 'emblazon' aloe vera on the front label but on examining the 'contents' section (on the back label) it appears the first ingredient is often 'aqua' or water. There is now absolutely no need for anyone, wherever they live, be it in the UK, the USA, Europe, the Far East, the Middle East, Australasia or Africa to buy such products. Why? Because there are other products – readily available to consumers in those areas – whose efficacy, purity and potency are guaranteed, and they are extremely price competitive. The vast disparity in the quality of aloe vera products that I first wrote about in 1996 has, in my opinion, become even worse.

> KEY TIP
> The proof of quality is in the tasting!
>
> A quality aloe vera drink should have a slightly vegetable flavour and smell and contain fibrous pulp. It should appear similar in texture or consistency to freshly squeezed orange juice – rather than a clear thin liquid.
>
> It undoubtedly has a very 'vegetable' taste (aloe vera is after all a vegetable!!) and some would say an 'acquired' taste!

Marks of quality

The IASC is still the only organisation that is involved in the development and implementation of quality standards for the aloe vera industry and aloe vera products on a global basis. Potential buyers of aloe vera products (whether for topical or internal use) should always ensure that such products carry the authentic IASC seal of approval before they make any purchase. Anyone who is confused about what type of products to buy can telephone, email or fax us at the Aloe Vera Centre or visit our website (see Appendix 1.1).

The quality issue will run and run

Many companies are still making claims about the benefits of highly concentrated aloe vera and my response to them is the same as it was four years ago:

> The natural balance of the nutrients in aloe vera and the synergistic way in which they work to provide the broad spectrum healing benefits has a proven track record dating back thousands of years.
>
> Processes used to concentrate any of the 'active ingredients' will unquestionably have an effect on that natural synergy and may result in a less potent healing mechanism than that found in the natural plant.

KEY TIP
Find a source of aloe vera that is 'as untampered with' as possible – even directly from the plant itself – but make sure that it is mature and that it grows naturally. Unfortunately, windowshelf or indoor grown aloe vera doesn't have the same rich concentrations of nutrients as outdoor grown aloe vera – though it can be useful for minor cuts, burns and stings.

Misleading labels

Whatever the label says, remember to make sure that when you look at the percentage of aloe vera content, it is given as a percentage by volume content, i.e. what percentage of the total content is aloe vera and if it is not listed ask the person or shop concerned. Many people are misled by the fact that labels very often refer to the percentage purity, i.e. they will have descriptions on the label such as '100 per cent pure aloe vera juice'. This has nothing to do with the percentage of aloe vera in the container – it relates only to the purity of the original aloe vera used. There could be as little as only ten to twenty per cent by volume of aloe vera in some drinks – which would obviously have little or no therapeutic benefit for the person taking it! Stabilised aloe vera should always be the number one ingredient in any aloe vera product.

It is impossible to encapsulate nearly 4,000 years of healing history in one book. Neither is it possible to condense the many scientific studies that have been undertaken and other papers that have been written by scientists from all over the world in the last seventy years or more. I have attempted to provide you with a concise and useful guide to aloe vera and its incredible healing properties, benefits and wide range of uses.

KEY TIP
If you are unsure, taste it. If it looks and tastes like water – or is a clear tasteless liquid – then it probably is mostly water. Don't buy it!

The original amber nectar

I call aloe vera my 'original amber nectar', and I would encourage you, whether you're health conscious or not, to just get high quality aloe vera on you or in you.

Don't mess about and don't delay, and in the words of a well known past global advertising slogan: 'Just do it' ...you'll soon see and appreciate the benefits.

Having read this book, you may begin to realise why I feel so passionately about this ancient plant and why I believe that it has such an important part to play in improved health and general well-being as we advance further into this high-tech twenty-first century. Aloe vera has stood the test of time over many centuries, it has a far longer track record of healing than any pharmaceutical medication and it has no toxic side effects.

Our future demands natural solutions

As scientists and the medical fraternity continue to struggle in the fight against new strains of killer bugs and diseases, maybe the 'answer really does lie in the soil' or with nature. Natural remedies and foods and plants such as aloe vera, and natural products such as bee propolis and honey from the beehive, could play a major role in this ongoing war! I firmly believe that high quality aloe vera products have an increasingly important role to play in the prevention of many diseases and disorders, as well as in the overall management of improved health and general well-being. Aloe vera is unquestionably one of nature's true legendary healers – working silently through the body – with a track record stretching back thousands of years. It really is something of an irony that in this highly electronic age, we have all the technology to communicate with someone on the other side of the world when walking along the street but we cannot find a cure for cancer or the common cold or eczema or IBS.

Companies and governments spend billions researching and paying for new and increasingly more expensive medications and equipment (all vital), and yet we are only now just beginning to rediscover the healing properties of many ancient plants. Many of these (and aloe vera is arguably one of the most important) were used successfully by past civilisations for their recognised healing and therapeutic properties and benefits.

Nutritional supplements – common sense, be your own best judge

The recent announcements by organisations like the Food Standards Agency (is this a truly independent organisation?) in the UK (and no doubt other such agencies in other countries in Europe) should be a warning sign to all of us that we must continue to subject the findings of any such government-linked agency to the utmost scrutiny. We, as consumers, really have no idea whether these findings are wholly objective and are in our 'best interests' or if they could be the first steps in a pan-European governmental initiative to 'ban' more and more nutritional supplements or have them classified as 'herbal medicines' that would then be subject to licensing fees that most suppliers and manufacturers could not afford to pay.

The only winners in this game would be the pharmaceutical companies, and yes, you've guessed it, the only losers would be us, the consumers. Our freedom of choice in yet another area would be seriously curtailed.

Be sensible when you take nutritional supplements and if necessary take advice from an independent nutritionist (or a doctor if with nutritional qualifications – most are not) or consult ION (see Appendix 1.15). Also remember that many recommended daily allowance (RDA) figures are generally wholly inadequate and take no account of the depletion in the nutritional quality of much of the so-called fresh fruit and vegetables available today and the health impact on our immune systems of the cocktail of pesticide, herbicide and other chemical residues that are often found on such produce.

Aloe vera – a wider role in improved health?

The growing body of scientific studies and knowledge and the years of anecdotal evidence gathered over the centuries provide a sufficient basis for advancing the potential role of aloe vera. Patrick Holford in his newsletter *100% Health*, issue one, lists aloe vera as one of the key recommended ingredients in his immune power plan. There are *sixteen* elements to his plan for people to build their immune systems, stay 'bug-free' and help combat specific infections. A case can be made that aloe vera can help to combat and manage some of the diseases and modern scourges of our time, such as cancer, asthma, arthritis, diabetes, heart disease and conditions like IBS, acne, eczema and psoriasis. I believe aloe vera's role in such healing initiatives is only just beginning.

I am however also convinced that pharmaceutical conglomerates and those directly and indirectly influenced by their financial resources (and this includes politicians and bureaucrats all over the world) will do all in their power to try and influence or indeed even prevent the growth and general use of products based on plants and other natural ingredients (e.g. products from the beehive such as honey, bee propolis, etc.). Such moves are nothing more than a cynical attempt by such organisations to extend their monopolistic practices and thus prevent the vast majority of the world's population that currently uses natural remedies from having a say in what they want to use. Everyone knows that pharmaceutical medicines are vital in many successful medical operations, procedures and treatments, but there must also be a recognition of the vital role that complementary therapies and/or natural products can play in many cases where either conventional medication has not worked or the individual has decided to use these alternatives.

There is now a significant increase in research programmes to study the role and effectiveness of natural products in the treatment of numerous diseases and illnesses. As these initiatives develop more momentum, and both the positive and negative outcomes are properly scrutinised and publicised, the public will be more informed, and will thus be able to make their own objective choices. It is vital that we continue to operate in a research and development environment that encourages both the scientists to unlock the powerful secrets that nature holds and the medical profession – at all levels – to remain independent and open minded.

I truly hope that you enjoy reading this book and find it a useful source of reference and that you decide to start using aloe vera products as an integral part of your health, nutrition, beauty, sport and fitness regimes. Aloe vera products are now an integral and essential part of our daily regime – make it yours. If you decide to make that decision, and I am confident you will, I am convinced you will both see and enjoy the benefits.

Good luck.

Alasdair Barcroft

Appendices

Appendix 1: References and sources of information/Useful addresses

In researching this book, we have used hundreds of references from many learned doctors (and other health professionals) and highly respected scientists, and we have visited many websites. All references to books, the scientific literature and the studies mentioned in this book are listed in Appendix 3 or are mentioned in Appendix 2. You can also determine, where relevant, how to obtain reprints of some of the papers listed in this book.

1.1 The Aloe Vera Centre

PO Box 19766
London
SW15 2WZ
UK
Contact: Alasdair and Mary Barcroft
Tel +44 (0) 20 8875-9915 or +44 (0) 8707-555800
Fax +44 (0) 20 8871-1798
Email alasdairaloevera@aol.com
Website www.aloeveracentre.com (UK, products), www.skyzthelimit.biz (UK, business), www.skyzthelimit.teamflp.com (USA)
Ebook/guide www.aloeveracentre.co.uk/avh

The Aloe Vera Centre was established as a UK retail mail order business selling direct to the public, as well as providing advice on aloe vera, its properties, uses and benefits. Now, by registering with the company – Forever Living Products or FLP (this procedure is free of charge) – anyone residing in one of the hundred or more countries in which FLP operates is able to purchase the products direct from FLP at the wholesale price (minimum order in UK, £50) and make a thirty per cent saving (for long-term users this is especially beneficial).

Please telephone, email or fax us for details on how to register and order products direct from the manufacturer. FLP also offers a business opportunity for people wishing to build a long-term residual royalty-based income, locally, nationally and internationally.

Various reprints of papers mentioned in this book are available through the Aloe Vera Centre (email alasdairaloevera@aol.com for details and prices).

Note, 'Aloe Vera Centre' is a registered trading name and the Aloe Vera Centre in London is the only organisation in the UK permitted to use 'Aloe Vera Centre' as its trading name.

1.2 Senter for LIVSHJELP/Norwegian Aloe Vera Centre

Integrated Medical and Health Centre
PO Box 7
N-1415 Oppegard
Norway
Contact: Dr Audun Myskja and Reidun Myskja
Tel 00 47 64-913990 / 66-99-1105
Fax 00 47 64-913991 / 66-99-3028
Email audun.myskja@organizer.net or info@livshjelp.no or aloevera@livshjelp.no
Website www.livshjelp.no

This centre was established as a multi-disciplinary medical centre and health clinic, offering a range of both conventional and complementary therapies. The centre also specialises in aloe vera and other nutritional products, music therapy, Tomatis therapy, flower remedies and other therapies.

Reidun Myskja is also a qualified reflexologist and homeopath.

1.3 Bimal

Medical and Sports Rehabilitation Clinic
The Hogarth Health Club/Clinic
Airedale Avenue
Chiswick
London
W4 2NW
Contact: Alan Watson
Tel +44 (0) 20 8742-1744
Fax +44 (0) 20 8747-0499
Email robyng@thehogarth.co.uk

One of the foremost and most innovative practitioners in his field, Alan Watson is often quoted in the media and has many sports and non-sports patients or clients in his practice, including many international sportsmen and women.

1.4 The International Aloe Science Council Inc

415 East Airport Freeway
Suite 260
Irving
Texas 75062
USA
Contact: Gene Hale, Managing Director
Tel 00 1 972-258-8772
Fax 00 1 972-258-8777
Email iasc@email.msn.com
Website www.iasc.org

1.5 The International Aloe Science Council

Q: What is the International Aloe Science Council?

A: It is a body set up to develop and monitor standards within the aloe vera industry worldwide.

Q: How is it funded?

A: The council is funded entirely by fees received. All members pay annual membership fees, and if a member wants to have a product certified, an analysis fee is charged. Members also pay an annual certification fee for every product that has been certified.

Q: Who are its members?

A: Its members include the following companies and many others:

Aloe Vera of America, Texas (this is a Forever Living Products Company)
Agro-Mar Inc, Nevada
Aloe Laboratories Inc, Texas
El Mar Enterprises Inc, California
Terry Laboratories Inc, Florida
Aloe Complete Inc, California
LODC, Texas
Univera Inc, Texas
Aloecorp, Texas
Aloe World Inc, Dominican Republican
Namyang Aloe Co, Korea

Q: What is the IASC seal of approval?

A: It is a certification of the quality of aloe vera products. It includes the auditing of the manufacturing facilities and processes, as well as an analysis of the product itself.

Q: How do you get the IASC seal of approval for your products?

A: All aloe vera suppliers are invited to submit their products for certification by the IASC. Once certified, and if their products contain the specified minimum amount of aloe vera, then the company is eligible to apply for the IASC seal of approval. Companies wanting to display the seal must have their products analysed by independent experts who use approved procedures developed by the IASC's Science and Technical Committee.

Q: How many aloe manufacturers genuinely hold the seal of approval?

A: FLP was the first company in the UK and Europe to receive the seal of approval on its products. There are now several other companies and brands in the UK and elsewhere in Europe that also meet the criteria laid down by the IASC.

Q: What can the IASC tell us about 'whole leaf aloe'?

A: As its name implies, whole leaf aloe is made by pulping the whole leaf, including rind and inner gel. As this would contain the aloin that acts as a strong purgative, the pulp is then passed through a carbon filter block, which absorbs the aloin, making the resulting product suitable for human consumption. However, the question of which other nutrients are absorbed by the filter has not yet been fully answered.

Q: What other definitions of aloe vera are there?

A: Aloe vera gel or juice is defined as the naturally occurring processed, undiluted (100 per cent), parenchymal tissue obtained from the aloe Barbadensis Miller plant, to which no more than five per cent additives (including preservatives) shall be added as part of the processing. An aloe vera beverage is defined as an ingestible product containing a minimum of fifty per cent aloe vera juice as defined in the reporting procedure adopted by the IASC. An aloe vera drink is defined similarly to the beverage, but the minimum content of aloe is only ten per cent. In addition, there are definitions for aloe vera spray dried, freeze dried, concentrate, pulp and oil.

1.6 David Urch (veterinary surgeon)

Urch, DL (1999), *Aloe Vera – Nature's Gift. Aloe Vera in Veterinary Practice.*
Blackdown Publications
Blackdown Farm
Lippiatt Lane
Shipham, Winscombe
Somerset
BS25 1QY
Email DLU3609@aol.com

Anyone who would like to order David Urch's book, *Aloe Vera – Nature's Gift. Aloe Vera in Veterinary Practice*, can do so by contacting him at the above street or email address.

1.7 Carrie Holmes

Carrie Holmes is the mother of Bronte who is featured in Chapter 5 and in Colour Plates 5, 6, 7, 8
Email carrieflp@hotmail.com
Mobile 07816-230158

1.8 Venetia Armitage (nutritionist)

71 York Mansions
Prince of Wales Drive
London
SW11 4BW
Tel 020 7720-2984
Email vlarmitage@aol.com

1.9 Tim and Sarah Page

Email timw.page@btopenworld.com, timwpage@msn.com
Website www.beehive.courier.co.uk/thechroniccrohnscampaignuk

Another website that may be of interest to those with allergies to dairy products is www.notmilk.com

1.10 PARA – Paratuberculosis Awareness and Research Association

PARA is an organisation set up to raise the awareness of the zoonotic (disease-causing) potential of the bacterium myobacterium avium subspecies paratuberculosis (MAP) in the national community of sufferers of Crohn's disease and to determine the role played by MAP in causing Crohn's disease. There is now a wide range of scientific evidence that implicates the bacterium known as MAP – a food- and water-borne bacterium in the causation of Crohn's disease.

Contact Karen Meyer
Website www.crohns.org

1.11 Glyconutrients/glyconutrition

Website www.GlycoInformation.com

1.12 Professor Michael F Kirkman

Intestinal Microbiology and Functional Probiotics (Bio Pathica Ltd)
Email ecnhs@hotmail.com

1.13 Rosemary Titterington (herbalist)

Iden Croft Herbs
Frittenden Road
Staplehurst
Kent
TN12 0DH
Tel 01580-891432
Fax 01580-89241

1.14 The Olivia Hodson Fellowship Fund

The Olivia Hodson Fellowship Fund was established in the memory of Olivia Hodson, who was two and a half years old when she died in April 1996. Olivia had a malignant germ cell tumour. She was a brave and happy child, who was healthy until her second birthday.

The fund was established by Olivia's family and is supported by the generosity of many friends. It primarily supports projects centred at Great Ormond Street Hospital and the Institute of Child Health (ICH).

Great Ormond Street Hospital is renowned for its care of sick children and houses the widest range of paediatric expertise, including the largest cancer centre, treating about ten per cent of all children with cancer in the UK. It also houses Britain's largest paediatric intensive care, neonatal and cardiac surgery units. It treats about 10,765 children as inpatients and 33,174 as outpatients each year.

The ICH has an international reputation in childhood cancer research, receiving a five-star A rating (the highest possible rating) in the UK's most recent review. The 'Cancer Theme' has programmes researching various leukaemias, neuroblastomas and brain tumours.

More than 1,000 children in the UK are diagnosed with cancer or leukaemia every year. Many children are now completely cured, as research has greatly improved survival rates. One in a thousand young adults are now survivors of malignancy but cancer still kills more children than any other group of disorders.

Deciding which charity to support is normally a challenging task. However, when we heard of the Olivia Hodson Fellowship Fund and met Olivia's mother, Christiane, and as parents ourselves, we felt it was something we really wanted to do. The greatest gift in life is to have a child and by supporting the charity we feel we are making a contribution to the improved health and well-being of someone else's child.

For more information about the Olivia Hodson Fellowship Fund, please contact Christiane Hodson on 020 8942-8400 or the fund secretary on 020 7813-8495, and please quote 'aloe vera'.

The Olivia Hodson Fellowship Fund is a special purpose fund of Great Ormond Street Hospital Children's Charity.

1.15 The Institute for Optimum Nutrition (ION)

ION offers personal consultations with qualified nutritionists, including a one-day optimum nutrition workshop, homestudy course and the nutrition consultants' diploma course. It also offers the British Association of Nutritional Therapists (BANT) directory of nutrition consultants to help you find a nutrition consultant in your area. For details of courses, consultations or publications and a free information pack, send an A5 SAE to:

ION
Blades Court
Deodar Road
London
SW15 2NU
Tel 020 8877-9993.

To subscribe to Patrick Holford's newsletter – *100% Health* – visit www.patrickholford.com.

1.16 The Haven Trust

The Haven Trust is dedicated to providing a network of welcoming and friendly support centres for people affected by breast cancer. Staffed by professionals, Haven offers information, advice, counselling and complementary therapies under one roof, free of charge and specifically designed to complement conventional medical treatment. The first Haven is in Fulham, South West London.

The Haven Trust
Effie Road
Fulham
London
SW6 1TB
Tel 020 7384-0000
Fax 020 7384-0001
Helpline 08707-272273

1.17 Ruth Dwornik

Ruth Dwornik
2 Willow Corner
Carbrooke
Norfolk
IP25 6SS
Tel 01953 884203

1.18 Ann Hayes

Rose Cottage
Marsh Lane
Hampton-in-Arden
Solihull
B92 0AH
Tel +44(0)1675-443826

1.19 Mary Peters

Tel 01189 287686
Email: mary@mayfairfarm.fsnet.co.uk

1.20 Philippa Jackson-Cox

The Pightle
Old School Lane
Stanford
Biggleswade
Beds
SG18 9JL
Tel 01462 814004

Appendix 2: Recommended reading

D L Urch (1999), *Aloe Vera – Nature's Gift. Aloe Vera in Veterinary Practice*, Blackdown Publications.

Hazel Courteney (2001), *500 Of The Most Important Health Tips You'll Ever Need*, Cico Books.

Hazel Courteney (2003), *500 Of The Most Important Ways To Stay Younger Longer*, Cico Books.

Patrick Holford (1996), *Living Food*, ION Press.

Patrick Holford (1997), *The Optimum Nutrition Bible*, Piatkus.

Patrick Holford (1999), *Say No To Cancer*, Piatkus.

Professor Jane Plant (2000), *Your Life In Your Hands*, Virgin.

Dr Lawrence G Plaskett, *The Health and Medical Use of Aloe Vera*, Aloe Vera Information Service.

Dr Peter Atherton (1997), *The Essential Aloe Vera.*

Julia Lawless and Judith Allan (2000), *Aloe Vera: Natural Wonder Cure*, Thorsons.

Janette Marshall (2000), *Eat to Beat Your Age*, Hodder and Stoughton.

Dr Gary Fischbach, MD, *Nature's Miracles – an MD's Experiences.*

Professor M F Kirkman, CBiol, FRIPH, FRSH, *Intestinal Microbiology and Functional Probiotics*, Bio Pathica Ltd.

I E Danhoff (1999), *Remarkable Aloe*, Grand Prairie Texas, Omnimedicus Press.

Linda Lazardes (2000), *The Amino Acid Report*, Waterfall.

Appendix 3: Bibliography and references

Agarwal, Dr O P (1984), 'Prevention of atheromatous heart disease', *Angiology*, 36 (8), 485–92.

Andersen, D C, Weber, N D, Wood, S G, Hughes, B G, Murray, B K, North, J A (1991), 'In vitro virucidal activity of selected anthraquinones and anthraquinone derivatives', Antiviral Research, September, 16 (2), 185–96.

Andersonn, B C (1983), 'Aloe vera juice: a veterinary medicament?', *The Compendium on Continuing Education for the Practising Veterinarian*, 5, S364–S368.

Atherton, Dr P (1997), *The Essential Aloe Vera.*

Atherton, Dr P (1998), 'Aloe vera: magic or medicine?', *Nursing Standard*, July 1–7, 41, 12.

Bland, J (1985), 'Effect of orally consumed aloe vera juice on gastrointestinal function in normal humans', Prevention.

Blitz, J, Smith, J W, Gerard, J H (1963), 'Aloe vera gel in peptic ulcer therapy', preliminary report, *The Journal of the American Osteopathic Association*, 62, April.

Bouthet, C F, Schirf, V R, Winters, W D (1995), 'Stimulation of neuron-like cell growth of aloe substances', Phytother, Res 9, 185–88.

Bradshaw, T W (1996), 'Aloe vera: its influence on the physiology of wound healing and inflammation, *Journal of British Podiatric Medicine*, 51 (2), 25–29, A7.

Brasher, W J, Zimmerman, E R, Collings, C K (1969), 'The effects of prednisolone, indomethacin and aloe vera gel on tissue culture cells', *Oral Surgery, Oral Medicine and Oral Pathology*, 27, 122–28.

Bruce, W G G (1987), 'Investigations of the anti-bacterial activity in the aloe', *South African Medical Journal*, 81, 984.

Buchman, D D (1983), *Herbal Medicine: The Natural Way to Get Well and Stay Well*, Rider.

Carpenter, R H, Yates, K M, Busbee, D, King, G, Tizard, I, McAnalley, B (1991), 'Clinical applications of a biological response modifier (acemannan) in veterinary clinical medicine', International Congress of Phytotherapy, October, Seoul, Korea, 62.

Chevalier, A (1996), *The Encyclopaedia of Medicinal Plants*, Dorling Kindersley.

Collins, C E, Collins, C (1935), 'Roentgen dermatitis treated with fresh whole leaf of aloe vera, *American Journal of Roentgenology and Radium Therapy*, 33, 396–97.

Collins, C (1935), 'Alvagel as a therapeutic agent in the treatment of radiation burns', *The Radiological Review*, 57, 6.

Courtney, H (1996), *What's the Alternative?*, second edition, Boxtree.

Danhof, I E, McAnalley, B H (1983), 'Stabilised aloe vera – effect on human skin cells', Drug and Cosmetic Industry, 133, 52, 54, 105–6.

Danhof, I (1996), *Remarkable Aloe*, video, Pro-Ma.

Danhof, I (1993), 'Potential reversal of chronological and photo-ageing of the skin by topical application of natural substances', Phytotherapy Research, special issue: *Proceedings of the International Congress of Phytotherapy*, 1991, S53–56.

Davis, R H, Agnew, P S, Shapiro, E (1986), 'Anti-arthritic activity of anthraquinones found in aloe for podiatric medicine', *Journal of American Podiatric Medical Association*, 76 (2), 61–66.

Davis, R H, Leitner, M E, Russo, J M (1987), 'Topical anti-inflammatory activity of aloe vera as measured by ear swelling', *Journal of American Podiatric Medical Association*, 77 (11), 610–12.

Davis, R H, Leitner, M G, Russo, J M, Byrne, M E (1989), 'Anti-inflammatory activity of aloe vera against a spectrum of irritants, *Journal of American Podiatric Medical Association*, 79 (6), 263–76.

Davis, R H, Leitner, M G, Russo, JM (1988), 'Aloe vera. A natural approach for treating wounds, edema and pain in diabetes', *Journal of the American Podiatric Medical Association*, 78 (2), 60–68.

Davis, R H, Maro, N P (1989), 'Aloe vera and gibberellin. Anti-inflammatory activity in diabetes', *Journal of the American Podiatric Medical Association*, January, 79 (1), 24–26.

Davis, R H, Rosenthal, KY, Cesario, L R, Omu, G A (1989), 'Processed aloe vera administered topically inhibits inflammation', *Journal of the American Podiatric Medical Association*, 79 (8), 395–97.

Davis, R H, Parker, W L, Murdoch, D P (1991), 'Aloe vera as a biologically active vehicle for hydrocortisone acetate', *Journal of the American Podiatric Medical Association*, 81 (1), 1–9, A3.

Davis, R H (1991), 'Influence of aloe on inflammation and wound healing', International Congress of Phytotherapy, October, Seoul, Korea, 29.

Davis, R H, Stewart, G J, Bregman, P J (1992), 'Aloe vera and the inflamed synovial pouch model', *Journal of the American Podiatric Medical Association*, March, 82 (3), 140–48.

Davis, R H, Didonato, J J, Hartman, G M, Haas, R C (1994), 'Anti-inflammatory and wound healing activity of a growth substance in aloe vera', *Journal of the American Podiatric Medical Association*, February, 84 (2), 77–81.

Davis, R H, Didonato, J J, Johnson, R W, Stewart, C B (1994), 'Aloe vera, hydrocortisone and sterol influence on wound tensile strength and anti-inflammation', *Journal of the American Podiatric Medical Association*, December, 84 (12), 614–21.

El Zawahry, M, Hegarty, M R, and Helal, M (1973), 'Use of aloe vera in treating leg ulcers and dermatoses', *International Journal of Dermatology*, 12, 68–73.

Filatov, V P (1945), 'Tissue therapy in Cutaneous leishmaniasis', *American Review of Soviet Medicine*, August.

Fine, A F, Brown, S (1938), 'Cultivation and clinical application of aloe vera leaf', *Radiology*, 31, 735–36.

Fulton, J E (1990), 'The stimulation of post-dermabrasion wound healing with stabilised aloe vera gel-polyethylene oxide dressing', *Journal of Dermatological Surgical Oncology*, 16, 5, 460–67.

Garnick, J, Hanes, P J, Hardim, J, Thompson, W (1994), 'Changes in root sensitivity with toothpastes containing aloe vera and allantoin', *Archives of Oral Biology*, 39 (suppl), 132S.

Gates, G (1975), 'Aloe vera – my favourite plant', *American Horticulturalist*, 54, 37.

Green, P (1996), 'Aloe vera extracts in equine clinical practice', *Veterinary Times*, 26, 9.

Grindlay, D, Reynolds, T (1986), 'The aloe vera phenomenon: A review of the properties and modern uses of the leaf parenchyma gel', *Journal of Ethnopharmacology*, 16, 117–51.

Gunther, R T (1934), *The Greek Herbal of Dioscorides*, Oxford University Press.

Hedendal, B E, *Whole Leaf Aloe Vera*, Beyond Nutrition Press, 17.

Heggers, J P, Winters, W (1993), 'Aloe and other topical anti-bacterial agents in wound healing', *Aloe Today/Aloecorp*, 8–11, A4.

Heggers, J P, Pelley, R P, Robson, M C (1993), 'Beneficial effects of aloe in wound healing', *Phytotherapy Research*, 7, 48–52.

Heggers, J P, Kucukcelebi, Ahmet, Listengarten, Dimitri, Stabenau, Catherine, J, Ko, Francis, Broemeling, Lyle, D, Winters, Wendell, Bouthet, Catherine and Robson, Martin, C (1992), 'Wound healing potential of aloe and other chemotherapeutic agents', presented at the sixth International Congress on Traditional and Folk Medicine, December, Kingsville, Texas.

Heinerman, J (1982), 'Aloe vera, the divine healer', in *Aloe Vera, Jojoba and Yucca*, Keats Publishing.

Hennessee, O M and Cook, B R (1989), 'Aloe: myth-magic', *Medicine*.

Holford, P (1992), *Optimum Nutrition*, ION Press.

Holford, P (1996), *Living Food*, ION Press.

Holford, P (1997), *The Optimum Nutrition Bible*, Piatkus.

Holford, P (1999), *Say No To Cancer*, Piatkus.

Jeong, H Y, Kim, J H, Hwang, S J, Rhee, D K (1994), 'Anti-cancer effects of aloe on sarcoma 180 in mice and on human cancer cell lines'.

Kahlon, J B, Kemp, M C, Carpenter, RH, McAnalley, B H, McDaniel, H R, Shannen, W M (1991), 'Inhibition of AIDS virus replication by acemannan in vitro', Mol, Biother, 3, 127–35.

Koo, M W L (1994), 'Aloe vera: anti-ulcer and anti-diabetic effects', *Phytotherapy Research*, 8 (8), 461–64.

Levenson, S, Somova, K (1956), 'Periodontitis treated with aloe extract', Irkukak Medical Institute.

Loveman, A B (1936), 'Leaf of aloe vera in treatment of roentgen ray ulcers', Archives of Dermatology and Syphilology, 36, 838–43.

Lorenzetti, L J, Salisbury, R, Beal, J L, Baldwin, J N (1984), 'Bacteriostatic property of aloe vera', *Journal of Pharmaceutical Science*, 53, 1287.

Lushbaugh, C C, Hale, D B (1953), 'Experimental acute radiodermatitis following beta radiation vs histopathalogical study of the mode of action of therapy with aloe vera', *Cancer*, 6, 690–98.

Mahmoud, Hazem, El-Sibaie, El-Borollosy, El-Kady (1986), 'Microbiological studies on the phyllospere of the desert plant aloe vera, extraction of anthraquinone glycosides and anthraquinone-aglycone from plant leaves tested as anti-microbial substances against six pathogenic and six non-pathogenic micro-organisms', *Egyptian Journal of Microbiology*, 21 (2), 229–38.

McDaniel, H R, McAnalley, B H (1987), 'Evaluation of polymannoacetate (carrisyn) in the treatment of AIDS', *Clinical Research*, 35, 483A.

Mandeville, F B (1939), 'Aloe vera in the treatment of radiation ulcers of mucous membranes', *Radiology*, 32, 598–99.

Morales, B L (nd), 'Aloe vera, the miracle plant', reprinted from *Let's Live, Health in Mind and Body*, Los Angeles, California.

Northway, R B (1975), 'Experimental use of aloe vera extract in clinical practice', *Veterinary Medicine/Small Animal Clinician*, 70, 89.

Ody, P (1997), *100 Great Natural Remedies*, Kyle Cathie.

Pelley, R P (1997), 'The story of aloe polysaccharides', extract from *Inside Aloe*, January, International Aloe Science Council.

Pietroni, P (1995), *The Family Guide to Alternative Health Care*, Simon and Schuster.

Plant, Dr J (2000), *Your Life in Your Hands*, Virgin.

Plaskett, Dr L G (1996), *The Health and Medical Use of Aloe Vera*, AVIS.

Ritter, L (1991), 'AIDS and aloe vera', *Health Consciousness*, April, 33.

Ritter, L (1993), *A Mission Discovered*, Triputic.

Robson, M C, Heggars, J P, and Hagstrom, W J (1982), 'Myth, magic, witchcraft or fact? Aloe vera revisited', *Journal of Burn Care and Rehabilitation*, 3, 157–63.

Rodriguez-Bigas, M, Cruz, N I, Suarez, A (1988), 'Comparative evaluation of aloe vera in the management of burn wounds in guinea pigs', *Plastic Reconstruction Surgery* (US), 81 (3), 386–89.

Sakai, R (1989), 'Epidemiology survey on lung cancer with respect to cigarette smoking and plant diet', *Japanese Journal of Cancer Research*.

Semionova, N (1998), 'Aloe vera: the natural healer', Moscow, Ripol Classic, 1998, orally translated from the Russian by Natasha Hull, 1999.

Sheets, M A, Unger, B A, Giggleman, G F, Tizard, I R (1991), 'Studies of the effect of acemannan on retrovirus infections: clinical stabilisation of feline leukaemia virus-infected cats', *Molecular Biotherapy*, 3, 41–45.

Sims, R M, Zimmerman, E R (1969), 'Report on effect of aloe vera on growth of certain micro-organisms', Baylon College of Dentistry, Dallas Microbial Assay Services, 1, 230–33.

Sims, R M, Zimmerman, E R (1971), 'The effect of aloe vera on mycotic organisms (fungi)', Aloe Vera of America Archives, Stabilised Aloe Vera, 241–42.

Sims, R M, Zimmerman, E R (1971), 'The effect of aloe vera on Herpes simplex and Herpes virus (strain zoster)', Aloe Vera of America Archives, Stabilised Aloe Vera, 1, 239–40.

Skousen, M B, *Aloe Vera Handbook*, Aloe Vera Research Institute, California.

Strickland, F M, Pelley, R P, Kripke, M L (1997), 'Prevention of ultraviolet radiation induced suppression of contact and delayed hypersensitivity of aloe Barbadensis gel extract', *Journal of Investigative Dermatology*, February, 102, 2.

Sudworth, R (1997), 'The use of aloe vera in dentistry', reprinted from *Positive Health*, 20, 8.

Sydiskis, R J, Owen, Lohr, Rosler, Blomster (1989), 'Inactivation of Herpes simplex virus by anthraquinones isolated from plants', *Journal Dental Research*, June, 68, 935.

Sydiskis, R J, Owen, Lohr, Blomster (1989), 'Inactivation of Herpes simplex virus by anthraquinones isolated from plants', *Journal of Dental Research*, June, 68, 935.

Syed, T A, Ashfaq, S, Holt, A H, Ahmad, S A, Ahmad, S H and Afzal, M (1996), 'Management of psoriasis with aloe vera extract in a hydrophilic cream: a placebo-controlled, double-blind study', *Tropical Medicine and International Health*, 1, 4, 505–9.

Taylor-Donald, L (1980), 'Aloe vera, "the wand of heaven"'.

Taylor-Donald, L (1981), 'A runner's guide to discovering the secrets of the aloe vera plant', *Runner's World*, December.

Tizard, I, Carpenter, R H, Kemp, M (1991), 'Immuno-regulatory effects of a cytokine release enhancer (acemannan)', International Congress of Phytotherapy, October, Seoul, Korea, 68.

Trattler, R (1987), *Better Health Through Natural Healing*, Thorsons.

Udupa, S L, Udupa, A L, Kulkarmi, D R (1994), 'Anti-inflammatory and wound healing properties of aloe vera', *Fitoterapia*, 65 (2), 141–45.

Urch, D (1999), *Aloe Vera – Nature's Gift*, Blackdown Publications.

Williams, M S, Bink, M, Loprimzi, C L, et al (1996), 'Phase III double-blind evaluation of the aloe vera gel as a prophylactic agent for radiation induced skin toxicity', *International Journal of Radiation* (Oncol-Biol-Phys), 36 (2), 345–49.

Winters, W D, Benavides, R, Clouse, W J (1981), 'Effects of aloe extracts on human normal and tumour cells in vitro', *Economic Botany*, 35: 89–95.

Wolfe, B, Iller, P (1988), 'Aloe vera: an ancient plant for modern dentistry'.

Womble, D, Heldermen, J H (1988), 'Enhancement of allo-responsiveness by human lymphocytes by acemannan', *International Journal of Immunopharmacology*, 10, 8, 967–74.

Womble, D, Helderman, J H (1992), 'The impact of acemannan on the generation and function of cytotoxic T-lymphocytes', *Immunopharmacology, Immunotoxicology*, 14, 63–77.

Wright, C S (1936), 'Aloe vera in the treatment of roentgen ulcers and telangiectasis', *Journal of the American Medical Association*, 106, 1363–64.

Yongchaiyudia, S, Rungpitakangsi, V, Bunyapraphatsaran et al (1996), 'Anti-diabetic activity of aloe vera juice I, clinical trial in new cases of Diabetes mellitus', 3 (3), 241–43.

Yongchaiyuda, S, Rungpitakangsi, V, Bunyapraphatsaran et al (1996), 'Anti-diabetic activity of aloe vera Juice II, clinical trial in new cases of Diabetes mellitus patients and combination with glibenclamide', *Phytomedicine*, 3 (3), 245–48.

Appendix 4: Glossary of terms

ALOIN Purgative compound found under the rind of the leaf.
ANALGESIC Ability to diminish pain by acting on the central nervous system.
ANTIBIOTIC Ability to slow down or stop the development of pathogenic microbes.
ANTI-INFLAMMATORY Ability to act against the inflammation of tissues caused by physical, chemical or biological aggression.
ASTRINGENT Ability to tighten tissues, to stop haemorrhages, diarrhoea, etc.
BACTERICIDAL Ability to destroy bacteria.
CATHARTIC Ability to purify, a mild laxative.
COLLAGEN Fibrous protein, principal constituent of the intercellular substance of conjunctive tissues.
DERMIS Conjunctive tissue that, together with the epithelium, forms the skin.
ELIXIR A liquid preparation usually made of aromatic vegetable substances in alcohol or wine.
EMOLLIENT Ability to soften, e.g. skin.
ENZYMES Proteins with great catalytic power, facilitating the metabolism of molecules produced by the genes.
EPITHILIUM A layer of cells covering the body, the skin or the lining of a cavity connected with it.
FIBROBLAST Cells of conjunctive tissue responsible for the fabrication of collagen fibres that form the skin and muscle tissues.
FUNGICIDAL Ability to destroy pathogenic fungus causing mycosis of the skin.
HAEMOSTATIC Substance that is coagulating and vasco-constricting, thus stopping bleeding.
LAXATIVE A substance that facilitates bowel movement and prevents or cures constipation.
METABOLISM The biological and chemical processes that take place in the cells to transform food into energy.
VIRUCIDAL Ability to destroy a virus.

CD-ROM 'Aloe Vera. Nature's Silent Healer'

We are planning to have a **'Read Only'** CD-ROM entitled *Aloe Vera, Nature's Silent Healer,* available from December 2003 for anyone who is interested in purchasing this book in a different format.

Customers will not be able to download information from this CD-ROM but will be able to use it to research particular topics. The cost of the CD-ROM will be circa £12.99 or the equivalent in US Dollars and Euros.

Further details from:

Alasdair Barcroft
Aloe Vera Centre
P.O. Box 19766
London
SW15 2WZ
UK
Tel +44(0)208-875-9915
Email alasdairaloevera@aol.com